Resolving Ethical Dilemmas
A Guide for Clinicians

Second Edition

Resolving Ethical Dilemmas
A Guide for Clinicians

Second Edition

Bernard Lo, M.D., F.A.C.P.
Professor of Medicine
Director, Program in Medical Ethics
University of California, San Francisco
Attending Physician, Moffitt-Long Hospital
School of Medicine;
San Francisco, California

LIPPINCOTT WILLIAMS & WILKINS
A **Wolters Kluwer** Company
Philadelphia · Baltimore · New York · London
Buenos Aires · Hong Kong · Sydney · Tokyo

Acquisitions Editor: Timothy Y. Hiscock
Developmental Editor: Glenda Insua
Production Editor: Frank Aversa
Manufacturing Manager: Kevin Watt
Cover Designer: Christine Jenny
Compositor: Circle Graphics
Printer: Vicks Lithograph

Library of Congress Cataloging-in-Publication Data

Lo, Bernard
    Resolving ethical dilemmas: a guide for clinicians / Bernard Lo.—2nd ed.
      p. ; cm.
    Includes bibliographical references and index.
    ISBN 0-7817-2219-5
      1. Medical ethics. I. Title.
      [DNLM: 1. Ethics, Medical. 2. Decision Making. 3. Life Support Care. 4. Physician-Patient Relations. W 50 L795r 2000]
    R724.L59 2000
    174′.2—dc21   99-059588

10 9 8 7 6 5 4 3

Contents

Preface to the First Edition vii

Preface xi

I. Fundamentals of Clinical Ethics

  1. An Approach to Ethical Dilemmas in Patient Care 3
  2. Overview of Ethical Guidelines 11
  3. Informed Consent 19
  4. Promoting the Patient's Best Interests: Responding to Patient's
      Refusals of Beneficial Interventions 30
  5. Confidentiality 42
  6. Avoiding Deception and Nondisclosure 52
  7. Keeping Promises 62

II. Shared Decision-Making

  8. An Approach to Decisions About Clinical Interventions 69
  9. Futile Interventions 72
 10. Decision-Making Capacity 80
 11. Refusal of Treatment by Competent, Informed Patients 89
 12. Standards for Decisions When Patients Lack Decision-Making Capacity . . . 94
 13. Surrogate Decision-Making 111

III. Decisions About Life-Sustaining Interventions

 14. Confusing Ethical Distinctions 121
 15. Patient or Surrogate Insistence on Life-Sustaining Interventions 128
 16. Physician Insistence on Life-Sustaining Interventions 135
 17. Ethics Committees and Case Consultations 140
 18. Do Not Resuscitate Orders 147
 19. Physician-Assisted Suicide and Active Euthanasia 156
 20. Tube and Intravenous Feedings 167
 21. The Persistent Vegetative State 173
 22. Determination of Death 177
 23. Legal Rulings on Life-Sustaining Interventions 181
 24. Myths About the Law on Life-Sustaining Interventions 189

IV. The Doctor–Patient Relationship

 25. Overview of the Doctor–Patient Relationship 195
 26. Refusal to Care for Patients 197

27. Gifts from Patients to Physicians 206
28. Sexual Contact Between Physicians and Patients 212
29. Secret Information about Patients. 219
30. Clinical Research 221

V. Conflicts of Interest

31. Overview of Conflicts of Interest 231
32. Bedside Rationing of Health Care 236
33. Incentives for Physicians to Increase Services 244
34. Incentives for Physicians to Decrease Services 248
35. Gifts from Drug Companies 258
36. Disclosing Mistakes 263
37. Impaired Colleagues 271
38. Ethical Dilemmas Facing Students and House Staff 277

VI. Ethical Issues in Clinical Specialties

39. Ethical Issues in Pediatrics 285
40. Ethical Issues in Surgery. 294
41. Ethical Issues in Obstetrics and Gynecology 302
42. Ethical Issues in Psychiatry 310

VII. Current Controversies

43. Transmission of HIV Infection in Health Care Settings 321
44. Ethical Issues in Organ Transplantation 328
45. Testing for Genetic Conditions. 337

Cases for Discussion 345

Subject Index 349

Preface to the First Edition

As a resident, I was paged by the intensive care unit late one night. I recognized the patient, a 17-year-old boy who had undergone bone marrow transplantation for leukemia and now had chronic interstitial fibrosis. The shy, bright smile I remembered from a previous admission was gone. According to the chart, he had developed progressive respiratory failure. His thin intubated body was squirming restlessly in the bed. The patient's father grabbed my hand and pointed to the ventilator, "Stop, it's enough. He doesn't want this." I phoned the attending physician, an eminent hematologist who said that the patient was expected to die in the next few days. I asked whether we should extubate the patient, as his father had requested, and sedate him. The hematologist said that the bone marrow transplant service wanted to continue intensive care; although he did not defend their decision, he deferred to it. We did agree on a DNR order. I gave some sedation to the patient, and tried to comfort him and his family. The boy died just before I went off duty the next morning, more comfortable perhaps, but by no means peaceful. The father asked me, "Why didn't they stop? Why?" Later the attending physician told me that after my phone call, he couldn't get back to sleep. He said that he wanted to call me back to tell me to extubate the patient.

Like this boy's father, I kept asking why? Why were we so insistent on imposing our medical technology on dying patients? Why were decisions driven by physicians' personalities, hospital politics, research priorities, or staffing problems, rather than by what was best for the patient? Why were we comfortable withholding CPR, but uneasy administering high doses of narcotics to a patient with intractable ventilatory failure? Although we spent much time on rounds talking about the use of immunosuppressive agents, antibiotics, ventilators, and a vast array of treatments, why did we avoid discussing what to do when such interventions were no longer helpful or appropriate?

My interest in medical ethics, and ultimately this book, grew from such perplexing cases as this, and from the illnesses of family members and friends. From visiting my favorite aunt, who had developed multi-infarct dementia, I learned how hard it is to say that life is no longer worth living. She had become almost immobile, dependent on others for all her needs, and would often moan and shout when moved. But she would smile when I held her hands or stroked her cheek. Although mute most of the day, she laughed when I showed her pictures of my son and would ask me, "How old?" We could spend an hour looking at the same pictures over and over, with her repeating the same questions. But even as her family and I despaired over her deteriorating condition, it was not yet time to let her go. Life was still a precious gift, not yet an intolerable burden.

As I began writing and speaking about medical ethics, I learned that many colleagues shared my concerns. At professional meetings, practitioners often tell me about cases whose ethical dilemmas still bother them. I have tried to keep in mind such physicians, struggling to do what was right in difficult situations. This book features realistic cases that physicians can relate to their own experience. The goal of *Resolving Ethical Dilemmas* is to help clinicians resolve the mundane ethical issues in patient care as well as the dilemmas that keep them awake at night. In some cases, there are persuasive reasons for a course of action, while in others the countervailing arguments are equally compelling. Yet even when the philosophical debate is closely balanced, physicians must act, choosing one plan of care or another.

This book grew in several ways beyond my initial work on decisions regarding life-sustaining interventions. First, over the years, I realized that physicians need help with many ethical issues. Friends and colleagues often asked me why no one has written about impaired colleagues, about patients' requests to deceive insurance companies, and about the ethical problems in managed care. Second, as the AIDS epidemic ravaged San Francisco, we grappled with new ethical dilemmas, such as the duty to provide care, access to experimental therapies, and the fear of nosocomial HIV infection. Third, the issues of this book were broadened by a personal calamity. On October 20, 1991, a firestorm raged through the Oakland hills. Our house and more than 2,000 others burned to the ground in a few hours. My wife and I felt sad, angry, frustrated, and overwhelmed by the task of putting our lives back together. It was hard to make any choices, much less informed or rational ones. Gradually I realized I was struggling with the same issues in this book as in life. Issues of autonomy, informed consent, and fiduciary responsibility took on increasing prominence. How can people make informed decisions when they are emotionally overwhelmed? Why must physicians act in the best interests of their patients, even to their personal financial disadvantage, when insurance companies and other businesses have no such obligation?

Colleagues sometimes ask me why I work on such "depressing" topics. While the issues are indeed somber, it is also a special privilege when patients and their families trust us with their grief, anger, and tranquillity and show us how to endure turmoil and sorrow. An elderly patient who had hidden for months the severity of her bone cancer pain was delighted when I made a home visit. "I am so glad I could show you my garden. Now you know why I want to die here, looking at my flowers." Another of my patients died from breast cancer and recurrent pleural effusions. She always cried and moaned as we tapped her effusions, even though she knew that her breathing would be easier. I wondered whether we were hurting her rather than helping her. After her death, I said to her son that it must have been hard for him to care for her. He replied softly, "Doc, it made me a better man." As physicians, we see the worst and the best of people. At times they are helpless and angry and make foolish decisions. But when confronting problems that are too large for them, people often become heroes. Ultimately I hope this book will help patients who struggle with such problems by guiding the physicians who care for them.

One of the nicest parts of writing a book is to thank the many people who have encouraged me, shaped my ideas, and pointed out my mistakes. While I was a young faculty member, Steven Schroeder had faith in my attempts to forge a new field. More recently, my dean, Joseph Martin, has been generous with his support and advice. William Kerr, the Director of Hospitals and Clinics at UCSF, has provided valuable support and encouragement. For years, Robert Steinbrook, Nancy Dubler, and Susan Tolle have been true friends and wonderful collaborators, who never hesitated to tell me when I was on the wrong track. My colleagues on the ethics committee at the American College of Physicians, the ethics committee at Moffitt-Long Hospital, and the White House Task Force on Health Care Reform have shared with me their wisdom. At UCSF, Ann Alpers, Lisa Backus, Jeffrey Burack, James Mittelberger, Thomas Prendergast, and James Tulsky have critiqued virtually all these chapters. Their thoughtful comments have greatly strengthened the book. Other colleagues have given valuable comments, including Deborah Aghib, Susan Barbour, Clarence Braddock, Gordon Brandt, Neal Cohen, Bill Detmer, Susan Folkman, Jan Gurley, James Kahn, Miriam Komaromy, Robert Layzer, Tracy Lieu, Stephen McPhee, Jackie Peterson, Rudi Schmid, Ashwini Sehgal, John Sharp, Miriam Shuchman, Robert Wachter, and Albert Wu. Mary Rose did an extraordinary job editing innumerable versions of the manuscript. She honed in on places where I was unclear, confused, or wrong and showed how to fix them. Lisa Gates' expert administrative skills made the office run smoothly and gave me the peace of mind to work on the book. Laura Evans provided valuable assistance during the final preparation of the manuscript. I am also grateful to the Robert Wood Johnson Foundation, the National Institutes of Mental Health (through

Center Grant MH42459), and the University of California Systemwide Biotechnology Research and Education Program for supporting my work.

Over the years my wife, Laurie Dornbrand, has been both my best friend and my toughest critic. She holds me to high standards of writing, keeps me focused on the human stories behind the dilemmas, and reminds me of the needs of physicians practicing on the front lines. Finally, my gratitude to my parents, Chien-Pen and Lucy Chu Lo, is enormous. They tried to instill in me their love of learning, their integrity, and their determination in the face of obstacles. Both my parents died as I was finishing this book. My mother faced her death with unforgettable dignity and calm. My father courageously strived for a little more time to complete his tasks. I dedicate this book to my parents and to my son Aaron, whose exuberance and ability to see the essentials brings me joy every day.

Bernard Lo, 1994

Preface

One night a few years ago, I was working late in the hospital, caring for a terminally ill patient. When I called home to explain that I would miss dinner, my son Aaron demanded to speak with me. He wanted to know if my patient was going to die. When I tried to explain that this patient's death was imminent and that my task was to ensure his comfort and dignity, Aaron exhorted me to keep trying. Had I asked doctors in other states for suggestions about my patient? Was I doing my best? And most plaintively, did I believe in myself? Even at age seven, my son believed that death is something to overcome and that a physician fails if his patient dies.

Dilemmas about care at the end of life remain prominent and difficult, although the shape of the issues has changed since the first edition of this book. Physician-assisted suicide grabs newspaper headlines. Our culture has become more willing to talk about death and the problems of end-of-life care. Empirical research has helped us to better understand how care is given at the end of life and how it might be improved. Physicians have rediscovered how disagreements over care at the end of life may be resolved through listening to the patient's and family's concerns and helping them find closure and meaning at this juncture. However, more families are insisting that invasive interventions be continued even though the patient's condition is worsening on maximal therapy. This second edition contains extensive revisions that reflect these new developments regarding life-sustaining interventions.

I have also revised the book to better cover the ethical issues raised by managed care. Physicians frequently complain that they spend as much time and energy dealing with managed care bureaucracy as they do caring for patients. In a recent office session, I had to spend time with all but one patient on such tasks: looking up which drugs were covered by the patient's insurance, responding to a suggestion from a pharmacy benefits manager that the patient be switched to another drug, finding the right form to obtain authorization for an MRI scan, and discussing whether the patient should pay out-of-pocket to see an out-of-network specialist. Since the first edition, the growth of managed care has raised additional concerns about conflicts of interest, the replacement of professionalism with entrepreneurism, and the erosion of patient trust. The coverage of these topics has been broadened in this edition.

New chapters have been added on ethical issues in obstetrics/gynecology, surgery, and pediatrics. These changes are intended to make the book more useful to medical students, who used the first edition widely. The book also includes cases for discussion, which have been developed as teaching cases for medical students at UCSF.

It is a pleasure to thank the colleagues and friends who have helped me better understand these difficult topics. I owe a special thanks to Ann Alpers, Steve Pantilat, and Leslie Wolf, who, through many discussions, have shared their clear thinking, common sense, and expertise. Claude Platton read each chapter, and his insightful suggestions made the manuscript clearer and more coherent. Collaborations with Tom Bodenheimer, Tom Gallagher, Timothy Quill, and James Tulsky have enabled me to explore new territory and fresh ideas. David Cox, Elena Gates, JanLori Goldman, and Kim Kirkwood have helped me better understand their respective specialties. Nancy Dubler has been an extraordinary friend and colleague, and the summer seminars we have taught together have been unforgettable experiences for me and my family. I have been fortunate to work with thoughtful colleagues on the National Bioethics Advisory Commission, the American College of Physicians–American Society of Internal

Medicine End-of-life Care Panel, and the Task Force on Confidentiality. I am grateful for the opportunity to learn from them. At UCSF, I have benefited from residents and students who asked hard questions and shared their tough cases. My chairman, Lee Goldman, has given on-going support and encouragement. I am grateful to the Robert Wood Johnson Foundation and the National Institutes of Mental Health (through Center Grant MH42459) for supporting my work.

To my family, I owe my greatest thanks. My parents, C.P. and Lucy Lo, and my aunt Edith Chu all died during the writing of the first edition of this book. I am continually grateful for the foundation and inspiration they gave me and wish they could be here to share my joy in trying to pass their values on to my children. The physicians in my family, my sister and brother-in-law, Anna and Peter Davol, and my wife, Laurie Dornbrand, have provided shining examples of dedication to patients, in the face of tightening managed care constraints. Laurie also keeps my ideas out of the clouds and grounded. I could not do what I do without her. Our son Aaron keeps the computers at home functioning smoothly and doesn't hesitate to give me answers to the questions I agonize over. He and his sister Maya, through their zest for life, make our world sparkle every day.

Bernard Lo

SECTION I

Fundamentals of Clinical Ethics

1

An Approach to
Ethical Dilemmas in Patient Care

"This case is really bothering me. I haven't been able to stop worrying about it. I'm just not sure what the right thing to do is." Ethical dilemmas may perplex physicians because strong reasons for a course of action may be balanced by powerful countervailing arguments. Common sense, clinical experience, being a good person, and having good intentions may not guarantee that physicians will know how to respond appropriately to such dilemmas. Ethical dilemmas provoke powerful emotional responses, and strong emotions often are a clue to the presence of an unresolved ethical issue. However, emotions alone are not a satisfactory way of resolving ethical dilemmas. The following cases illustrate the range of ethical issues in clinical medicine.

CASE 1.1. DECISIONS ABOUT LIFE-SUSTAINING INTERVENTIONS. *An elderly woman with severe dementia develops pneumonia. Her daughter insists that hospitalization and antibiotics would be pointless and that the patient would not want such "heroics." However, her son demands that she be treated, because he believes that life is sacred. In this case, the physician can be criticized no matter what she does, either for imposing unwanted interventions or for withholding beneficial therapy.*

CASE 1.2. CONFIDENTIALITY OF HIV TEST RESULTS. *A 32-year-old man with a positive test for human immunodeficiency virus (HIV) antibodies refuses to notify his wife. "If she finds out, it would destroy our marriage." Should the physician notify the wife despite the patient's objections? Although maintaining patient confidentiality is important, it seems cruel not to warn the wife that she is at risk for a fatal infection.*

CASE 1.3. REFERRALS IN A MANAGED CARE SYSTEM. *A high school basketball star suffers a knee injury and probable meniscus tear. She belongs to a particular health maintenance organization (HMO) whose orthopedic surgeons have little experience with arthroscopic surgery. Should the physician tell the patient that more experienced surgeons are available outside the HMO? In this situation, the financial interest of the HMO and the self-interest of the physician conflict with the physician's obligation to act in the patient's best interests.*

In such cases, physicians cannot avoid difficult decisions. Doing nothing or delaying action are also choices, which may have momentous consequences. This chapter describes how clinical ethics can help physicians deal with such dilemmas and presents an approach to resolving them. Specific ethical problems are discussed in detail in subsequent chapters.

WHAT IS CLINICAL ETHICS?

Sources of Moral Guidance

Personal Moral Values

Physicians, like all people, draw on many sources of moral guidance, including parental and family values, cultural traditions, and religious beliefs. These are the roots of a person's moral values and create a disposition to do the right actions. They also instill virtues, such as altruism, compassion, and truthfulness. However, there are several reasons why they cannot be the only guidance for dilemmas in clinical ethics.

First, these personal moral values often do not resolve such dilemmas. They may not address important issues in clinical ethics: often doctors face many difficult ethical issues for the first time during their training and clinical practice. In Case 1.1, laypeople have little education about such topics as life-sustaining treatment or surrogate decision-making. In addition, personal moral values may offer conflicting advice on a particular situation. Individuals often hold several fundamental beliefs that are in conflict. A physician may want both to alleviate the suffering of a dying patient and to respect the sacredness of life. For physicians to be perplexed about a dilemma in clinical ethics is not a blot on their character or background.

Second, physicians have role-specific ethical obligations that differ from their obligations as good citizens and good persons. Doctors have special duties to maintain confidentiality in Case 1.2 and to disclose information to patients during the informed consent process in Case 1.3. The moral values and upbringing that guide physicians' personal lives usually do not address professional roles.

Third, physicians need to persuade others of their plans to resolve ethical dilemmas. Other health care workers, patients, and family members may have different religious or cultural backgrounds. Patients and relatives may not agree with the physician's professional codes of behavior. Clinical ethics analyzes the reasons that justify a particular course of action. People can be persuaded by cogent arguments, and individuals with different world views can reach agreement in specific cases. Frequently positions on ethical issues can be shown to be untenable because they are internally inconsistent or do not take into account countervailing arguments.

We next discuss the general types of justifications commonly offered for actions. Subsequent chapters analyze specific justifications for actions in various situations.

Claims of Conscience

Sometimes people explain their actions as a matter of conscience: to act otherwise would make them feel ashamed or guilty or violate their sense of wholeness or integrity. Conscience involves self-reflection and judgment about whether an action is right or wrong (1). For example, in Case 1.2, a physician might declare, "I couldn't live with myself if I didn't notify his wife."

Deeply held claims of conscience generally are honored. It would be dehumanizing to compel people to act in ways that violate their sense of integrity and responsibility. Claims of conscience, however, may not always resolve a dispute. Other people may cite their own conscience as a countervailing argument. Also people may use appeals to conscience to rationalize a selfish or immoral action.

Claims of Rights

To explain their positions on ethical issues, people often appeal to rights, such as a "right to die," or a "right to health care." To philosophers, rights are justified claims that a person can make on others or on society (1). The language of rights is widespread in U.S. culture, yet appeals to rights are often controversial. Other people may deny that the right exists or may assert conflicting rights. For example, in Case 1.2, even if the seropositive patient has a right to confidentiality, the wife may have a countervailing right to know that she is at risk for a fatal infectious disease. Finally, claims of rights often are used to end debates; however, the crucial issue is whether there are persuasive arguments that support the existence of the right.

Distinguishing Morality and Ethics

The terms "morality" and "ethics" are often used interchangeably to refer to standards of right and wrong behavior. However, it is helpful to draw some distinctions. Moral choices ultimately rest on values or beliefs that cannot be proved but are simply accepted. Morality usually refers to conduct that conforms "to the accepted customs or conventions of a people" (2). What a particular culture or group regards as correct is usually learned as a child from parents and religious leaders and may be accepted without deliberation. Ultimately, such fundamental moral beliefs are part of a person's character. Yet ordinary moral rules, which usually provide an adequate guide for daily conduct, may fail to provide clear direction in many clinical situations. For instance, moral precepts to respect the sanctity of life can be used in Case 1.1 to justify both continuing and withholding antibiotics.

In contrast to morality, ethics connotes deliberation and explicit arguments to justify particular actions. Ethics also refers to a branch of philosophy that deals with the "principles governing ideal human character" or to a professional code of conduct (2). To philosophers, ethics focuses on the reasons *why* an action is considered right or wrong. It asks people to justify their positions and beliefs by rational arguments.

How Does Clinical Ethics Differ From Law?

The law, through statutes, regulations, and decisions in specific cases, also provides guidance on what physicians may and may not do. On many issues the law reflects an ethical consensus in society. Moreover, rulings by courts give reasons for decisions and therefore provide an analysis of pertinent issues. Hence physicians should be familiar with what the law says regarding issues in clinical ethics. However, the law cannot provide definitive answers to ethical dilemmas.

First, the law, particularly the criminal law, sets only a minimally acceptable standard of conduct. It indicates what acts are so *wrong* that the physician will be held legally liable. In contrast, ethics focuses on the *right* or best decision in a situation. From a legal perspective, pediatricians need only obtain the authorization of the parent or guardian to treat a child. However, professional ethics requires pediatricians to provide pediatric patients with pertinent information in ways that are developmentally appropriate and to obtain their assent for care (*see* Chapter 39). Furthermore, ethical standards require pediatricians to act with compassion and integrity; it is impossible for the law to enforce such standards. Second, the law explicitly grants physicians discretion in some situations. For instance, most states allow physicians to determine when a patient lacks decision-making capacity and thus when a surrogate should take over the role of making decisions with the physician (*see* Chapter 10). In these states, physicians must act on ethical and clinical considerations, not legal ones. Third, the law may provide no clear guide to action on certain topics. For example, the law provides scant guidance on the issue of disclosing genetic information to relatives when the patient objects to disclosure. Finally, law and ethics may conflict. Abortion is legal throughout the United States, and physician-assisted suicide is legal in the state of Oregon. However, both practices continue to be controversial ethically.

Furthermore, actions that are prohibited by law may be regarded as ethical by many persons. In a few states, the courts have rejected family decision-making for incompetent patients who have not provided written advance directives. Ethically, however, the consensus is to respect surrogate decision-making by concerned family members (*see* Chapter 13). In such conflicts, most physicians feel uncomfortable about following the letter of the law.

How Does Clinical Ethics Differ from Professional Oaths and Codes?

Many physicians seek ethical guidance from professional codes, such as the Hippocratic Oath or the modern codes of ethics of the American Medical Association or the American College of Physicians–Society for Internal Medicine (3,4). Although professional oaths and codes may provide helpful guidance for physician behavior, they have several shortcomings (5). First, they are unilateral declarations by groups of physicians, without any input from patients or the public. Codes of ethics and professional oaths do not acknowledge that society has granted autonomy and privileges to physicians and therefore has the right to insist on certain expectations. Second, the content of professional codes has been criticized. The Hippocratic tradition is highly paternalistic, granting patients little role in making decisions. For instance, it does not require physicians to disclose information to patients or allow them to make informed choices. Nor does the Hippocratic Oath enjoin physicians to be truthful with patients. Third, oaths and codes are often terse documents that fail to cover many important ethical issues. Frequently they articulate a position without giving a detailed analysis of the issues.

HOW CLINICAL ETHICS CAN HELP PHYSICIANS

Certain situations commonly recur in clinical practice. Physicians learn to recognize individual cases as examples of syndromes, such as "angina" or "hyponatremia" (6). Placing cases into categories allows physicians to organize relevant data and draw on experiences with similar cases. For each type of case, the physician learns to gather additional information, to anticipate associated problems or complications, and to develop an approach to the class of cases. To be sure, the approach needs to be modified in specific cases, because no two cases are identical and there are always exceptional cases. Nonetheless, the vast majority of cases can be managed by a standard approach. The more categories of cases physicians have studied, the better prepared they are for clinical practice.

Learning about clinical ethics can help physicians to identify, understand, and resolve common ethical issues in patient care. By studying "teaching cases," physicians can gain vicarious experience in resolving specific dilemmas (7,9). Doctors can learn how to interpret ethical guidelines in particular situations, how to identify features of a case that distinguish it from other apparently similar cases, and when exceptions to guidelines are justified.

Identify Ethical Issues

By studying realistic cases that illustrate common ethical problems, physicians may better recognize the ethical issues in their own cases. In some cases, physicians may have only a vague uneasiness that important ethical issues are at stake. In other situations, health care workers may be perplexed about difficult decisions but fail to identify problems as specifically ethical in nature, as opposed to issues of clinical management or interpersonal conflict. Thus, physicians need to be able to identify such fundamental ethical issues as assessment of decision-making capacity, advance directives, or confidentiality and to develop an approach to each issue.

Understand Areas of Ethical Consensus and Controversy

On many issues, physicians, philosophers, and the courts agree on what should be done (1,4,5,9). Such agreement is often possible even when people disagree on the reasons for their actions (10). For example, it is well established that competent, informed patients may refuse interventions recommended by their physicians and that certain exceptions to confidentiality of medical information are appropriate both ethically and legally. Subsequent chapters point out areas of widespread ethical agreement as well as those areas of ongoing controversy.

Clinical ethics can indicate which actions are clearly right or wrong and which are controversial. Philosophers distinguish among actions that are obligatory, permissible, and wrong (1). In Case 1.3, it would be *obligatory* for physicians to tell the patient about other options for care (*see* Chapter 40). At the other extreme, it would be *wrong* for physicians to lie and tell the patient that the orthopedic care in this HMO is as good as care elsewhere. Still other actions might be ethically *permissible* but not required. Some acts may be optional because the arguments for and against them are so evenly balanced that reasonable people may disagree. Other actions are optional in a different sense: it would be praiseworthy to perform them, but failure to do so would not be blameworthy. For instance, it would be heroic for the physician in Case 1.3 to devote extensive time to convince the HMO to pay for orthopedic care outside the system, but he could not be blamed if he merely wrote a letter and made some phone calls on her behalf.

AN APPROACH TO ETHICAL DILEMMAS IN CLINICAL MEDICINE

A systematic approach to ethical problems helps to ensure that no important considerations are overlooked and that similar cases are resolved consistently. The approach outlined in Table 1-1 includes three general steps: gathering information, clarifying ethical issues, and resolving the dilemma. For any particular case, an experienced physician may modify the general approach.

Gather Information

Physicians first need to gather pertinent information about the patient and the case.

What Is the Clinical Situation?

Sound ethical decision-making requires accurate clinical information about the patient's diagnosis and prognosis, the options for care, and the benefits and risks of each alternative. In ad-

TABLE 1-1. *An approach to ethical dilemmas in patient care*

Gather information
  What is the clinical situation?
  Who is the primary decision-maker?
  What are the views of the health care team and other stakeholders?
Clarify the ethical issues
  What are the pertinent ethical issues and conflicts?
  Understand the best thinking on the pertinent issues.
Resolve the dilemmas
  What pragmatic issues complicate the case?
  Hold a team meeting.
  Meet with the patient or family.
  Deal with psychosocial issues directly.
  Seek assistance as needed.

dition, psychosocial information is essential, such as the relationship between the brother and sister in Case 1.1 or between the husband and wife in Case 1.2.

Who Is the Primary Decision-Maker?

The patient is the focus of clinical care. If the patient is competent, he or she makes decisions jointly with the physician, choosing among feasible alternatives. If the patient lacks decision-making capacity, an appropriate surrogate needs to be identified. Generally this will be a family member, such as the parents of a child or the spouse of a patient with severe dementia. Case 1.1 illustrates how disagreements may arise over who is the appropriate surrogate. Physicians need to understand the preferences of the patient or surrogate, as well as the reasoning behind their choices.

What Are the Views of the Health Care Team and Other Stake-Holders?

Other health care workers who provide direct care to the patient need to be involved in decisions. Nurses, house staff, and medical students are responsible for their actions when carrying out the attending physician's "orders." In addition, these health care workers have close relationships with patients and families, answer their questions, and explain plans for care.

Other people may also have a stake in decisions. In Case 1.2, the patient's wife will be directly affected by the decision. Her viewpoint needs to be taken into account.

Clarify the Ethical Issues

What Are the Pertinent Ethical Issues and Conflicts?

As with clinical medicine, how a case is framed often determines how it is resolved. Case 1.1 could be framed as a family disagreement. However, it is more fruitful to focus on more specific ethical issues:

- Has the patient provided trustworthy advance directives (*see* Chapter 12)?
- Who should serve as surrogate decision-maker for incompetent patients (*see* Chapter 13)?

Framing the issues in this way leads the physician to gather more information and raises points to consider.

It is helpful to clarify the nature of the ethical disagreements in a case. Often different ethical guidelines are in conflict. In Case 1.2 maintaining patient confidentiality conflicts with preventing harm to another person. In other cases, people may agree on ethical guidelines but disagree over how to interpret them. In Case 1.1 the son might agree with respecting the patient's choices but argue that her previous statements were too ambiguous to direct care. Clarifying a disagreement is a necessary first step in trying to resolve it.

Understand the Best Thinking on the Pertinent Issues

After reviewing the pertinent literature on the ethical issues, the physician can often develop an approach to resolving the dilemmas. In Case 1.1, if the patient had given trustworthy advance directives, they should be respected. There are well-accepted arguments in the published literature for following such directives (*see* Chapter 12). Similarly, in Case 1.3, if the physician's arrangement with a managed care plan includes a "gag clause" that forbids her from disclosing interventions not covered by the plan, the physician needs to understand why such clauses are considered unethical (*see* Chapter 34).

Resolve Dilemmas

In real cases, physicians benefit from practical suggestions as well as philosophical clarity.

What Pragmatic Issues Complicate the Case?

Emotions, interpersonal conflicts, poor communication, and time pressures often complicate clinical dilemmas. Physicians need to appreciate and acknowledge this context. Health care workers may feel powerful emotions, such as frustration and anger. The emotions of patients or family members may also be significant. In Case 1.2, the seropositive patient may feel guilty, or ashamed, or afraid. Finally, institutional factors may be important. Hospital policy or insurance coverage may conflict with what the physician believes is ethically correct.

Hold a Team Meeting

Such meetings provide additional information about the patient's choices and values. Physicians clarify their thinking when they have to provide reasons for their decisions. People with different personal values, religious and cultural backgrounds, and clinical experience frequently can point out hidden assumptions and value judgments, call attention to neglected issues, and suggest fresh alternatives.

Meet with the Patient or Family

Physicians must elicit and respond to the concerns and needs of patients or surrogates. Open-ended questions help patients or surrogates articulate their concerns. In Case 1.1, the physician can ask, "As you think about your mother's condition, what concerns you the most? What do you hope for?" If such concerns can be addressed directly, the patient or family often accepts, the physician's recommendations.

Patients or families may become confused if they hear mixed messages from different clinicians. If the health care team cannot agree on recommendations, the areas of agreement and disagreement need to be articulated carefully.

Deal with Psychosocial Issues Directly

If emotional reactions or interpersonal conflicts are acknowledged and discussed explicitly, the discussion of ethical issues is generally more straightforward. Indeed, many "ethical" dilemmas are settled by paying attention to emotional reactions and interpersonal conflicts, rather than through philosophical debate. Conversely, unless such psychosocial issues are addressed directly, agreement on the ethical issues usually will be difficult.

Seek Assistance as Needed

In difficult cases, the physician may seek assistance from the hospital ethics committee or an ethics consultant (*see* Chapter 17). A second opinion from another physician not directly involved in the case may also be helpful. A chaplain, social worker, or nurse may have better rapport with the patient or family than the physician and be able facilitate discussions.

In summary, physicians commonly face difficult ethical issues in clinical practice. Reading about such issues, thinking about them, and discussing them with colleagues can help physicians resolve ethical dilemmas. As with any clinical problem, following a systematic approach helps ensure that all pertinent considerations are taken into account. The important steps include gathering information about the medical situation and the preferences of the patient or surrogate and clarifying the salient ethical and pragmatic issues.

REFERENCES

1. Beauchamp TL, Childress JF. *Principles of biomedical ethics,* 4th ed. New York: Oxford University Press, 1994:69–77,211,474–483.
2. *Webster's new dictionary of synonyms.* Springfield, MA: Merriam-Webster, 1984:547.
3. Council on Ethical and Judicial Affairs. *Code of medical ethics: current opinions with annotations.* Chicago: American Medical Association, 1998.
4. American College of Physicians. American College of Physicians Ethics Manual. *Ann Intern Med* 1998; 128:576–594, 947–960.
5. Veatch RM. *A theory of medical ethics.* New York: Basic Books, 1981.
6. Kassirer JP. Diagnostic reasoning. *Ann Intern Med* 1989;110:893–900.
7. Lo B, Jonsen AR. Ethical dilemmas and the clinician. *Ann Intern Med* 1980;92:116–117.
8. Lo B, Quill T, Tulsky J. Discussing palliative care with patients. *Ann Intern Med* 1999;130:744–749.
9. President's Commission for the Study of Ethical Problems in Medicine and Biomedical Behavioral Research. *Deciding to forego life-sustaining treatment.* Washington: U.S. Government Printing Office, 1983.
10. Jonsen AR, Toulmin S. *The abuse of casuistry: a history of moral reasoning.* Berkeley: University of California Press, 1988.

2

Overview of Ethical Guidelines

In clinical medicine, ethical problems arise because there are sound reasons for conflicting courses of action. In resolving ethical dilemmas, physicians need to refer to general maxims that inform choices and justify actions. This chapter provides an overview of guidelines in clinical ethics. Subsequent chapters in the book discuss these ethical guidelines in detail and apply them to specific cases.

RESPECT FOR PERSONS

Treating patients with respect entails several ethical obligations. First, physicians must respect the medical decisions of persons who are autonomous (1). The term *autonomy* literally means "self-rule." Autonomous people act intentionally, are informed, and are free from interference and control by others. They should be allowed to shape their lives and control their destinies. The concept of autonomy includes the ideas of self-determination, independence, and freedom. In addition to respecting the decisions of autonomous patients, doctors should take steps to promote patient autonomy, as by disclosing information and helping patients deliberate.

With regard to health care, autonomy justifies the doctrine of informed consent (*see* Chapter 3). Informed consent has several specific aspects. Informed, competent patients may refuse unwanted medical interventions. Such refusals respect patients' bodily integrity; patients may not be subjected to invasive interventions without their consent. In addition, patients may choose among medically feasible alternatives. Important clinical choices may not involve major bodily invasion. For instance, choosing whether to have an x-ray or choosing among several drugs for a condition do not implicate the patient's bodily integrity in a manner similar to surgery. Competent, informed patients have the right to make choices that conflict with the wishes of family members or the recommendations of their physicians.

A person's autonomy is not absolute and may be justifiably restricted for several reasons. If a person is incapable of making informed decisions, trying to respect her autonomy may be less important than acting in her best interests. Autonomy may also be constrained by the needs of other individuals or society at large. A person is not free to act in ways that violate the autonomy of other people, harm others, or impose unfair claims on society's resources.

A second meaning of respect for persons goes beyond respecting autonomy. Many patients are not autonomous because their decision-making capacity is impaired by illness or medications. Physicians should still treat them as persons with individual characteristics, preferences, and values. Decisions should respect their preferences and values, so far as they are known. In addition, all patients, whether autonomous or not, should be treated with compassion and dignity. Thus respect for persons includes responding to the patient's suffering with caring, empathy, and attention.

Third, respect for persons is related to other ethical guidelines, such as avoiding misrepresentation, maintaining confidentiality, and keeping promises. Breaches of these other guidelines show disrespect for patients and also compromise their self-determination. There are additional reasons for these other guidelines, as we now discuss.

AVOID DECEPTION AND NONDISCLOSURE

Truth telling—avoiding lies—is a cornerstone of social interaction. If people could not depend on others to tell the truth, no one would make agreements or contracts. Physicians also may mislead patients without technically lying. Doctors may give partial information that is literally true but deceptive. Deception violates the autonomy of people who are deceived because it causes them to make decisions based on false premises. To cover these broader issues, this book uses the term "deception" rather than "lying." In addition, physicians may withhold from patients information about their diagnosis or prognosis. Physicians may withhold information to protect patients from bad news. However, patients cannot make informed decisions about their medical care if they do not receive information about their condition that they would like to have.

MAINTAIN CONFIDENTIALITY

Maintaining the confidentiality of medical information respects patient privacy. It also encourages people to seek treatment and to discuss their problems frankly. In addition, confidentiality protects patients from harms that might occur if information about psychiatric illness, sexual preference, or alcohol or drug use were widely known. Patients and the public expect physicians to keep medical information confidential. Maintaining confidentiality, however, is not an absolute duty. In some situations, the physicians need to override confidentiality in order to protect third parties from harm (*see* Chapter 5).

KEEP PROMISES

Promises generate expectations in other people, who in turn modify their plans on the assumption that promises will be kept. The very concept of promises is undermined if people are free to break them. It is unfair for someone to expect others to honor their promises, but to break his or her own. Keeping promises also enhances trust in both the individual physician and the medical profession. Furthermore, promises relieve patients' anxiety about the future, by providing reassurance that doctors will not abandon them.

ACT IN THE BEST INTERESTS OF PATIENTS

The guideline of nonmaleficence, or "do no harm," forbids physicians from providing ineffective therapies or from acting selfishly or maliciously (2). This oft-cited precept, however, provides only limited guidance, because many beneficial interventions also entail serious risks and side effects.

The guideline of *beneficence* requires physicians to take positive actions for the benefit of patients (*see* Chapter 4). Because patients do not possess medical expertise and may be vulnerable because of their illness, they rely on physicians to provide sound advice and to promote their well-being. Physicians encourage such trust. For these reasons, physicians have a fiduciary duty to act in the best interests of their patients.

Unwise Decisions by Patients

Acting in patients' best interests may conflict with respecting their informed choices, as when patients' refusals of care may thwart their own goals or cause them serious harm. For example, a young man with asthma may refuse mechanical ventilation for reversible respiratory failure. Simply accepting such refusals, in the name of respecting autonomy, would constitute a constricted view of responsibility. Physicians need to listen to patients, educate them, try to persuade them to accept beneficial treatment, or negotiate a mutually acceptable compromise. If disagreements persist, the patient's informed choices and view of best interests should prevail.

Patients Who Lack Decision-Making Capacity

The choices and preferences of many such patients are unknown or unclear. In this situation, respecting autonomy is not pertinent. Instead, physicians should be guided by the best interests of the patient (*see* Chapter 4).

Conflicts of Interest

Physicians should act in the best interests of the patient when conflicts of interest occur (*see* Chapters 31–38). Patients trust their physicians to act on their behalf and feel betrayed if that trust is abused. In a potential conflict of interest, physicians should consider how patients, the public, and colleagues would react if they knew about the situation. Even the appearance of a conflict of interest may damage trust in the individual physician and in the profession.

ALLOCATE RESOURCES JUSTLY

The term "justice" is used in a general sense to mean fairness, that is, people should receive what they deserve. In addition, people who are situated equally should also be treated equally. It is important to act consistently in cases that are similar in ethically relevant ways. Otherwise, decisions would be arbitrary, biased, and unfair. More precisely, people who are similar in ethically relevant respects should be treated similarly, and people who differ in ethically significant ways should be treated differently. To make this formal statement of justice operational, the physician would need to specify what counts as an ethically relevant distinction and what it means to treat people similarly.

In health care settings, "justice" usually refers to the allocation of health care resources. Allocation decisions are unavoidable because resources are limited and could be spent on other social goods, such as education or the environment, instead of on health care. Ideally, allocation decisions should be made as public policy and set by government officials or judges, according to appropriate procedures. Physicians should participate in public debates about allocation and help set policies. In general, however, rationing medical care at the bedside should be avoided because it may be inconsistent, discriminatory, and ineffective. At the bedside, physicians usually should act as patient advocates within constraints set by society and sound practice (*see* Chapter 32). In some cases, however, two patients may compete for the same limited resources, such as physician time or a bed in intensive care. When this occurs, physicians should ration their time and resources according to patients' medical needs and the probability and degree of benefit.

THE USE OF ETHICAL GUIDELINES

Having summarized guidelines for clinical ethics, we next discuss how physicians should use guidelines in specific cases. This book uses the term *guidelines* to connote that ethical generalizations cannot be mechanically or rigidly applied but need to be used in particular cases with discretion and judgment. Guidelines are derived from decisions made in specific cases as well as from moral theories (3,4). In turn, guidelines shape decisions in similar cases in the future. However, guidelines may be difficult to apply in new cases for several reasons.

Guidelines Need to be Interpreted in the Context of Specific Cases

The meaning or force of a guideline may not be clear in a particular case. Uncertainty and case-by-case variation are inherent in clinical medicine. Furthermore, patients have different priorities and goals for care. A crucial issue is whether the case to be decided can be distinguished in ethically meaningful ways from previous cases to which the guideline was applied. Unforeseen or novel cases may point out the shortcomings of existing guidelines and suggest that the guideline needs to be modified or an exception made.

Exceptions to Guidelines May be Appropriate

Guidelines are not absolute. A particular case may have distinctive features that justify making an exception to a guideline (3). To ensure fairness, physicians who make an exception to a guideline should justify their decision. The justification should apply not only to the case under consideration but also to all similar cases faced by other physicians. Some philosophers regard guidelines simply as rules of thumb that provide advice but are not binding, but if people can set aside guidelines too easily, decisions may be inconsistent, and planning for the future may be impossible. Many philosophers regard ethical guidelines as *prima facie* binding: they should be followed unless they conflict with stronger obligations or guidelines, or unless there are compelling reasons to make an exception (5). *Prima facie* guidelines are more binding than mere rules of thumb. The burden of proof is on those who claim that an exception to the guideline is warranted. Furthermore, when *prima facie* guidelines are overridden, they are not simply ignored. People often experience regret or even remorse that guidelines are being broken. Thus people should minimize the extent to which *prima facie* guidelines are violated and mitigate the adverse consequences of doing so.

Different Guidelines May Conflict

In many situations, following one ethical guideline would require the physician to compromise another guideline. Respecting a patient's refusal of treatment may clash with acting in his best interests. Maintaining confidentiality may conflict with protecting third parties from harm. Allocating resources equitably may conflict with doing what is best for an individual patient. The practice of medicine would be much easier if there were a fixed hierarchy of ethical guidelines, for example, if patient autonomy always took priority over beneficence. However, life is not so simple. In some clinical situations, respecting a patient's wishes should be paramount, whereas in others a patient's best interests should prevail. Physicians need to understand why an ethical guideline should take priority in some situations but not in others.

The ability to make prudent decisions in specific situations has been described as discernment or practical wisdom. Discernment involves an understanding of how ethical guidelines are relevant in a variety of situations and to the particular case at hand (1).

PRINCIPLES, RULES, AND DUTIES

This book uses the term guidelines to refer to ethical generalizations that guide action, because other terms, such as principles, rules, and duties, have undesirable connotations. According to the dictionary, *principle* connotes a "basis for reasoning or a guide for conduct or procedure" (6). Many philosophers, however, use the term in a more restricted sense, to refer only to a comprehensive ethical theory that explains how to resolve conflicts among different precepts (1,7). A unified theory would also presumably provide clear, specific rules for action and a justification of those rules (7).

Philosophers have devoted considerable effort to developing comprehensive ethical theories. The two main types of ethical theory are consequentialist and deontological. *Consequentialist* theories judge the rightness or wrongness of actions by their consequences. Utilitarianism, the most prominent consequentialist theory, considers actions and rules appropriate when the overall benefits to all parties outweigh the overall harms. For instance, a utilitarian would consider it justified to tell a lie, breach confidentiality, or break a promise if on the whole the benefits of doing so outweighed the harms. In contrast, *deontological* theories claim that the rightness or wrongness of an action depends on more factors than the consequences of an action. To a deontologist, actions such as telling a lie, breaching confidentiality, and breaking promises are inherently wrong. They would be morally suspect even if they produced no harmful consequences or led to beneficial ones.

Comprehensive theories of clinical ethics, however, are problematic (10). Utilitarian theories are flawed because they condone seemingly harmful actions that are not detected. For example, utilitarians might condone breaking a promise when no one else knows it is broken. Furthermore, acts that maximize the benefits for society as a whole may impose grave harms on individual persons. Although society may benefit if a promise is broken, the person to whom the promise was made may suffer great detriments. Often people change their plans in the expectation that promises will be kept. Such an inequitable distribution of benefits and harms may be unfair.

In a similar way, deontological theories can be criticized because they cannot provide a satisfactory account of which principles or rules take priority over others in cases of conflict. For example, deontological theories would have difficulty determining whether beneficence or confidentiality would prevail when a patient with human immunodeficiency virus (HIV) infection refused to notify his wife that she is at risk.

Detailed and lucid expositions of ethical theories as well as critiques of them are available (1). Many writers, myself included, believe that a comprehensive and consistent theory of clinical ethics cannot be developed (8). This book avoids reference to ethical theories and to the term "principle" not only because of these conceptual problems but also because ethical theories and principles are too abstract to provide guidance to physicians in specific cases.

The term *rule* is used in ethics to refer to generalizations that are narrower in scope than principles. The term is helpful because it focuses on individual conduct in specific situations, rather than abstract generalizations. However, rules are generally regarded as binding, often prohibiting certain behaviors (3). In common language, "rule" may imply restrictions on individual conduct in order to maintain order in the group or for the sake of a goal (6). For example, we speak of rules for a game or for an institution. The implication may be that rules can be applied in a straightforward manner, as when disputes in a game are settled by referring to the rules. In this sense, rules may be arbitrarily imposed in order to establish clear expectations for everyone. For example, rules for visiting hours may be established in a hospital to provide clear guidance for conduct, without any claim that one choice of hours is superior to another. However, the term "rule" is misleading in clinical ethics, because exceptions need to be made and because guidelines are not arbitrary conventions but reflect deeply held values.

Finally, this book avoids the term *duty*, which may connote legal as well as ethical obligations. Ethical obligations, however, differ from legal duties imposed by legislation, regulations, or court rulings, as Chapter 23 discusses.

OTHER APPROACHES TO ETHICS

Because ethical theories and principles often do not help people resolve conflicts, other approaches to clinical ethics have been suggested (1,8).

Casuistry

Instead of constructing or relying on theories, some writers focus on how to resolve specific cases (3,9–11). According to these writers, in everyday life people resolve dilemmas by "looking at the concrete details of particular cases" (10). In this view, moral rules are not absolute; they merely create presumptions that may be rebutted depending on the particular circumstances. The strategy is to compare a given case with clear-cut, paradigmatic cases. The key issue is whether the given case so closely resembles the paradigmatic case that it should be resolved in a similar manner, or whether it can be distinguished (3). In some cases, the application of ethical maxims will be clear-cut. In more difficult cases, it may be unclear whether a guideline applies, or different guidelines may provide conflicting advice. Proponents of case-based ethics emphasize the need for what Aristotle called practical wisdom, the ability to make appropriate decisions given the particular circumstances of the case. The essential issue is "how closely the present circumstances resemble those of the earlier precedent cases for which this type of argument was originally devised" (10). In educational terms, casuistry teaches by case analyses, starting with paradigmatic cases in which principles clearly apply and moving to complex, ambiguous cases over which reasonable people may disagree.

A case-based approach to clinical ethics takes into account the complexity of real-life decisions and offers readers a vicarious experience in resolving ethical problems (12). Dilemmas in clinical ethics generally present as specific decisions in patient care, not as clashes of abstract philosophical principles. This book emphasizes how to approach difficult cases and how to weigh different considerations in reaching a decision.

Case-based analyses, however, face a serious challenge: to provide a convincing basis for weighing some factors more heavily than others in reaching a decision. Indeed, casuistry runs the risk of *ad hoc* reasoning and inconsistent decisions. To avoid such pitfalls, this book will continually refer back to the ethical guidelines described in this chapter and explain why particular factors will be decisive in some situations, whereas different considerations will weigh most heavily in other circumstances.

An Ethic of Caring

Feminist writers argue that principles and rules provide an incomplete and inadequate conception of ethics (13,14). In this perspective, rule-based morality gives insufficient attention to maintaining or restoring relationships among individuals and avoiding interpersonal conflicts. In this view, responding to the needs and welfare of specific individuals may be more important than acting in accord with abstract standards. For example, when family members make decisions for an incompetent patient, traditional ethics may undervalue the need for the family members to get along with each other and live with the consequences of their decisions (15). In some situations, it may be more important to prevent serious family disputes than to follow the patient's prior directives. Such caring and responsiveness is often claimed to be a typically "feminine" orientation, as contrasted with a "masculine" orientation toward rules and principles. Empirical studies, however, do not support the hypothesis of gender-related orientations to ethics (16).

The emphasis on caring and on the well-being of others is welcome in medicine and other helping professions. No one denies that caring is essential in the doctor–patient relationship and that sympathy and compassion may be more important in clinical practice following ethical guidelines. But it is also important to move beyond a sensitivity to these issues to a detailed description of how caring should impact on decisions in specific clinical situations. Furthermore, attending to the welfare of others may conflict with other important ethical imperatives, such as respecting the patient's autonomy.

Virtue Ethics

Some writers point out that following guidelines may lead to a thin view of ethics. Physicians may do the right actions but lack the spirit that should animate the medical profession. Virtue ethics emphasizes that the characteristics of the physician ultimately are more important than the doctor's specific actions and their congruence with ethical principles (17). In this perspective, the essential questions are: Is the doctor a good physician? Is she a good person? In one such view, the virtues of a good physician include fidelity, compassion, fortitude, temperance, integrity, and self-effacement (17).

Virtue ethics is helpful because it emphasizes the importance of such qualities as compassion, dedication, and altruism in physicians. Furthermore, in some extremely complicated or unique situations, the physician's integrity may be a crucial factor in resolving dilemmas. However, virtue ethics also has serious limitations because it lacks specifics on what the doctor should do in particular circumstances. A virtuous person may still commit wrong actions. Virtues may also conflict with each other. In a given case, some people may believe that following a general guideline demonstrates the physician's integrity, while others believe that it would be compassionate to make an exception to the guideline.

In summary, ethical guidelines include showing respect for persons, avoiding deception, maintaining confidentiality, keeping promises, acting in the best interests of patients, and allocating resources justly. These guidelines need to be applied to particular cases with discretion and judgment. Subsequent chapters discuss these guidelines in detail.

REFERENCES

1. Beauchamp TL, Childress JF. *Principles of biomedical ethics,* 4th ed. New York: Oxford University Press, 1994:3–43, 44–119, 120–132, 468–469.
2. Jonsen AR. Do no harm. *Ann Intern Med* 1978;88:827–832.
3. Sunnstein CR. *Legal reasoning and political conflict.* New York: Oxford University Press, 1996.
4. Beauchamp TL, Childress JF. *Principles of biomedical ethics.* 4th ed. New York: Oxford University Press, 1994:3–43.
5. Beauchamp TL, Childress JF. *Principles of biomedical ethics.* 4th ed. New York: Oxford University Press, 1994:33–34.
6. *Webster's new dictionary of synonyms.* Springfield, MA: Merriam-Webster, 1984:638.
7. Clouser KD, Gert B. A critique of principlism. *J Med Philos* 1990;15:219–236.
8. Pellegrino ED. The metamorphosis of medical ethics: a 30-year retrospective. *JAMA* 1992;269:1158–1162.
9. Toulmin S. The tyranny of principles. *Hastings Center Rep* 1981;11:31–39.
10. Jonsen AR, Toulmin S. *The abuse of casuistry: a history of moral reasoning.* Berkeley: University of California Press, 1988:30, 35.
11. Arras JD. Getting down to cases: the revival of casuistry in bioethics. *J Med Philos* 1991;16:29–51.
12. Lo B, Jonsen AR. Ethical dilemmas and the clinician. *Ann Intern Med* 1980;92:116–117.
13. Gilligan C. *In a different voice: psychological theory and women's development.* Cambridge: Harvard University Press, 1982.
14. Gilligan C, Ward JV, Taylor JM, eds. *Mapping the moral domain: a contribution of women's thinking to psychological theory and education.* Cambridge: Harvard University Press, 1988.
15. Alpers A, Lo B. Avoiding family feuds: responding to surrogates' demands for life-sustaining treatment. *J Law Med Ethics* 1999;27:69–73.

16. Bebeau MJ, Brabeck M. Ethical sensitivity and moral reasoning among men and women in the professions. In: Brabeck MM, ed. *Who cares? Theory, research, and educational implications of the ethic of care.* New York: Praeger, 1989:144–163.
17. Pellegrino ED, Thomasma DG. *The virtues in medical practice.* New York: Oxford University Press, 1993.

ANNOTATED BIBLIOGRAPHY

1. Beauchamp TL, Childress JF. *Principles of biomedical ethics*, 4th ed. New York: Oxford University Press, 1994.
   Comprehensive and lucid presentation of the philosophical foundations of biomedical ethics. Excellent references for further reading in the philosophical literature.
2. Pellegrino ED. The metamorphosis of medical ethics: a 30-year retrospective. *JAMA* 1992;269:1158–1162.
   Insightful review and critique of various approaches to medical ethics.
3. Jonsen AR, Toulmin S. *The abuse of casuistry: a history of moral reasoning.* Berkeley: University of California Press, 1988.
   Offers a cogent rationale for a case-based approach to ethics and provides an overview of the accomplishments and downfall of casuistry.

3

Informed Consent

Informed consent requires physicians to share decision-making power with patients. Many physicians, however, are skeptical about informed consent or even hostile to it. Some believe that it is impossible because patients can never understand medical situations as well as doctors. Other physicians regard informed consent as a meaningless legal ritual because they can almost always persuade patients to follow their recommendations. In addition, some patients do not want to participate in decision-making, as in the following case.

CASE 3.1. RELUCTANCE TO MAKE A DECISION. *Mr. T. was an 88-year-old man with severe chronic obstructive pulmonary disease (COPD), coronary artery disease, and peptic ulcer disease. He developed a adenocarcinoma of the lung, which could be treated with surgery or radiation therapy. His physician was reluctant to recommend surgery because of the patient's increased operative risk. In addition, his COPD was so severe that he might be dyspneic after a pneumonectomy. When his doctor discussed alternatives for treatment, Mr. T. said, "Do what you think is best. You're the doctor."*

In this case, only Mr. T. can determine if the chance of being cured of cancer is worth the risk of severe dyspnea, but Mr. T. apparently does not want to make decisions. How should the physician proceed? This chapter discusses the definition of informed consent, its justification, its requirements, problems with informed consent, and ways in which physicians can promote shared decision-making with patients.

WHAT IS INFORMED CONSENT?

Discussions about informed consent are often confusing because people use this term in different senses.

Agreement With the Physician's Recommendations

Patients usually agree with physicians' recommendations. Such agreement is particularly common in an acute illness, when the goals of care are clear, one option is superior, the benefits are great, and the risks are small. For example, a patient who suffers a wrist fracture almost always agrees to a cast. In such situations, informed consent seems tantamount to obtaining the patient's agreement to the proposed intervention. Physicians often speak of "consenting the patient," implying that it is a foregone conclusion that the patient will agree.

Right to Refuse Interventions

Another view of informed consent is that patients have an ethical and legal right to be free of unwanted medical interventions. Hence competent patients have the power to reject their physicians' recommendations about care.

Choice Among Alternatives

A broader view of informed consent holds that patients should have the positive right to choose among feasible options, in addition to the negative right to refuse unwanted interventions. For instance, Case 3.1 involves not only the right to refuse surgery but also a choice between surgery and radiation therapy.

Shared Decision-Making

A still more comprehensive view is that informed consent is a process of shared decision-making by the physician and patient (1). Both parties need to discuss the issues and reach a mutually acceptable decision. Through repeated discussions, physicians can educate patients about their condition and the alternatives for care, help them deliberate, make recommendations, and to try to persuade them to accept the recommendations (2).

REASONS FOR INFORMED CONSENT AND SHARED DECISION-MAKING

Several ethical and pragmatic reasons justify a broader conception of informed consent (3–5).

Respect Patient Self-Determination

People want to make decisions about their bodies and health care in accordance with their individual values and goals. Decision-making power in health care is important because the stakes can be high. One court expressed this idea in sweeping terms, declaring, "Every human being of adult years and sound mind has a right to determine what shall be done with his own body" (6).

Patient choice should be promoted because in most clinical settings different goals and approaches are possible, outcomes are uncertain, and an intervention may cause both benefits and harms (7). Individuals place different values on health, medical care, and risk. Some patients are wary about the side effects of medication, while others want to try risky therapies that promise better outcomes. Lung cancer patients are generally concerned about the short-term morbidity and mortality of surgery as well as long-term survival and cure (8). Older patients often prefer radiation therapy, which has a lower 5-year survival rate but also a lower likelihood of death during treatment. Physicians cannot accurately predict patient's preferences. For example, patients with newly diagnosed cancer are more likely to prefer intensive chemotherapy with little chance of cure than are physicians, nurses, and the general public (9).

Enhance the Patient's Well-Being

The goal of medical care is to enhance patient well-being, which can be judged only in terms of the patient's own goals and values. The patient's values are particularly important when there are major differences between possible outcomes or complications, when choices involve tradeoffs between short-term and long-term outcomes, when one of the options carries a small chance of a grave outcome, and when the patient has unusual aversions toward risk or certain outcomes (10). The choice between surgery and radiation in Case 3.1 has many of these characteristics. Similarly, for men with benign prostatic hyperplasia, the values they place on current symptoms and the prospect of postoperative sexual dysfunction determine whether surgery is the preferred option (11).

In addition, participation in decisions generally has other beneficial consequences for patients, such as an increased sense of control, self-efficacy, and adherence to plans for care.

Fulfill Legal Requirements

Physicians may consider informed consent "a nuisance, an alien imposition of the legal system that must be tolerated . . . but can be dealt with in relatively mechanical ways, such as making sure patients sign consent forms before major procedures" (4). Similarly, many patients are cynical about informed consent. In one study, fully 80% of patients said that the purpose of informed consent was to protect the physician (12).

REQUIREMENTS FOR INFORMED CONSENT

Ethically and legally, informed consent requires discussions of pertinent information, obtaining the patient's agreement to the plan of care, and freedom from coercion (4).

Information to Discuss with Patients

Physicians need to discuss with patients information that is relevant to the decision at hand (Table 3-1). Most court decisions and legal commentaries use the term "disclose," and when summarizing legal doctrine, this book uses this term. In general, however, we prefer the term "discuss," to emphasize that a dialogue between the physician and patient is preferable to a monologue by the physician.

Patients need to know the *nature* of the intervention, the expected *benefits*, the *risks*, and the likely *consequences*. In general, risks that are common knowledge, already known to the patient, of trivial impact, or very infrequent do not need to be discussed. For instance, patients do not need to be told about the nature of venipuncture, the rare risk of infection, or the minor discomfort of hematomas. On the other hand, for invasive interventions, courts have ruled that physicians need to discuss serious but rare risks, such as death or stroke. In Case 3.1, the physician should discuss with Mr. T. the risks of surgical mortality, prolonged hospitalization, and long-term shortness of breath following surgery.

The risks of an intervention may include psychosocial as well as biomedical risks. For human immunodeficiency virus (HIV) and genetic testing, the pertinent risks are not the risks of venipuncture, but the risks of stigma and discrimination in employment or health insurance. Many states have enacted special provisions requiring written informed consent and pretest counseling for HIV testing (13).

Patients also need to understand the *alternatives* to the proposed test or treatment and their risks, benefits, and consequences. In particular, the alternative of no intervention needs to be discussed. If a patient declines the recommended intervention, the physician needs to explain

TABLE 3-1. *Information to discuss with patients*

The nature of the test or treatment
The benefits, risks, and consequences of the intervention
The alternatives and their benefits, risks, and consequences

the adverse consequences of the refusal. In one case, a court ruled that when a woman refuses a Pap smear, the physician needs to discuss how the test could diagnose cancer at an early stage and avert death through early treatment (14).

Physicians must take the initiative in discussing information, rather than waiting for patients to ask questions. Patients, who have far less medical knowledge than physicians, may not even know what questions to pose.

It is controversial whether physicians need to inform patients of alternatives for care that they do not believe are medically indicated. Obviously physicians do not need to mention treatments that have no scientific rationale, would provide no medical benefit, or are known to be ineffective or harmful, such as laetrile for cancer. Nor do physicians need to discuss complementary or alternative medicines that they do not accept as valid. However, physicians should inform patients of alternatives that other reasonable physicians would recommend. Thus a physician who believed that surgery was the best approach to Mr. T.'s lung cancer still ought to inform him about the option of radiation therapy.

Discussions about the proposed test or treatment and the alternatives should be conducted by the attending physician or the physician performing the intervention (15). Such discussions should not be delegated to nurses, medical students, or house officers. Some busy physicians who have already discussed an intervention with the patient during an office visit ask a nurse or house officer to obtain the patient's signature on a consent form in the hospital. Although this approach is understandable because it saves time, it may be problematic if the patient has questions that an inexperienced physician or a nurse cannot answer.

Patient Agreement With the Treatment Plan

Patients must agree with the intended plan of care. For major interventions, such as surgery, obtaining explicit written authorization is standard. Written consent signals the patient that the decision is important. In ambulatory care, oral agreement to the plan of care is usual because the risks are lower and because patients can choose to discontinue medications (16,17).

Agreement Should Be Voluntary

Coercion and manipulation invalidate consent because they preclude free choices by patients. Coercion involves threats that are intended to control patients' behavior and that patients find irresistible (18). An example is a threat to discharge the patient from the hospital if he does not agree with the recommended care. Manipulation of information may also thwart informed decisions. For example, physicians may misrepresent the patient's condition or the nature of the proposed intervention. Coercion and manipulation contrast with persuasion, which is an attempt to convince the patient to act in a certain way by providing rational arguments and accurate data (18). Persuasion respects patient autonomy and indeed enhances it by improving the patient's understanding of the situation and the options.

Certain constraints on patients' choices are not coercive (5). The patient's prognosis may be so grim that all alternatives are undesirable and the patient has no "real choice." Warnings by the physician about the outcomes of choices or about the natural history of the illness are also not coercive because the physician makes no threat to bring about undesirable outcomes. Indeed, physicians would be remiss if they did not point out to patients the consequences of unwise choices.

Patients may lack the capacity to make informed decisions, as is discussed in Chapter 10. For such patients, decisions should be guided by advance directives or by appropriate surrogates (*see* Chapters 12 and 13).

OBJECTIONS TO INFORMED CONSENT

Patients Do Not Understand Medical Information

Patients often do not recall information they have discussed with physicians, even basic information about the proposed treatment. In a study of cancer patients who had just consented to treatment, only 60% understood the purpose and nature of the treatment, 55% could name any complications, and 27% could name an alternative treatment. Furthermore, just 40% had read the consent form carefully (19). Many physicians have had similar experiences with patients and conclude that patients are unable to make decisions in an informed way.

Physicians, however, are partly to blame for patients' poor comprehension. Doctors often use technical jargon that is incomprehensible to laypeople. Informed consent forms are usually difficult to read and understand (20). More importantly, physicians often fail to provide patients with information about interventions (21). In a study of hospitalized patients, physicians discussed the rationale for tests or treatments in 43% of cases, the benefits in 34% of cases, the risks in 14% of cases, and alternatives in 12% of cases (22). In a study of outpatients, physicians discussed alternatives in 14% of cases, discussed the pros and cons in 9%, and elicited the patient's preferences in 19% (16). As a result, patients are "simply not recognized"; they are "ignored," "patronized," or "taken for granted" (23).

Patients Do Not Want to Make Decisions

As in Case 3.1, some patients may not want to make decisions, but instead defer to physicians or family members. Several empirical studies indicate that although patients generally want information about their condition and treatment, many do not want to make decisions. In one study, almost all hospitalized patients regarded the physician as the decision-maker (21). Patients wanted information about plans for care in order to know what was going to happen and how to carry out those plans effectively. However, the only patients playing an active role in decision-making were those with chronic diseases who needed to take medications regularly and to report changes in their condition. In ambulatory settings, while most patients want information about their illness, approximately one-half of patients want to defer decisions to physicians (12,24). Many patients, however, want to play a more active role in decisions later, after they have experience with the prescribed medications (24). Doctors underestimate patients' desire for information and for discussions about therapy, and overestimate their desire to participate in decision-making.

More recent studies suggest that many patients want to share with physicians the choice among options. In one study, almost one-half of subjects wanted to decide with the doctor what treatment option is selected, and only about one-fourth wanted to turn this decision over to the physician (25). Another study found that 68% of patients wanted to share with physicians decision-making about invasive procedures (26).

Patients Make Decisions That Contradict Their Best Interests

A common criticism of informed consent is that patients may make unwise or harmful choices. Some physicians fear that information about risks may cause patients to refuse medically beneficial interventions. Empirical studies, however, do not support these concerns. In one study of 104 refusals of inpatient treatment, none were attributed to disclosure of information (27). Fourteen patients, however, refused care because of inadequate information about tests or treatments. Another benefit of informed consent is that patients may be more likely to decline interventions that have a low likelihood of success, are unproven, or are not recommended (28,29).

LEGAL ASPECTS OF INFORMED CONSENT

Court rulings have shaped the doctrine of informed consent, with particular focus on what information must be disclosed to patients.

Malpractice

Physicians who do not obtain informed consent may be found liable in civil suits for battery or negligence (4). *Battery* is harmful or offensive touching of another person. Physicians may commit battery if they carry out surgery without the consent of the patient, or if the surgery exceeds the scope of patient consent (30). For instance, a physician may be liable for performing a mastectomy on a patient who had consented only to a biopsy. Such legal liability may occur even if the intervention was medically appropriate, skillfully performed, and beneficial to the patient. This battery model, however, fits medicine poorly. Many cases do not involve physical touching of the patient, as when physicians prescribe drugs, fail to consider alternative approaches, or do not disclose information to the patient. In addition, battery requires that the physician intended to provide care without the patient's consent. Most cases of malpractice, however, involve unintentional actions.

The modern approach to malpractice, which has supplanted the battery model, is to hold physicians liable for *negligence*. To be found negligent, the physician must breach a duty to the patient, the patient must suffer a harm, and the breach of duty must cause the harm. With regard to informed consent, the patient needs to prove that the physician failed to disclose a risk that should have been disclosed, that he would not have consented had the risk been discussed, and that the risk occurred and harmed him. A crucial issue in malpractice law, therefore, is what risks should be discussed.

Standards for Disclosure

Full or complete disclosure of all information that physicians know about a particular condition is impossible. Thus the issue is not *whether* physicians should limit the amount and types of information they discuss with patients, but rather *what* information should be discussed or omitted.

Courts have used several standards to determine what information to disclose to the patient (4,31). A slight majority of states have adopted a *professional standard*: the physician must disclose what a reasonable physician of ordinary skill would disclose in the same or similar circumstances. This is equivalent to providing the information that colleagues customarily provide. The professional standard has been criticized because patients generally want more information than physicians customarily discuss.

Many states have adopted a patient-oriented standard for disclosure: physicians should disclose what a *reasonable patient* in the same or similar situations would find relevant to the medical decision. Generally this standard requires more disclosure than the professional standard, and it is more in keeping with the goal of promoting patient decision-making and choices.

Some individuals, however, may desire more information than the standard "reasonable" patient. For example, a carpenter may be particularly concerned that a new medication might impair her dexterity or alertness. To accommodate individual patient needs fully, a few states have adopted a subjective standard for disclosure: the physician must provide information that the *individual patient* would find pertinent to the decision. This subjective standard for disclosure is problematic in malpractice litigation. If a rare, undisclosed complication occurs, the patient may claim that he would not have consented to the intervention if the physician had mentioned that particular risk. In hindsight, it may be difficult to decide whether this assertion is plausible.

In some states, statutes specify that certain risks need to be disclosed, for example, "brain damage," or "loss of function of any organ or limb" (4). State courts have also ruled on issues of disclosure. A California court ruled that a physician did not have to give a quantitative estimate of life expectancy to a patient with pancreatic cancer. His widow claimed that if he had known such information he would have declined chemotherapy and arranged his business affairs (32).

Consent Forms

The consent form documents that the patient agreed to treatment. In some states, a signed consent form provides a legal presumption of valid consent (33). However, a signed consent form is not tantamount to informed consent because the discussion of the risks, benefits, alternatives, and consequences may be inadequate (4).

EXCEPTIONS TO INFORMED CONSENT

Several exceptions to informed consent illustrate how acting in the patient's best interests may supersede patient self-determination. These exceptions need to be carefully limited, so that they do not undermine informed consent.

Lack of Decision-Making Capacity

When patients lack decision-making capacity, an appropriate surrogate should give consent or refusal, following the patient's previously stated preferences or his best interests (*see* Chapter 4).

Emergencies

In an emergency, delaying treatment to obtain informed consent might jeopardize the patient's health or life. Legally, the courts have recognized a doctrine of *implied consent*: since reasonable persons would consent to treatment in such emergency circumstances, physicians may presume that the patient in question would also consent. Few people would object to treating life-threatening emergencies, such as an impending airway obstruction in anaphylaxis, without the patient's explicit consent. It is often possible to abbreviate the process of disclosure and consent in an urgent situation, rather than dispense with it altogether. In addition, the process of informed consent often can be initiated while the treatment is being started.

The emergency exception should not be used when informed consent is feasible or if it is known that a particular patient does not want the treatment. For example, terminally ill patients may have indicated that they do not want cardiopulmonary resuscitation (CPR). If such patients seek emergency care, the usual presumption that CPR should be initiated in case of cardiac arrest would not be valid.

Some physicians claim that consent is implied when a patient seeks care from a hospital or signs a general consent form upon admission. The implication is that informed consent for specific tests or treatments is unnecessary. However, this use of "implied consent" is unacceptable, because it allows physicians to administer any type of care they choose. When patients come to a hospital, they do not give physicians *carte blanche*. Most patients would probably agree to certain interventions, such as diagnostic testing, but want to base further decisions on new information.

Therapeutic Privilege

Physicians may withhold information when disclosure would severely harm the patient or undermine informed decision-making by the patient (1). For example, a patient may be depressed and have a history of previous suicide attempts in response to serious medical diagnoses. Telling such a patient he has cancer might provoke another suicide attempt. However, the concept of therapeutic privilege needs to be sharply circumscribed. The likelihood that the patient will feel sad does not justify withholding a serious diagnosis. Therapeutic privilege also does not allow the physician to "remain silent simply because divulgence might prompt the patient to forego therapy the physician feels the patient really needs" (34).

Waiver

Patients like Mr. T. in Case 3.1 may not want to participate in making decisions about their care. Ethically and legally, patients' requests to waive the right of informed consent should be respected. Self-determination would be undermined if patients were forced to participate in decision-making against their wishes. Shared decision-making entitles patients to participate actively in health care decisions but does not require them to do so (5). To be ethically valid, a waiver of informed consent must itself be informed. Patients must appreciate that they have the right to receive information and to make decisions about their care. Physicians can give patients the option not to receive information or make a decision, without thereby suggesting that they should do so. Physicians must keep in mind that patients may later want to participate more actively in decisions.

PROMOTING SHARED DECISION-MAKING

The process of shared decision-making generally requires multiple discussions between the physician and patient (Table 3-2).

Encourage the Patient to Play an Active Role in Making Decisions

Physicians can encourage patient involvement in decisions, even with patients like Mr. T. in Case 3.1. Patients who have never made decisions about their medical care may need considerable assistance from their physicians.

Elicit the Patient's Perspective About the Illness

Physicians can elicit the patient's concerns, expectations, and values regarding medical care through open-ended questions. Mr. T.'s physician might ask, "What is the most important thing for you over the next few years?" Another useful question is "What concerns you the most about your health?"

TABLE 3-2. *Promoting shared decision-making*

Encourage the patient to play an active role in decisions.
  Elicit the patient's perspective about the illness.
  Interpret the alternatives in light of the patient's goals.
Ensure that patients are informed.
  Provide comprehensible information.
  Try to frame issues without bias.
  Check that patients have understood information.
Protect the patient's best interests.
  Make a recommendation.
  Try to persuade patients.

Interpret the Alternatives in Light of the Patient's Goals

Patients need to understand that alternatives exist, with different benefits and burdens. When asked about his views, Mr. T. said that he wanted to continue to care for his sister, who had stomach cancer. Knowing these concerns, the physician explained that while surgery offered the best chance for long-term survival, Mr. T. might die after the operation and also would be unable to care for his sister while recuperating from surgery.

Ensure that Patients Are Informed

Provide Comprehensible Information

To enhance patient understanding, physicians should use simple language and avoid medical jargon. Innovative ways of presenting information include videotapes, interactive videodiscs, and discussions with patients who have had the intervention (11).

Try to Frame Issues Without Bias

People are more likely to accept a treatment if the outcomes are phrased in terms of survival, rather than in terms of death (35). Lung cancer patients are more likely to prefer surgery to radiation therapy if outcomes are framed as the probability of living rather than the probability of dying (35). Moreover, surgery is more attractive when survival data are presented as the average number of years lived rather than as the probability of surviving a given time period. To minimize bias, Mr. T.'s physician should describe the likelihood of both surviving and dying after surgery and radiation therapy.

Physicians also need to consider how to frame the disclosure of rare but serious risks, such as the risk of an anaphylactic reaction to radiographic contrast material (36). Patients might infer incorrectly that a risk is significant because the physician has mentioned it. Physicians should put the risk in context, for example, by saying, "I believe that this is a very small risk, compared with the information we would gain from the test."

Check that Patients Have Understood Information

Disclosure by the physician is not equivalent to comprehension by the patient. It is helpful to ask patients to repeat the information in their own words.

Promote the Patient's Best Interests

The guideline of beneficence requires physicians to help patients make decisions that are in their best interests (*see* Chapter 4). In addition to providing information, physicians should help patients deliberate about their choices.

Make a Recommendation

Physicians should not merely list the alternatives and leave it up to the patient to decide (37,38). Patients seek a recommendation regarding what plan is most likely to fulfill their goals. Mr. T.'s physician recommended against surgery, in light of Mr. T.'s desire to care for his sister.

Try to Persuade Patients

Physicians also should try to dissuade patients from choices that are contrary to their best interests (2).

In summary, shared decision-making respects patient self-determination. In order for patients to make informed choices, physicians must discuss with them the alternatives for care and the benefits, risks, and consequences of each alternative. Physicians also need to encourage patients to play an active role in decision-making and to ensure that patients are informed.

REFERENCES

1. Meisel A, Kuczewski M. Legal myths about informed consent. *Arch Intern Med* 1996;156:2521–2526.
2. Emanuel EJ, Emanuel LL. Four models of the physician-patient relationship. *JAMA* 1992;267:2221–2226.
3. President's Commission for the Study of Ethical Problems in Medicine and Biomedical and Behavioral Research. *Making health care decisions.* Washington: U.S. Government Printing Office, 1982.
4. Appelbaum PS, Lidz CW, Meisel A. *Informed consent: legal theory and clinical practice.* New York: Oxford University Press, 1987:35–67, 175–189.
5. Brock DW. *Life and death.* New York: Cambridge University Press, 1993:21–54.
6. Schloendorff v. Society of New York Hospitals. 211N.Y.125,105 N.E.92 (1914).
7. Shultz MM. From informed consent to patient choice: a new protected interest. *Yale Law J* 1985;95:219–299.
8. McNeil BJ, Weichselbaum R, Pauker SG. Fallacy of the five-year survival in lung cancer. *N Engl J Med* 1978;299:307–401.
9. Slevin ML, Stubbs L, Plant HJ, et al. Attitudes toward chemotherapy: comparing views of patients with cancer with those of doctors, nurses, and general public. *BMJ* 1990;300:1458–1460.
10. Kassirer JP. Incorporating patient preferences into medical decisions. *N Engl J Med* 1994;330:1895–1896.
11. Barry MJ, Fowler FJ, Mulley AG, et al. Patient reactions to a program designed to facilitate patient participation in treatment decisions for benign prostatic hyperplasia. *Med Care* 1995;33:771–782.
12. Cassileth BR, Zupkis RV, Sutton-Smith K, et al. Information and participation preferences among cancer patients. *Ann Intern Med* 1980;92:832–836.
13. Lo B, Steinbrook RL, Coates T, et al. Voluntary HIV screening: weighing the benefits and harms. *Ann Intern Med* 1989;110:727–733.
14. Truman v. Thomas, 27 Cal.3d 285, 165 Cal.Rptr. 308, 611 P.2d 902.
15. Rozovsky FA. *Consent to treatment: a practical guide*, 2nd ed. Boston: Little, Brown, 1990:721–727.
16. Braddock CH, Fihn SD, Levinson W, et al. How doctors and patients discuss routine clinical decisions: informed decision making in the outpatient setting. *J Gen Intern Med* 1997;12:339–345.
17. Diem SJ. How and when should physicians discuss clinical decisions with patients? *J Gen Intern Med* 1997;12:397–398.
18. Faden RR, Beauchamp TL. *A history and theory of informed consent.* New York: Oxford University Press, 1986:337–381.
19. Cassileth BR, Zupkis RV, Sutton-Smith K, et al. Informed consent—why are its goals imperfectly realized? *N Engl J Med* 1980;302:896–900.
20. Grundner TM. On the readability of surgical consent forms. *N Engl J Med* 1980;302:900–902.
21. Lidz CW, Meisel A, Osterweis M, et al. Barriers to informed consent. *Ann Intern Med* 1983;99:539–543.
22. Wu WC, Pearlman RA. Consent in medical decision-making: the role of communication. *J Gen Intern Med* 1988;3:9–14.
23. Katz J. *The silent world of doctor and patient.* New York: The Free Press, 1984.
24. Strull WM, Lo B, Charles G. Do patients want to participate in decision making? *JAMA* 1984;252:2990–2994.
25. Deber RB, Kraetschmer N, Irvine J. What role do patients wish to play in treatment decision-making? *Arch Intern Med* 1996;156:1414–1420.
26. Mazur DJ, Hickam DH. Patients' preferences for risk disclosure and role in decision making for invasive medical procedures. *J Gen Intern Med* 1997;12:114–117.
27. Appelbaum PS, Roth LH. Patients who refuse treatment in medical hospitals. *JAMA* 1983;250:1296–1301.
28. Murphy DJ, Burrows D, Santilli S, et al. The influence of the probability of survival on patients' preferences regarding cardiopulmonary resuscitation. *N Engl J Med* 1994;330:545–549.
29. Wolf AMD, Nasser JF, Wolf AM, Schorling JB. The impact of informed consent on patient interest in prostate-specific antigen screening. *Arch Intern Med* 1996;156:1333–1336.
30. Rozovsky FA. *Consent to treatment: a practical guide,* 2nd ed. Boston: Little, Brown, 1990:24–29.
31. Meisel A. *The right to die,* 2nd ed. New York: John Wiley & Sons, 1995:81–110.
32. Annas GJ. Informed consent, cancer, and truth in prognosis. *N Engl J Med* 1994;330:223–225.
33. Annas GJ, Law SA, Rosenblatt RA, et al. *American health law.* Boston: Little, Brown, 1990:601–612.
34. Canterbury v. Spence, 464 F.2d 772 (D.C. Cir. 1972).
35. McNeil BJ, Pauker SG, Sox H, et al. On the elicitation of preferences for alternative therapies. *N Engl J Med* 1982;306:1259.

36. Brody H. *The healer's power*. New Haven: Yale University Press, 1992.
37. Ingelfinger FJ. Arrogance. *N Engl J Med* 1980;303:1507–1511.
38. Quill TE, Brody H. Physician recommendations and patient autonomy: finding a balance bewteen physician power and patient choice. *Ann Intern Med* 1996;126:763–769.

ANNOTATED BIBLIOGRAPHY

1. Appelbaum PS, Lidz CW, Meisel A. *Informed consent: legal theory and clinical practice*. New York: Oxford University Press, 1987.
   Comprehensive and lucid book, covering ethical, legal, and practical aspects of informed consent. Stresses the need for dialogue between doctors and patients.
2. President's Commission for the Study of Ethical Problems in Medicine and Biomedical and Behavioral Research. *Making health care decisions*. Washington: U.S. Government Printing Office, 1982.
   Thoughtful discussion of shared decision-making by physicians and informed, competent patients.
3. Lidz CW, Meisel A, Osterweis M, et al. Barriers to informed consent. *Ann Intern Med* 1983;99:539–543.
   Empirical study that illustrates how informed consent may be absent in clinical practice.
4. Meisel A, Kuczewski M. Legal and ethical myths about informed consent. *Arch Intern Med* 1996;156:2521–2526.
   Corrects several common misunderstandings about informed consent.

4

Promoting the Patient's Best Interests: Responding to Patients' Refusals of Beneficial Interventions

Patients may reject the recommendations of their physicians, refusing beneficial interventions or insisting on interventions that are not indicated. In such cases, physicians are torn between respecting patient autonomy and acting in patients' best interests. If physicians simply accept unwise patient decisions in the name of respecting patient autonomy, their role seems morally constricted. This chapter discusses how physicians can protect the well-being of patients, while avoiding the pitfalls of paternalism.

PATIENT REFUSAL OF BENEFICIAL INTERVENTIONS

The following case illustrates how patients may refuse beneficial interventions.

CASE 4.1. REFUSAL OF SURGERY FOR CRITICAL AORTIC STENOSIS. *Mrs. N. is a 76-year-old widow with aortic stenosis. For several years she has refused further evaluation, saying that she would not want surgery. After an episode of near-syncope, she agrees to echocardiography, mostly to humor her physician. Critical aortic outflow obstruction is found. Her primary care physician strongly recommends valve replacement. The risks of surgery are unacceptable to her, particularly the risk of prolonged hospitalization or neurological or cognitive impairment. Having lived a full life, she says she welcomes a sudden death rather than a prolonged decline. In the past, she has been reluctant to visit physicians, undergo tests, or take medications. She leads an active life, writing a resource book for senior citizens, leading several volunteer organizations, and enjoying concerts.*

Mrs. N.'s physicians believe that her refusal conflicts with her best interests. With valve replacement, she is likely to live longer and avoid debilitating symptoms such as chest pain and dyspnea. Refusal of surgery may result in what she most fears: progressive decline and loss of independence.

How can physicians respond to Mrs. N.'s refusal? On the one hand, it would be disrespectful and impractical to override Mrs. N.'s refusal and operate without her consent. At the other extreme, accepting her refusal without further discussion may result in an adverse outcome that could have been averted. What attempts by physicians to persuade Mrs. N. to agree to surgery are warranted? To address these issues, physicians need to understand the ethical guidelines of doing no harm and acting in their patients' best interests.

DOING NO HARM TO PATIENTS

The ethical guideline of nonmaleficence requires people to refrain from inflicting harm on others. Prohibiting harmful actions is the core of morality (1). For instance, the Ten Commandments prohibit killing, lying, and stealing. In medicine, harms may include suffering and death, as well as infringements on liberty and privacy. Avoiding harm is generally considered a more stringent ethical obligation than providing benefit (1).

The widely quoted maxim, "Do no harm," has several distinct meanings (2). First, physicians should not provide interventions that are known to be ineffective. Second, physicians should not act maliciously, as by providing substandard care because they dislike the patient's ethnic background or political views. Third, doctors should also act with due care and diligence. Fourth, the maxim sometimes is cited as "Above all, do no harm," or, more impressively in Latin, *Primum non nocere*. If physicians cannot benefit patients, they at least should not harm them or make the situation worse. Fifth, when benefits and burdens are evenly balanced, physicians should err on the side of not intervening.

However, the precept "do no harm" provides only limited guidance. Many medical interventions, such as the aortic valve replacement mentioned in Case 4.1, offer both great benefits and serious risks and side effects. Literally doing no harm would preclude such interventions, yet some patients may accept substantial risks to gain medical benefits (3). Furthermore, as we next discuss, merely doing no harm seems a limited view of the physician's role (4).

PROMOTING THE PATIENT'S BEST INTERESTS

The ethical guideline of beneficence requires physicians to promote patients' "important and legitimate interests" (4). This guideline arises from the nature of the doctor–patient relationship and of medical professionalism.

The Fiduciary Nature of the Doctor–Patient Relationship

Physicians have special responsibilities to act for the well-being of patients because patients are often impaired in significant ways by their illness (5,6). Furthermore, the stakes are high; poor decisions may place patients' health or lives at risk.

Reasons for the Fiduciary Relationship

Patients Are Vulnerable

Because illness may undermine patients' independence and judgment, people may be less able to look after their own interests when they are sick. Furthermore, patients often have no previous experience in making medical decisions. Because of this vulnerability, patients often depend on physicians for advice and trust their recommendations.

Physicians Have Expertise That Patients Lack

Physicians know the benefits, risks, and likely outcomes of different approaches to the patient's care. Physicians also have experience and judgment, which allow them to apply their knowledge to the patient's individual circumstances.

Patients Rely on Their Physicians

It is difficult for patients to obtain information and advice other than through physicians. In serious illness, patients may have little time to seek second opinions. Similarly, it is hard for laypeople to determine whether a physician's advice is sound or to evaluate a physician's skills. Hence, patients rely on the advice of their physicians.

Definition of a Fiduciary Relationship

Legally, relationships between professionals and clients are characterized as fiduciary. The term fiduciary is derived from the Latin word *fidere*, to trust. Fiduciaries hold something in trust for another. They must act in the best interests of their patients or client, subordinating their self-interest. Fiduciaries are held to higher standards than ordinary citizens and business-people, who use their knowledge and skill for their own self-interest, rather than for the benefit of their customers (6). Ordinary business relationships are characterized by the phrase *caveat emptor*, "let the buyer beware," not by trust and reliance.

The fiduciary nature of the doctor–patient relationship is challenged by many arrangements in managed care (*see* Chapter 34). Financial incentives under managed care encourage physicians to act in their own self-interest or in the interest of third parties such as hospitals, physician groups, or managed care plans, rather than in the best interests of patients. Utilization review and practice guidelines may also undermine patient trust and limit physicians' freedom to act on behalf of their patients. Patients may fear that physicians no longer exercise independent clinical judgment, but simply carry out bureaucratic policies set by administrators.

The Nature of Professionalism

In professional codes of ethics, physicians promise to serve the best interests of patients. Literally, physicians "profess" to use their skills to heal and comfort the sick, encouraging patients to rely on them and promising to act in a fiduciary manner (7).

Professional codes and oaths have limitations. They are a generous but gratuitous acceptance of responsibilities and do not recognize the numerous benefits that physicians receive from society (8). Society grants physicians a great deal of autonomy. Physicians select applicants for medical school and postgraduate training, establish standards for certification, and discipline practitioners who do not meet these standards. In addition, during their training, physicians benefit when patients agree to serve as teaching subjects. Hence acting for the best interests of patients is something physicians owe patients and society in exchange for the privileges and benefits that society grants them (8).

Problems with Best Interests

The idea that physicians should act in the best interests of patients is indisputable. However, in any given case, the actions that are in the patient's best interests may be controversial.

Disagreements Over What Is Best for a Patient

People may disagree over the goals of care or the assessment of the benefits and burdens of an intervention. In Case 4.1, the physicians' goal is to increase the patient's likelihood of survival. However, the patient's goal is to avoid physical and mental decline, particularly in the perioperative period. Furthermore, the physicians and patients may weigh the risks and benefits of surgery differently (9). Physicians focus on the prospect of long-term survival, while Mrs. N. is more concerned about the short-term risks of surgery and her quality of life (10).

Quality of Life

The term *quality of life* is used in many different ways. Factors that might be considered include the following:

- The symptoms of the illness and the side effects of treatment
- The patient's functional ability to perform basic activities of living such as walking, shopping, and preparing meals
- The patient's experiences of happiness, pleasure, pain, and suffering
- The patient's independence, privacy, and dignity

Competent patients usually consider their quality of life as well as duration of life when making health care decisions. In some situations, a patient with a serious illness may decide that his quality of life is so poor that interventions are unacceptably burdensome. The principle of autonomy requires respect for a patient's judgments about quality of life, when that patient is competent and informed. More controversy exists if other persons are making the judgments.

Others Tend to Underestimate Patients' Quality of Life

Persons with chronic illness such as coronary artery disease and chronic obstructive lung disease rate their quality of life higher than do their physicians (11). Similarly, elderly patients who have survived a hospitalization in the intensive care unit view their quality of life higher than their family members do (12). Such discrepancies are not surprising. Many patients learn to cope with chronic illness over time, develop support systems, and continue to find substantial pleasure in life.

Discrimination May Occur

Assessments of quality of life may be discriminatory if they are based on the patient's economic value to society or social worth. Furthermore, quality of life may improve substantially if in-home assistance or adaptive devices are provided. Thus decisions based on quality of life may mask problematic value judgments.

Particularly Controversial Quality of Life Judgments

When a person cannot communicate with others, such judgments can be controversial. Consider a patient with severe Alzheimer's disease, who usually appears comfortable and smiles when music is played or when someone gives him a back rub. However, he has catastrophic reactions, shouting and striking people when asked to take a bath. How can other people determine whether such a patient has an acceptable quality of life?

Some writers argue that a patient's quality of life falls below a minimal acceptable level if he lacks qualities that are considered essential to being a person (13,14). In this view, patients in a persistent vegetative state or who never survive outside an intensive care unit have an unacceptable quality of life (13). These authors contend that such lives are "useless" and "not worth living and that it is not a goal of medicine to sustain biological existence in such situations" (13).

Others reject such quality of life considerations. Advocates for persons with disabilities fear that such considerations will lead to discrimination against people with disabilities. Proponents of a "right to life" believe that biological life should be prolonged, regardless of prognosis or quality of life. This position is often based on fundamentalist religious beliefs about the sacredness of life. Some states have adopted this position as public policy (15).

Medical Paternalism

Historically, beneficence rather than respect for persons was the dominant ethical principle for physicians. Doctors made decisions for the patient based on what they believed was the patient's best interests. This approach to decision-making has been termed medical paternalism (1), in analogy to how parents similarly make decisions for their children, rather than letting children decide for themselves. Deferring to the physician's recommendations is reasonable in many acute illnesses or emergencies, when cure is possible, the benefits of therapy far outweigh the risks, and treatment must be started promptly.

Philosophers define paternalism as intentionally overriding a person's known preferences or actions, in order to benefit that person (1). They further distinguish two types of paternalism. In weak or soft paternalism, the patient's decisions are not informed or not voluntary (1). If a patient's autonomy is impaired or in doubt, it is appropriate for physicians to intervene, at least temporarily. The justification is that patients should be protected from harming themselves through nonautonomous decisions and actions (16). Intervening to determine whether a patient is competent and informed is a minimal imposition on patient autonomy, compared with the possible harms of allowing an incompetent patient to act unwisely.

In strong or hard paternalism, a patient's autonomous choices are overridden. An example is withholding a diagnosis or test result requested by a patient because the physician believes the information will upset the patient greatly. When writing about paternalism, philosophers generally mean strong or hard paternalism (1). Strong or hard paternalism has been sharply criticized, as we next discuss.

Problems with Medical Paternalism

Critics of (strong) paternalism raise several objections (1). First, value judgments are unavoidable in clinical medicine, and patients, not physicians, should make them. Physicians can define the burdens and benefits of an intervention, but only Mrs. N. can decide whether the surgical risk and side effects are worth the chance for long-term survival and relief of symptoms.

Second, if strong paternalism were accepted, it would be difficult to set limits and avoid abuses. The concern is that physicians would override patient decisions that they considered unreasonable, even if the individual patient had strong reasons for the decision.

Third, the belief that patients cannot make wise medical decisions is a self-fulfilling prophecy. If patients are not informed, they will not be able to make meaningful choices. Similarly, patients who sense that they have no decision-making power will become passive. In contrast, if patients are empowered to make decisions, they generally ask questions, seek information, and take responsibility for difficult choices.

Fourth, physicians may seek to override a patient's wishes because of their own psychological and emotional reactions to the case. Some physicians are affronted if patients reject their recommendations. "Refusal of treatment is seen by physicians as a rejection of an offer of help, which in turn may be seen as a rejection of the person making the offer. . . . As a result physicians may feel angry, frustrated, and unwilling to explore the underlying basis of refusal" (16). Furthermore, some physicians have difficulty accepting that a patient is terminally ill or has little hope for meaningful recovery.

PATIENT INSISTENCE ON INTERVENTIONS

Patients sometimes insist on medical interventions that physicians consider far more harmful than beneficial. Such insistence may frustrate and anger physicians.

Disagreements over patient requests are often framed as conflicting rights: the patient claims the right to decide about his medical care, while the physician asserts a countervailing right to follow her professional judgment. Framing the issues in this way, however, generally leads to stalemate. A more fruitful approach is to examine the benefits and burdens for the patient.

CASE 4.2. REQUEST FOR CONTROLLED DRUG FOR PAIN. *A 56-year-old man has been disabled by chronic back pain for 10 years. Extensive evaluations, including a magnetic resonance (MR) scan, have been negative. Exercises and physical therapy have provided only minor improvement. After changing health insurance plans, the patient visits a new physician and requests a refill of a prescription for eight tablets of oxycodone (Percodan) daily. He says that he has not changed the dosage in several years. His new physician does not prescribe narcotics at this strength and dosage for chronic pain. She wants to wean the patient off narcotics and to help him live an active life despite the pain. The patient refuses a referral to a pain clinic. "I know that Percodan works. Nothing else helps me."*

Respecting Patient Autonomy

The ethical guideline of respecting patient autonomy and the legal doctrine of informed consent give patients the *negative* right to refuse unwanted treatments (*see* Chapter 3). However, this patient claims the *positive* right to receive a specific drug. Some countries allow patients to buy many drugs, including antibiotics, without a physician's prescription. In the United States, however, only physicians are licensed to order tests or prescribe medications.

Prescriptions for narcotics such as oxycodone require special physician registration numbers and triplicate forms. These restrictions address the concern that narcotics may be diverted to illegal uses or used to maintain an addiction. In California, a physician may prescribe narcotics and other controlled substances only if "in good faith he believes" that the patient's medical condition requires it" (17).

Respecting Physician Autonomy

Physicians claim the right to be free of inappropriate control by others. Doctors argue that their own autonomy would be undermined if they were forced to provide care that they regard as clinically inappropriate or substandard (18). However, doctors have different practice styles, and often no clear standard of care exists. In Case 4.2, many physicians would be willing to prescribe codeine, but almost no physician would fill a request for dilaudid. The issue is whether oxycodone in this situation is more similar to codeine or dilaudid. Many experts in pain management believe that the regular use of narcotics for chronic pain syndromes rarely leads to addiction and is effective in relieving pain and enhancing function (19).

Because claims of patient autonomy and counterclaims of professional autonomy often end in stalemate, a more promising approach is to examine the benefits and burdens of the requested intervention.

Acting for the Patient's Benefit

According to the guideline of beneficence, physicians should benefit patients, or at least not harm them. However, the patient and physician may disagree over what the goals of care should be, what should be considered a benefit or harm, and how much weight to place on various outcomes.

CASE 4.3. INTERVENTION WITH NO BENEFIT AND SERIOUS RISKS. *A 34-year-old woman is receiving adjuvant chemotherapy for breast cancer. She had six nodes positive for cancer and was estrogen receptor negative. She decides to discontinue chemotherapy because of side effects and to take laetrile. She asks her physician to monitor her while she receives the drug from another practitioner.*

In Case 4.3, the patient's goal is fewer side effects. For physicians, however, the goal is long-term survival. The patient regards the side effects of chemotherapy as intolerable, while physicians regard them as an unavoidable aspect of therapy that prolongs survival.

Laetrile, an unapproved drug derived from the kernels of apricots or peaches or from bitter almonds, is an alternative cancer "remedy." A rigorous clinical trial showed that laetrile is not effective against advanced cancer (20,21). Moreover, laetrile may have serious toxicity, such as cyanide poisoning. Physicians should not cooperate in the care of a patient taking laetrile because it is known to have no clinical benefit and serious risks.

Case 4.3 needs to be distinguished from alternative or complementary therapies in other situations. If the patient has not responded to standard medical therapy, she has little to lose by trying an alternative therapy that has no serious side effects. The use of alternative therapies is beyond the physician's control. In a 1997 survey, 42% of patients reported that they were taking complementary therapies, such as chiropractic manipulation, herbal remedies, and megavitamins (22). Doctors should continue to see patients who receive care from alternative healers, such as chiropractors, homeopaths, or herbalists, whose interventions are known not to present serious risk (23).

CASE 4.4. INTERVENTION WITH SMALL BENEFIT AND NO RISK TO PATIENT. *A 41-year-old bus driver has episodes of crampy abdominal pain and alternating diarrhea and constipation. One year ago, after an evaluation that included colonoscopy, she was diagnosed with irritable bowel syndrome. Dietary manipulations have been ineffective. On the advice of a friend, she asks her doctor to order an abdominal computed tomography (CT) scan because when the cramps are severe, she fears something serious has been missed. She also says that "if doctors could only find out what is causing this, they would be able to do something about it." She refuses to discuss psychosocial issues about her illness, saying that "my problems aren't in my head."*

The physician's goal in Case 4.4 is to help the patient cope with a chronic medical condition and live an active life despite her symptoms. However, the patient's goals are relief of her symptoms and reassurance that her condition is not dangerous. Because of their divergent goals for care, it is understandable that the patient and physician disagree on weighing the benefits and burdens of the CT scan.

To the patient in Case 4.4, a scan has great benefit and little risk. A negative scan would provide reassurance. In the unlikely event that the scan is abnormal, her course of care would be dramatically changed. Furthermore, the scan has no medical risk. In contrast, from the physician's perspective, a negative scan result is unlikely to lead to reassurance. Patients who seek "just another test" for reassurance often request further tests in a fruitless quest for a definitive diagnosis. Articles on irritable bowel syndrome advise against additional diagnostic tests if a thorough initial work-up is negative and the clinical course is typical (24,25).

In other cases, the medical risks of the requested therapy may be serious. If the patient in Case 4.4 had requested exploratory surgery to establish a definitive diagnosis, the physicians should certainly have demurred.

Allocating Resources Fairly

Given the soaring cost of health care, physicians have a duty to allocate health care resources fairly. They cannot ignore the costs of patient requests. Expensive high-technology procedures such as the CT scans noted in Case 4.4 drive up the cost of medical care. In addition, CT scans may reveal lesions that require further costly evaluation but ultimately prove to be clinically insignificant.

Cost, however, should not be the main reason for refusing patient requests. Under the current health care system, physicians have no explicit societal mandate to limit care in order to control costs. In managed care systems, potential conflicts of interest make it problematic to limit highly beneficial care on the basis of cost (*see* Chapter 34).

The primary consideration should be the benefits and risks to the patient, rather than costs. If the medical risks of the intervention outweigh any benefits for the patient, the patient's request can be refused without reference to costs. Cost may determine how much time and effort physicians should spend on trying to dissuade the patient. The physician should spend more time trying to discourage an expensive CT scan than in discouraging inexpensive tests. If the patient with irritable bowel syndrome in Case 4.4 wanted a simple blood test that offered no benefit, few physicians would strongly object.

Maintaining the Doctor–Patient Relationship

Physicians may fear that agreeing to a patient's requests will set a precedent for subsequent requests and create expectations about future care. For example, the physician may fear that the patient with back pain in Case 4.2 may ask for increasing doses of narcotics for pain relief, or that the patient with irritable bowel syndrome in Case 4.4 might want other studies if the CT scan is negative. We next discuss how physicians might continue a partnership with patients who insist on specific interventions.

REACHING AGREEMENTS ON BEST INTERESTS

The guidelines of beneficence and autonomy offer contrasting views of patients. Beneficence assumes that patients are vulnerable, medically ignorant, and in need of protection. In contrast, autonomy assumes that patients are active, informed, and capable of determining what is best for themselves. Both views have some truth. In some situations, physicians need to assist patients and protect them from unwise decisions. In other situations, patients know better than physicians what is appropriate for them.

In Case 4.1, it is appropriate for physicians to continue to talk with Mrs. N. to ensure that she understands the benefits and risks of surgery and that her decision-making capacity is intact. In addition, physicians can promote the best interests of patients, while recognizing patients' ultimate power to decide (Table 4-1).

TABLE 4-1. *Promoting the patient's best interests*

Understand the patient's perspective.
Address misunderstandings and concerns.
Try to persuade the patient.
Negotiate a mutually acceptable plan of care.
Ultimately let the patient decide.

Understand the Patient's Perspective

Before trying to persuade patients, physicians first should try to elicit the patient's perspective, including her understanding of the illness, goals and expectations for care, and concerns (26,27). Open-ended questions are helpful. In Case 4.1, the physician might ask:

- "What bothers you the most about your health?"
- "What about your condition causes you the most concern?"
- "What do you believe will happen with your condition if you do not have the surgery?"
- "What concerns you most about surgery?"

Empathic statements may facilitate discussions. For example, the physician might say, "It sounds frustrating to live with such back pain for so many years."

Address Misunderstandings and Concerns

The physicians may identify specific concerns or misunderstandings that can be addressed. These might include practical problems such as convalescence, psychosocial factors such as fear of loss of control, religious or cultural beliefs about illness, the experiences of relatives or friends, or their own past experiences (26,28,29). If such concerns can be addressed directly, patients may agree to the physician's recommendations. Often simply making feelings conscious helps dispel unwarranted fears and untangle past experiences that may "have no relevance to the present situation" (29).

Try to Persuade the Patient to Accept Beneficial Interventions

Physicians can help patients clarify their goals and choices for care (30). In Case 4.1, Mrs. N. has conflicting goals: to be active, retain her independence, and also avoid hospitalization. Many patients work out their general goals and preferences only through making specific decisions about an illness.

Physicians should recommend what they believe is best for the patient, taking into account the patient's values and preferences. In shared decision-making, physicians should not merely present patients with a list of alternatives and leave them to decide.

Physicians should try to dissuade patients from unwise decisions. Persuasion respects patients and fosters their autonomy. Persuasion may include talking to the patient on several occasions and asking her to talk to family members, friends, other physicians, or other patients who have had the intervention.

When patients decline beneficial interventions, physicians should acknowledge that patients may view the goals, risks, and benefits of interventions differently. In Case 4.1, the physicians should try to help Mrs. N. understand how her decision is likely to thwart her own goal of an active life. In other cases, doctors may need to encourage patients to reconsider what they regard as an acceptable benefit or risk.

When a patient requests ineffective or harmful interventions, the physician should acknowledge that it is natural to desire more effective therapy. The doctor should explain why testimonials and uncontrolled trials do not reliably prove that a therapy is effective. Most patients withdraw their request for such interventions after these discussions.

Persuasion needs to be distinguished from deception or threats. The latter are wrong because they undermine the patient's autonomy. Persuasion also must be distinguished from badgering the patient. Continual attempts to convince patients to change their minds may be counterproductive. It might be better to acknowledge that the choices are difficult, allow patients more time to decide, and give them more control over the decision-making process.

Negotiate a Mutually Acceptable Plan of Care

In negotiations, conflicting parties try to reach a mutually acceptable plan (27,31).

Focus on Problems, Not on Positions

Rather than disputing the patient's specific request, the physician might address the underlying problems in other ways. Thus, in Case 4.1 the doctor can address Mrs. N.'s concerns about the risks of surgery. In Case 4.3, the doctor can focus on the patient's concerns about the side effects of chemotherapy.

Think of Innovative Approaches to the Problem

In Case 4.3, the physician might modify the chemotherapy regimen or suggest that the patient take a "holiday" from chemotherapy. In Case 4.4, the physician might give the patient some articles on irritable bowel syndrome and cancer screening, to help the patient understand why the tests are not advisable.

Find Common Ground for Ongoing Care

The process of negotiation requires that both sides are willing to compromise. For example, in Case 4.2, the patient and physician might agree to continue oxycodone while attempting other methods of pain control, including such nonpharmacological approaches as stress management. In Case 4.4, the physician and patient might agree to obtain a CT scan but perform no further tests unless symptoms dramatically change. In addition, they might explore why the patient is so worried about a serious condition and how to cope with the uncertainty of clinical diagnosis.

The physician's efforts to persuade and negotiate should be proportional to the balance of benefits and burdens for the patient. If a patient refuses an intervention, the greatest efforts at persuasion are needed when the benefits of an intervention are highly likely, of great magnitude, and long-lasting and the side effects are rare, mild, and brief. If the patient insists on an intervention, physicians should be most persistent if the intervention has little benefit and great risk.

Strategies When Patients Refuse a Beneficial Intervention

The physician should take one step at a time. The doctor initially might ask the patient simply to talk with a specialist or a patient who has undergone the procedure. The doctor can emphasize that the patient is free to continue to refuse the intervention after this discussion. Major interventions, such as colostomy, amputation, renal dialysis, and transplantation, require patients to accept changes in self-image and learn new coping skills. Patients who initially refuse may change their minds with more information, more time to accept their new condition, and greater understanding of how many patients cope with their new situation.

When disagreements persist after repeated discussions, the competent patient's informed choices and definition of best interests should prevail. Appropriate follow-up care should be arranged to allow them to change their mind.

Strategies When Patients Insist on Interventions

Acknowledge Emotional Reactions to the Patient

Patients' insistence on interventions may lead to interpersonal conflict with physicians. Physicians may feel personally and professionally threatened if a patient seeks unorthodox remedies

(32). In addition, physicians may find persistent patients disagreeable or even obnoxious (33). Dislike for patients, however, is not an ethical justification for denying their requests. To guard against bias, physicians should ask themselves how they would respond to the request if it came from a favorite patient.

Set Limits

The physician is not obligated to provide futile care that has no pathophysiological rationale or has already failed (*see* Chapter 9). In addition, physicians should not prescribe medications merely to give patients hope or a sense of control if the drug is known to be ineffective and to have significant medical risks.

Involving Patients in Discussions

Some patients decline to discuss their refusal of the doctor's recommendations. In the hospital, patients may keep silent or turn their backs on physicians. In ambulatory settings, they may not keep return appointments. A physician's instinct not to accept the patient's refusal to talk is sound: the patient may be conflicted and ambivalent, and unconscious forces may be involved (29).

Several strategies may encourage patients to talk about their decisions. First, a sense of crisis or confrontation only makes things worse. Second, physicians need to acknowledge that patients may have good reasons to keep silent. They may be tired of people asking them questions, or they may be sleepy or hungry. The physician might say, "You have good reason to feel annoyed that people aren't allowing you to get any rest." Third, giving patients control is usually more helpful than trying to force patients to talk. In such cases, the physician might say, "I'm not here to force you to do anything. I am very concerned about your decision. What I ask is that you let me know your point of view and then let me know that you understand mine" (34). Fourth, other persons may be able to engage the patient. A nurse, social worker, psychiatrist, religious advisor, or family member may be able to induce patients to explain their reasoning.

In summary, physicians need to respect patient autonomy and act in the patient's best interests simultaneously. Physicians have a fiduciary obligation to act for the well-being of patients, as patients would define it. Physicians can satisfy the ethical guidelines of beneficence and autonomy by understanding the patient's perspective, by trying to persuade patients, and by negotiating a mutually acceptable plan.

REFERENCES

1. Beauchamp TL, Childress JF. *Principles of biomedical ethics*, 4th ed. New York: Oxford University Press, 1994:189–258, 271–287.
2. Jonsen AR. Do no harm. *Ann Intern Med* 1978;88:827–832.
3. Delaney M. The case for patient access to experimental therapy. *J Infect Dis* 1989;159:416–419.
4. Beauchamp TL, Childress JF. *Principles of biomedical ethics*, 3rd ed. New York: Oxford University Press, 1989:194–227.
5. Hall MA, Berenson RA. Ethical practice in managed care: a dose of realism. *Ann Intern Med* 1998;128:395–402.
6. Rodwin MA. *Medicine, money, and morals: physicians' conflicts of interest*. New York: Oxford University Press, 1993.
7. Pellegrino ED, Thomasma DG. *For the patient's good: the restoration of beneficence in health care*. New York: Oxford University Press, 1988.
8. Veatch RM. *A theory of medical ethics*. New York: Basic Books, 1981.
9. Slevin ML, Stubbs L, Plant HJ, et al. Attitudes toward chemotherapy: comparing views of patients with cancer with those of doctors, nurses, and general public. *BMJ* 1990;300:1458–1460.

10. McNeil BJ, Weichselbaum R, Pauker SG. Fallacy of the five-year survival in lung cancer. *N Engl J Med* 1978;299:307–401.
11. Pearlman RA, Uhlmann RF. Quality of life in chronic diseases: perceptions of elderly patients. *J Gerontol* 1988;43:M25–30.
12. Danis M, Patrick DL, Southerland LI, et al. Patients' and families' preferences for medical intensive care. *JAMA* 1988;260:797–802.
13. Schneiderman LJ, Jecker NS, Jonsen AR. Medical futility: its meaning and ethical implications. *Ann Intern Med* 1990;112: 949–954.
14. Schneiderman LJ, Jecker NS, Jonsen AR. Medical futility: response to critiques. *Ann Intern Med* 1996; 125:669–674.
15. Cruzan *v.* Harmon, 760 S.W.2d 408.
16. Appelbaum PS, Lidz CW, Meisel A. *Informed consent: legal theory and clinical practice.* New York: Oxford University Press, 1987:196.
17. California Health & Safety Code. §11210.
18. Brett AS, McCullough LB. When patients request specific interventions. *N Engl J Med* 1986;315:1347–1351.
19. Rosenthal E. Patients in pain find relief, not addiction, in narcotics. *New York Times* 1993 Mar 28:Al.
20. Moertel CG, Fleming TR, Rubin J, et al. A clinical trial of amygdalin (laetrile) in the treatment of human cancer. *N Engl J Med* 1982;306:201–206.
21. Relman AS. Closing the books on laetrile. *N Engl J Med* 1982;307:236.
22. Eisenberg DM, Davis RB, Ettner SL, et al. Trends in alternative medicine use in the United States, 1990–1997: results of a follow-up national survey. *JAMA* 1998;280:1569–1575.
23. Eisenberg DM. Advising patients who seek alternative medical therapies [see comments]. *Ann Intern Med* 1997;127:61–96.
24. Drossman DR. Irritable bowel syndrome. In: Dornbrand L, Hoole AJ, Pickard CG, eds. *Manual of clinical problems in adult ambulatory care.* Boston: Little, Brown, 1992:206–209.
25. Longstreth GF. Irritable bowel syndrome: diagnosis in the managed care era. *Dig Dis Sci* 1997;42:1105–1111.
26. Kleinman A, Eisenberg L, Good B. Culture, illness and care: clinical lessons from anthropologic and cross cultural research. *Ann Intern Med* 1978;89:251–258.
27. Quill TE. Partnerships in patient care: a contractual approach. *Ann Intern Med* 1983;98:228–234.
28. Jackson DL, Younger S. Patient autonomy and "death with dignity". *N Engl J Med* 1979;301:404–408.
29. Katz J. *The silent world of doctor and patient.* New York: The Free Press, 1984:122,156–163.
30. Emanuel EJ, Emanuel LL. Four models of the physician-patient relationship. *JAMA* 1992;267:2221–2226.
31. Fisher R, Ury W. *Getting to Yes,* 2nd ed. New York: Penguin, 1991.
32. Campion EW. Why unconventional medicine? *N Engl J Med* 1993;328:282–283.
33. Groves JE. Taking care of the hateful patient. *N Engl J Med* 1978;298:883–887.
34. Cassem NH, Hackett TP. The setting of intensive care. In: Cassem NH, ed. *Massachusetts General Hospital handbook of general hospital psychiatry.* St. Louis: Mosby Year Book, 1991:373–400.

ANNOTATED BIBLIOGRAPHY

1. President's Commission for the Study of Ethical Problems in Medicine and Biomedical and Behavioral Research. *Making health care decisions.* Washington: U.S. Government Printing Office, 1982.
   Lucid and thoughtful exposition of shared decision-making by physicians and patients.
2. Quill TE. Partnerships in patient care: a contractual approach. *Ann Intern Med* 1983;98:228–234.
   Practical suggestions on how to negotiate mutually acceptable decisions with patients.
3. Pellegrino ED, Thomasma DG. *For the patient's good: the restoration of beneficence in health care.* New York: Oxford University Press, 1988.
   Comprehensive exposition of the importance of beneficence in the doctor–patient relationship.

5

Confidentiality

Patients reveal to physicians sensitive information about their medical and emotional problems, alcohol and drug use, and sexual activities. The presumption is that physicians should maintain confidentiality of patient information. However, exceptions to confidentiality may be warranted to prevent serious harm to third parties or to the patient (Table 5-1). The human immunodeficiency virus (HIV) epidemic and the development of computerized medical records have sharpened controversies over confidentiality.

THE IMPORTANCE OF CONFIDENTIALITY IN MEDICINE

Reasons for Confidentiality

Keeping medical information confidential shows respect for patients (Table 5-1) (1,2). Patients want to control access to sensitive personal information and expect physicians to maintain confidentiality. Maintaining confidentiality also has beneficial consequences for patients and for the doctor–patient relationship. It encourages people to seek medical care and discuss sensitive issues candidly with health care professionals, issues such as psychiatric illness, sexually transmitted diseases, and substance abuse. In turn, treatment benefits both the individual patient and the public health. Furthermore, maintaining confidentiality prevents harmful consequences to patients, such as stigmatization and discrimination. Breaches of confidentiality have caused HIV-infected persons to lose jobs, housing, and schools, even though there was no risk of transmission in those settings (3). Patients who have employer-based health insurance may fear that the employer will gain access to their health information and use it to discriminate against them (4).

Respect for confidentiality is a strong tradition in medicine. The Hippocratic Oath enjoins physicians, "What I may see or hear in the course of the treatment . . . , which on no account one must spread abroad, I will keep to myself, holding such things shameful to be spoken about" (5). Modern professional codes similarly urge physicians to maintain confidentiality. The legal system may also hold physicians liable for unwarranted disclosure of medical information (6).

Difficulties Maintaining Confidentiality

Maintaining confidentiality has become increasingly difficult in modern medicine. Many people have access to medical records, including the attending physician, house staff, students, consultants, nurses, social workers, pharmacists, secretaries, medical records personnel, insurance company employees, and quality of care reviewers (7).

TABLE 5-1. *Exceptions to confidentiality*

Exceptions to protect third parties
  Reporting to public officials
    Infectious diseases
    Impaired drivers
  Injuries caused by weapons or crimes
  Partner notification by public health officials
  Warnings by physicians to persons at risk
  Violence by psychiatric patients
  Infectious diseases
Exceptions to protect patients
  Child abuse
  Elder abuse
  Domestic violence

Computerized medical records, which improve access to medical information, also allow more serious breaches of confidentiality (8). Confidentiality can be violated at any computer station, and information on a large number of patients can be accessed at once (9). Other new communication technologies, such as fax or e-mail, also present opportunities for confidentiality to be broken (10).

Although these structural changes in medical practice make confidentiality harder to maintain, many breaches of confidentiality result from health care workers' indiscretions. Caregivers may discuss patients by name at parties or even in hospital elevators or cafeterias (11,12). Although many physicians take such discussions for granted, patients object to such breaches of confidentiality (11). As a court ruling pointedly asked, "What policy would be served by according the physician the right to gossip about a patient's health?" (6).

Physicians often discuss patients by name at conferences in informal discussions with colleagues. However, the objectives of education and patient care can be achieved without disclosing the patient's identity. During such discussions physicians should obscure details that would identify patients. Patients expect such discretion (11).

Waivers of Confidentiality

Patients commonly give physicians permission to disclose information about their condition to others. For example, patients routinely sign forms to authorize releases of information to other physicians or to insurance companies. Insurers often require clinical information before they reimburse physicians or hospitals. Patients may not appreciate that signing a general release allows the insurance company to disseminate the information further. Insurance companies generally place patients' diagnoses in a computerized database that is accessible to other insurance companies or to employers without further permission from the patient (4).

DISCLOSING THE PATIENT'S CONDITION TO CONCERNED PERSONS

Disclosure of information about a patient's illness to family members, friends, or the press may raise ethical issues.

Disclosure to Relatives and Friends

Relatives, friends, and other concerned persons often ask about the patient's condition. Most patients want the physician to talk to their family, and usually physicians do not even ask the patient's permission to do so. In some cases, however, the relationship between the patient and the relative is rancorous.

CASE 5.1. ESTRANGEMENT FROM RELATIVES. *A 32-year-old woman is admitted to the hospital after a serious automobile accident. She is disoriented and confused. The patient's sister requests that the patient's husband not be given any information. The patient has previously told the physician about her hostile divorce proceedings. The husband, however, learns that she is hospitalized and inquires about her condition.*

In Case 5.1, the physician believes that the patient would want to limit her husband's involvement in her care, yet without an explicit directive from her to withhold information, it is appropriate to inform the husband. Legally, he has authority to serve as his wife's surrogate, unless she has appointed someone else as health care proxy (*see* Chapter 13). Ethically, the physician should acknowledge the divorce proceedings in discussions with both the husband and the sister and should explain to the sister why the husband should have access to information.

Information about Public Figures

The press may seek information about patients who are public figures or celebrities. The public and the news media may have legitimate reasons to know medical information about a public figure. For instance, a political candidate's health is an important concern to voters (13), yet famous people have a right to confidentiality, as do all people. The physician and hospital should ask the patient or appropriate surrogate what information, if any, should be released.

OMITTING SENSITIVE INFORMATION FROM THE MEDICAL RECORD

Patients who are concerned about breaches of confidentiality may ask physicians to omit sensitive information from their medical record.

CASE 5.2. OMISSION OF INFORMATION FROM THE MEDICAL RECORD. *A nurse who is in excellent health has a routine checkup at the hospital where he works. He asks his physician not to write in the medical record that he had been severely depressed several years ago. He knows that many people in the hospital might see his record, and he does not want colleagues to know his psychiatric history. He also fears that he will have difficulty changing jobs in the future if his history is known, even if he has no symptoms at the time.*

Physicians may fear that omitting medical information from patient records may compromise the quality of care. Important clinical information may not be available in an emergency. In addition, documentation of the patient's current condition and treatment may be required for insurance payment or authorization for services. Furthermore, in some health care organizations, laboratory tests and prescriptions may be ordered only by computer. Thus patients who wish to exclude information on active problems from their record may need to pay out of pocket or seek care elsewhere.

The purpose of the medical record is to enhance patient well-being and quality of care. Generally the patient is the best judge of his best interests. Some patients may regard breaches of confidentiality as more threatening than the risk of suboptimal care resulting from incomplete medical records.

Therefore, patients may choose to withhold information about an inactive medical problem, but not an ongoing condition for which they are receiving therapy, and a patient's informed preferences to exclude sensitive information from the medical record should be respected if feasible. Sympathetic to such patient concerns, many psychiatrists already keep their detailed psychotherapy notes separate from the rest of the patient's medical record.

OVERRIDING CONFIDENTIALITY TO PROTECT THIRD PARTIES

Overriding patient confidentiality may prevent serious harm to third parties, as the following case illustrates.

CASE 5.3. RISK OF HIV TRANSMISSION. *A 32-year-old accountant reveals to his physician that he had a positive test for HIV antibodies at an anonymous testing center. He asks his physician not to disclose the test results to anyone, because he is concerned about losing his job and health insurance. His physician encourages him to notify his wife, so that she can be tested. After several discussions, the patient continues to refuse to notify his wife or allow others to do so. He declares, "If she finds out, it would destroy our marriage." Should the physician notify the wife despite the patient's objections?*

Infected persons have a moral duty not to harm others and to notify persons whom they have placed at risk. This duty is particularly strong when trust is expected, as in marriage. The common law may also impose on infected persons a legal duty to notify partners whom they place at risk (14). In Case 5.3, the patient abrogates this responsibility. Physicians caring for infected persons also have an ethical duty to prevent serious harm to third parties, as we discuss next.

Justifications for Overriding Confidentiality

The balance between preventing harm to third parties and protecting confidentiality may be set by society through statutes, public health regulations, and court decisions. Setting this balance as public policy allows all points of view to be represented and is preferable to decisions by the individual physicians in their offices or at the bedside. Laws on confidentiality vary from state to state. In general, exceptions to confidentiality are warranted when all the following conditions are met (Table 5-2):

- The potential harm to identifiable third parties is serious.
- The likelihood of harm is high.
- There is no less invasive alternative means for warning or protecting those at risk.
- Breaching confidentiality allows the person at risk to take steps to prevent harm.
- Harms to the patient resulting from the breach of confidentiality are minimized and acceptable. Disclosure should be limited to information essential for the intended purpose, and only those persons with a need to know should receive information.

TABLE 5-2. *Situations in which overriding confidentiality is warranted*

The potential harm to third parties is serious.
The likelihood of harm is high.
No alternative for warning or protecting those at risk exists.
Breaching confidentiality will prevent harm.
Harms to the patient are minimized and acceptable.

In these circumstances, the overall harm to the third parties at risk is judged to be greater than the harm to the index case resulting from overriding confidentiality (1).

Confidentiality can be overridden in several ways. Physicians need to distinguish reporting to public officials, partner notification by public health officials, and direct warnings to third parties at risk.

Reporting to Public Officials

In certain situations, physicians are legally required to break confidentiality and to report the name of a patient to appropriate public officials (Table 5-1).

Infectious Diseases

Physicians, clinical laboratories, and hospitals are required to report to public health officials the names of patients with specified infectious diseases, such as tuberculosis and gonorrhea. Such reporting allows accurate epidemiologic statistics and public health planning and facilitates partner notification. Physicians, however, may be reluctant to report such patients to public health officials (15). In one study, over 60% of physicians were willing to allow a patient with gonorrhea to tell his wife that he had nonspecific urethritis (15). This strategy is ethically problematic. The wife would not know the nature of the infection, her long-term risk of infertility, or the need for follow-up tests for cure. In addition, feminist critics contend that male physicians apply an unfair double standard, protecting the man's interests rather than the woman's health.

HIV Infection

Earlier in the HIV epidemic, public health policies about HIV infection differed from policies regarding other infectious and sexually transmitted diseases. It was feared that standard public health policies, such as reporting of cases by name and partner notification, might deter HIV-infected patients from being tested or seeking care. In turn, such reluctance would undermine public health efforts. Alternative test sites were established where people could be tested for HIV antibodies anonymously. Many states passed laws to strengthen the confidentiality of HIV test results and to require written informed consent for HIV testing (16). Studies indicate that more high-risk persons will seek HIV testing if confidentiality is ensured (17–19). Furthermore, although the Centers for Disease Control and Prevention (CDC) required that acquired immunodeficiency syndrome (AIDS) cases be reported, HIV infection was not reportable in many states (3).

Recently, reporting of HIV infection to public health officials has become more similar to reporting of other infectious diseases. Reporting of persons with HIV infections by name, in addition to persons with AIDS, is now required in most states and has been recommended nationally (20–22). There are several reasons for this policy change (20,22). Because prognosis has improved dramatically with highly active antiretroviral therapy, AIDS reporting gives an inaccurate picture of the epidemic, undermines public health planning, and leads to inequitable distribution of funding based on caseload. However, because name reporting may keep some patients at risk from testing, continuation of anonymous testing is also recommended (23). This compromise illustrates how public policies must take into account both the importance of confidentiality and the benefits of reporting.

Impaired Drivers

Many states require physicians to report to the department of motor vehicles persons with specified medical conditions that impair their ability to drive safely. Such conditions include epilepsy, syncope, dementia, sleep apnea, and other conditions that impair consciousness (24–26). Even if the underlying condition is treated, the patient may not be able to drive safely. For example, after placement of an implantable cardiac defibrillator, about 10% of patients experience syncope or near-syncope associated with defibrillation in the first year (27). The physician's role is not to stop the patient from driving or to decide whether the patient should be permitted to drive. Such determinations are properly made by the department of motor vehicles. The physician only informs officials of persons who warrant investigation. Reporting is particularly important for patients who drive commercially and present greater risks because they spend more hours on the road, are responsible for third parties, and drive heavy vehicles (26,27).

Injuries Caused by Weapons or Crimes

Almost all states require physicians to report injuries involving a deadly weapon or criminal act (28). The rationale is to protect the public from further violence.

Partner Notification by Public Health Officials

In partner notification, persons at risk for an infectious disease are warned that they have been exposed. More partners are notified when notification is carried out by public health officials than when done by patients themselves (29). In the AIDS epidemic, the term *partner notification* has replaced the traditional term *contact tracing*. Many contagious diseases, such as tuberculosis, are spread through aerosolized particles and can be transmitted by casual contact. Many casual contacts may be located without the cooperation of the index case, as by going to the index case's workplace.

"Mandatory" Partner Notification

For all practical purposes, partner notification in HIV and other blood-borne and sexually transmitted diseases must be voluntary (30). In many cases, sexual or drug-sharing partners cannot be identified without the cooperation of the infected person. If patients do not wish to cooperate, they can deny that they have partners or give inaccurate names and addresses. Attempts to make partner notification "mandatory" are misguided and counterproductive. Any perception that partner notification programs are punitive or disrespectful to index cases will further reduce cooperation.

Minimizing Harms during Partner Notification

In partner notification, partners should be told only that they have been exposed. The identity of the index case is not revealed (30). However, index cases cannot be promised anonymity, because partners can often infer their identity.

Warnings by Physicians to Persons at Risk

In addition to notifying public officials, physicians may have a legal duty or the legal option to warn identifiable persons whom a patient places at risk (Table 5-1).

Violence by Psychiatric Patients

Physicians have a legal responsibility to override confidentiality to protect potential victims of violence by psychiatric patients (*see* Chapter 42). The landmark Tarasoff ruling declared, "Protective privilege ends where public peril begins" (31). Although many physicians believe that the law requires them to *warn* the potential victim, in fact the law requires a broader duty to *protect* the potential victim from harm. This duty to protect victims may involve more intensive therapy, voluntary or involuntary hospitalization, convincing the patient to give up weapons, or notifying the police. Many other states have similar requirements.

Infectious Diseases

Courts may require physicians to warn patients with infectious diseases to take precautions to prevent their infectious disease from afflicting others (32). In addition, some courts require physicians to notify identified persons whom their infected patients place at risk (33,34). These court rulings involved such conditions as hepatitis, tuberculosis, and Rocky Mountain spotted fever. Generally physicians can fulfill this duty by notifying public health officials, but dilemmas may occur, as we discuss next.

HIV Infection

Some jurisdictions allow physicians discretion regarding partner notification, permitting but not requiring notification (35,36). For example, in California, physicians are not *required* to notify partners of HIV-infected patients (or notify public health officials), but *may* notify (37). Physicians who notify cannot be held liable in civil or criminal proceedings (37).

If faced with a situation like Case 5.3 and no mandate to report, physicians may try to compromise. For example, the index case may promise to use condoms but refuse to notify his wife. This approach, however, does not give her the options of being tested, seeking antiretroviral therapy if infected, and deciding to discontinue the relationship.

Sound medical ethics might require notification even though the law does not. In Case 5.3, the criteria in Table 5-2 for overriding confidentiality are fulfilled: the risk is serious and likely, notification may prevent harm by allowing the wife to take precautions or seek antiretroviral therapy, there are no alternative means to warn such unknowing partners, and harm to the patient can be minimized if the physician discusses with him how notification might best be carried out. In Case 5.3, the husband also contravenes a reasonable expectation of trust and disclosure.

OVERRIDING CONFIDENTIALITY TO PROTECT PATIENTS

In several situations, physicians are required to override confidentiality to protect the patient, rather than third parties (Table 5-1).

Child Abuse

All states require health care workers to report suspected child abuse or neglect to child protective services agencies (38). The privacy of the parents is overridden in order to protect vulnerable children from the possibility of serious harm. Over 1000 children die of neglect and abuse each year, most of whom are under the age of 5 (38). Health care workers may be the only people outside the family to have close contact with preschool children. Physicians need only reasonable suspicion of abuse and neglect, not definitive proof, to justify a fuller investigation. To encourage reporting, most states grant immunity from civil and criminal liability when reporting is done in good faith. Intervention may enable parents to obtain enough assistance and support to prevent further abuse. In extreme cases, the child may be removed from parental custody. In evaluating possible child abuse, pediatricians should treat parents with respect, keeping in mind that most parents are trying their best to deal with the challenges of childrearing.

Elder Abuse

Most states require health care workers to report cases of elder abuse to adult protective services (39). The goal is to identify persons who are incapable of seeking assistance on their own and to offer them help. Elderly persons who are dependent on their caretakers may be unwilling or unable to complain about physical or psychological abuse or neglect (40). Patients might not be aware of available in-home supportive services or might feel intimidated by caretakers. Patients may fear that if they complain, they will be worse off, perhaps placed in a nursing home. Most elder abusers are family members, who are overwhelmed by caring for a frail elderly person. Thus reporting and intervention may provide resources that allow the elderly person to continue to live safely at home. Elderly persons who are truly capable of making informed decisions, free of intimidation or coercion, are free to decline offered assistance.

Specific laws for reporting elder abuse vary from state to state. Generally, reasonable suspicion of abuse is sufficient to trigger reporting. Health care workers must report abuse only when they obtain information about a patient in their professional role. Thus, while a physician as a private citizen *may* report a neighbor whom she suspects is a victim of elder abuse, she is not *required* to do so. Health care workers receive legal immunity when they make reports of suspected abuse in good faith.

Reporting of elder abuse has been criticized because it presumes that elderly persons are incapable of making decisions about their life. Furthermore, resources for protective services are often inadequate. Thus many health care workers may consider reporting elder abuse an empty or counterproductive formality. Instead of disregarding reporting laws, however, health care workers should report the case and also make patients aware of available support and help them gain access to it.

Domestic Violence

Domestic violence is physical, sexual, or psychological assault against intimate partners. The vast majority of victims are women. Many states require health care workers to report suspected domestic violence or abuse (28). Reporting is intended to protect the victim and to hold perpetrators of violence accountable. However, it may be ineffective or even counterproductive (28). Mandatory reporting may put battered patients at risk for retaliation by their perpetrators. Furthermore, victims may hesitate to seek medical care or disclose abuse because they fear that reporting will place them and their children in greater danger. The police and courts often respond poorly to reports of abuse. Thus physicians may face conflicting obligations: a legal mandate to report, their judgment that reporting is not in the woman's best interests, and the patient's desire not to report the abuse. Physicians should provide emotional support and refer patients to shelter, legal services, and counseling. In addition, doctors should discuss with the patient the possibility of reprisal and the need for shelter or protective orders and should communicate concerns about retaliation when making a report (28). Whenever possible, physicians should promote the victim's autonomy, for example, respecting her request to delay reporting until she can find shelter.

In conclusion, physicians should maintain confidentiality unless there are compelling reasons to override it. Physicians need to understand why society has determined that in some situations it is appropriate to override confidentiality.

REFERENCES

1. Beauchamp TL, Childress JF. *Principles of biomedical ethics*, 4th ed. New York: Oxford University Press, 1994: 226–269, 282–284, 418–429.
2. Bok S. *Secrets*. New York: Pantheon Books, 1982.
3. Gostin LO. The AIDS litigation project: a national review of court and human rights commission decisions, part I: the social impact of AIDS. *JAMA* 1990;263:1961–1970.
4. Donaldson MS, Lohr KN, ed. *Health data in the information age*. Washington: National Academy Press, 1994.
5. Beauchamp TL, Childress JF. *Principles of biomedical ethics,* 3rd ed. New York: Oxford University Press, 1989:329–341.
6. Horne *v*. Patton, 287 So.2nd 824 (Ala. 1974).
7. Siegler M. Confidentiality in medicine—a decrepit concept. *N Engl J Med* 1982;307:1518–1521.
8. Gostin LO, Turek-Brezina J, Powers M, et al. Privacy and security of personal information in a new health care system. *JAMA* 1993;270:2487–2493.
9. Committee on Maintaining Privacy and Security in Health Care Applications of the National Information Infrastructure. *For the record: protecting electronic health information*. Washington: National Academy Press, 1997.
10. Rind DM, Kohane IS, Szolovits P, et al. Maintaining the confidentiality of medical records shared over the Internet and the World Wide Web. *Ann Intern Med* 1997;127:138–141.
11. Weiss BD. Confidentiality expectations of patients, physicians, and medical students. *JAMA* 1982;247: 2695–2697.
12. Ubel PA, Zell MM, Miller DJ, et al. Elevator talk: observational study of inappropriate comments in a public space. *Am J Med* 1995;99:190–194.
13. Annas GJ. The health of the President and presidential candidates: the public's right to know. *N Engl J Med* 1995;333:945–949.
14. Kathleen K. *v*. Robert B, 150 Cal. App. 3d 992, 198 Cal Rptr. 273 (1984).
15. Novack DH, Detering BJ, Arnold R, et al. Physicians' attitudes toward using deception to resolve difficult ethical problems. *JAMA* 1989;261:2980–2985.
16. Rennert S. *AIDS/HIV and confidentiality: model policy and procedures*. Washington: American Bar Association, 1991.
17. Fehrs LJ, Fleming D, Foster LR, et al. Trial of anonymous versus confidential human immunodeficiency virus testing. *Lancet* 1988;ii:379–382.
18. Judson FN, Vernon TM. The impact of AIDS on state and local health departments: issues and few answers. *Am J Public Health* 1988;78:387–393.
19. Bindman AB, Osmond D, Hecht FM, et al. Multistate evaluation of anonymous HIV testing and access to medical care. Multistate Evaluation of Surveillance of HIV (MESH) Study Group. *JAMA* 1998;280:1416–1420.
20. Gostin L, Ward JW, Baker AC. National HIV case reporting in the United States—a defining moment in the history of the epidemic. *N Engl J Med* 1997;337:1162–1167.
21. Gostin LO, Webber DW. HIV infection and AIDS in the public health and health care systems. *JAMA* 1998;279:1108–1113.
22. CDC. Draft guidelines for national HIV case surveillance, including monitoring for HIV infection and acquired immunodeficiency syndrome. http://search.cdc.gov/search97cgi. December 12, 1998.
23. CDC. HIV testing among populations at risk for HIV infection—nine states, November 1995–December 1996. *MMWR* 1998;47:1086–1091.
24. Strickberger SA, Cantillon CO, Friedman PL. When should patients with lethal ventricular arrhythmia resume driving? *Ann Intern Med* 1991;115:560–563.
25. Drachman DM. Who may drive? Who may not? Who shall decide? *Ann Neurol* 1988;24:787–788.
26. Suratt PM, Findley LJ. Driving with sleep apnea. *N Engl J Med* 1999;340:881–882.
27. Epstein AE, Miles WM, Benditt DG, et al. Personal and public safety issues related to arrhythmias that may affect consciousness: implications for regulation and physician recommendations. *Circulation* 1996;94:1147–1166.
28. Hyman A, Schillinger D, Lo B. Laws mandating reporting of domestic violence: do they promote patient well-being? *JAMA* 1995;273:1781–1787.
29. Landis SE, Schoenbach VJ, Weber DJ, et al. Results of a randomized trial of partner notification in cases of HIV infection in North Carolina. *N Engl J Med* 1992;326:101–106.
30. Bayer R, Toomey KE. HIV prevention and the two faces of partner notification. *Am J Public Health* 1992; 82:1158–1164.
31. Tarasoff *v*. Regents of the University of California, 551 P2d 334 (Cal 1976).
32. Areen J, King PA, Goldberg S, et al., eds. *Law, science and medicine,* 2nd ed. Westbury, NY: The Foundation Press, 1996.

33. Furrow BR, Johnson SH, Jost TS, et al. *Health law: cases, materials, problems,* 3rd ed. St. Paul, MN: West Publishing, 1997:385–388.
34. Bradshaw *v.* Daniel, 854 S.W.2d 865 (Tenn. 1993).
35. Edgar H, Sandomire H. Medical privacy issues in the age of AIDS: legislative options. *Am J Law Med.* 1990;16:155–222.
36. Gostin LO, Lazzarini Z, Flaherty KM. Legislative survey of state confidentiality laws, with special emphasis on HIV and immunization. www.epic.org/privacy/medical/cdc_survey.html
37. Cal. Health and Safety Code, §§120975–121020 (www.leginfo.cagove/cgi—bin).
38. Wissow LS. Child abuse and neglect. *N Engl J Med* 1995;332:1425–1431.
39. Lachs MS, Pillemer K. Abuse and neglect of elderly persons. *N Engl J Med* 1995;332:437–443.
40. Diagnostic and treatment guidelines in elder abuse and neglect. *Arch Fam Med* 1993;2:371–388.

ANNOTATED BIBLIOGRAPHY

1. Siegler M. Confidentiality in medicine—a decrepit concept. *N Engl J Med* 1982;307:1518–1521.
   Confidentiality is difficult in modern medicine because so many people have access to a patient's medical record.
2. Lo B, Alpers A. The uses and abuses of personal health information in pharmacy benefits management. *JAMA* 2000;283:801–806.
   Analyzes dilemmas regarding confidentiality and use of personal health information in computerized databases in health care organizations.
3. Bayer R, Toomey KE. HIV prevention and the two faces of partner notification. *Am J Public Health* 1992; 82:1158–1164.
   Argues that failure to distinguish between contact tracing and the duty to warn has led to serious confusion. Contact tracing cannot be compulsory and has traditionally protected the anonymity of the index case.
4. Hyman A, Schillinger D, Lo B. Laws mandating reporting of domestic violence: do they promote patient well-being? *JAMA* 1995;273:1781–1787.
   Recent laws mandating reporting of domestic violence may place physicians in a dilemma if reporting is likely to lead to retaliation by the perpetrator.
5. Gostin L, Ward JW, Baker AC. National HIV case reporting in the United States—a defining moment in the history of the epidemic. *N Engl J Med* 1997;337:1162–1167.
   Argues that in the era of highly active antiretroviral therapy, name reporting of persons with HIV infecftion is appropriate provided that confidentiality is adequately safeguarded.

6

Avoiding Deception and Nondisclosure

All children are taught to tell the truth and avoid lies. The distinction between telling the truth and lying, however, may seem simplistic in clinical medicine. Doctors who condemn outright lying may consider withholding a grave diagnosis from a patient or using deception to gain benefits for a patient. This chapter analyzes the ethical considerations regarding lying, deception, misrepresentation, and nondisclosure. Such actions may mislead either the patient or a third party, such as an insurance company or disability agency.

DEFINITIONS

The following case illustrates the various ways physicians may provide misleading information.

CASE 6.1. FAMILY REQUEST NOT TO TELL THE PATIENT THE DIAGNOSIS OF CANCER. A 70-year-old Chinese-speaking man with a change in bowel habits and weight loss is found to have a carcinoma of the colon. The daughter and son ask the physician not to tell their father he has cancer. They say that patients in his generation are not told they have cancer and that if he is told, he will lose hope.

Physicians may provide misleading information in a number of different ways.

Lying: A lie is a statement (a) that the speaker knows is false or believes to be false and (b) that is intended to mislead the listener. For example, the physician may tell the patient that the tests were normal.

Deception is broader than lying. It includes statements and actions that are intended to mislead the listener, whether or not they are literally true. An example would be telling the patient that he has a "growth," hoping that the patient will believe there is nothing seriously wrong. Other examples include using technical jargon to confuse a patient, omitting important qualifying information, and presenting misleading statistics.

Misrepresentation is a still broader category, which includes unintentional as well as intentional statements and actions. The statements may or may not be literally true. Unintentional misrepresentation may result from inexperience, poor interpersonal skills, or lack of diligence. For instance, the physician may not check the patient's appreciation of the situation and thereby not appreciate that the patient has misunderstood.

Nondisclosure means that the physician does not provide information about the diagnosis, prognosis, or plan of care. For example, a physician may not tell the patient his diagnosis unless he specifically asks.

Many writers on medical ethics use terms such as "truth-telling" or "veracity." This book, however, uses the terms deception and misrepresentation, because ethically difficult cases usually involve deception or nondisclosure, rather than outright lies.

DECEPTION OR NONDISCLOSURE TO THE PATIENT

Traditional codes of medical ethics did not require physicians to be truthful or forthcoming to patients (1). The writings of Hippocrates urge physicians to conceal "most things from the patient while you are attending him." Until recently, many physicians in the United States either did not tell patients about serious diagnoses such as cancer or deceived them (2). There are several reasons for this practice.

Reasons for Deception or Nondisclosure

Deception and Nondisclosure Prevent Serious Harm to Patients

Physicians may fear that disclosing a serious diagnosis may cause a patient to lose hope, refuse medically beneficial treatment, or become depressed. Few patients, however, refuse recommended treatment after learning a serious diagnosis (3). While sadness and anxiety may be common, major depression or suicide attempts are rare. Some patients, however, already have major depression or have attempted suicide previously. In such cases, it would be justified to withhold the diagnosis while obtaining psychiatric consultation and assessing the likelihood of harm. In exceptional cases, the risk of harm may be so serious that it would be justified to withhold the diagnosis until the patient's mental health improves.

Disclosure Is Not Culturally Appropriate

In many cultures, patients traditionally are not told they have cancer or other serious diagnoses. Although 87% of European-American patients and 89% of African-American patients want to be told if they have cancer, 65% of Mexican-Americans and 47% of Korean-Americans would not want to be told (4). Furthermore, although 69% of European-American patients and 63% of African-American patients want to be told a terminal prognosis, only 48% of Mexican-Americans and 35% of Korean-Americans would want to be told (4). In some cultures, disclosure of a grave diagnosis is believed to cause patients to suffer, while withholding information causes serenity, security, and hope (5). Being direct and explicit may be considered insensitive and cruel. Families and physicians may try to protect the patient by taking on decision-making responsibility (6). It would be unfair to impose American standards of disclosure on patients who do not want it. However, the crucial ethical issue is whether the individual patient wants to know his diagnosis, not what most people in the culture would want.

Patients Do Not Want to Be Told

If the patient does not want to know his diagnosis, it would be autocratic to force him to receive information against his will, even in the name of promoting informed decisions. Indeed, it would violate patient autonomy to do so.

Reasons Against Deception and Nondisclosure

Lying and Deception Are Morally Wrong

Lying and deception are considered prima facie wrong; the presumption is that they are inappropriate (7). There are numerous reasons why this is so. Traditional religious and moral codes forbid lying. The Old Testament, for example, exhorts people not to bear false witness. Lying and deception show disrespect for other people. Those who are lied to or deceived generally feel betrayed, even if the liar has benevolent motives. Lying also undermines social trust. The issue is whether general prohibitions on lying also apply to deception and nondisclosure.

Most Patients Want to Know Their Diagnosis and Prognosis

The vast majority of patients in the United States want to know if they have a serious diagnosis. In one survey, 94% of the public report that they "would want to know everything" about their medical condition, "even if it is unfavorable" (8). Ninety-six percent want to know a diagnosis of cancer (8). The desire to be told a serious diagnosis is so strong in the United States that over 90% of patients want radiologists to tell them of abnormal results at the time of the imaging study, rather than waiting for their primary physician to give them the results (9). Even among patients from cultures in which nondisclosure is traditional, many want to be told their diagnosis (4).

Patients Need Information for Decisions

For patients to make informed decisions, physicians need to disclose pertinent information (see Chapter 3). Doctors are expected to disclose such information without patients having to ask for it.

Disclosure Has More Beneficial than Harmful Consequences

Disclosure of the diagnosis and prognosis can benefit patients. Patients are more likely to adhere to treatment regimens that they understand and have agreed to. Furthermore, many patients with a serious diagnosis already suspect it. If physicians and family members remain silent, patients might imagine a worse situation than is actually the case. Often patients feel relieved when their illness is explained and they can focus on treatment options.

Deception and Nondisclosure Require More Deception

Deception and nondisclosure usually require additional, more elaborate deceptions. If a patient is not told the diagnosis of cancer, deception is needed to explain the reasons for surgery or other treatments.

Deception and Nondisclosure May be Impossible

In the long run, it may be unrealistic to keep the patient from knowing his diagnosis. A nurse, house officer, or x-ray technician might disclose it. When patients belatedly find out their diagnosis, they may feel angry and betrayed. Thus the practical issue may not be whether to tell the patient the diagnosis, but rather how to tell him.

Resolving Dilemmas About Misrepresentation and Nondisclosure to Patients

Physicians can respond to dilemmas about informing patients of serious diagnoses, without resorting to misrepresentation or nondisclosure (Table 6-1).

TABLE 6-1. *Resolving dilemmas about deception and nondisclosure to patients*

Anticipate problems with disclosure.
Determine what the patient wants.
Elicit the family's concerns.
Focus on how to tell the diagnosis, not whether to tell.
If you are withholding information, plan for future contingencies.

Anticipate Dilemmas Regarding Disclosure

Dilemmas can often be anticipated, for example if the patient is from a culture in which serious diagnoses traditionally are not disclosed. When ordering tests, physicians can ask patients whether they wish to be informed of the results. "Many patients want to know their test results, while other patients want the doctor to tell a family member. I will do whatever you prefer. Do you want me to tell you the test results?" After the physician receives the test results, asking a question may signal that the results are abnormal, because there is no reason to withhold normal results from the patient.

Determine What the Patient Wants

When the family requests that the patient not be told, the physician should assess whether this is the patient's wish or the family's. Has the patient explicitly said that he would not want to be told a serious diagnosis? Convincing evidence that the patient himself would not want to be told should be respected.

Elicit the Family's Concerns

The physician should elicit the family's concerns. "What do you fear most about telling your father he has cancer?" In such discussions, the physician needs to validate the family's feelings as the natural reactions of loving relatives. The physician also needs to explain to the family how disclosure is usually beneficial, as discussed previously.

Focus on How to Tell the Diagnosis, Not Whether to Tell

Disclosing bad news usually can be done in supportive ways that help patients to cope. Physicians can soften bad news by being compassionate, responding to the patient's concerns, offering empathy, and helping to mobilize support (10–15). The Appendix discusses how to break bad news to patients.

If Withholding Information, Plan for Future Contingencies

If the physician deems it appropriate to withhold the diagnosis, the doctor should discuss plans for care with an appropriate surrogate, usually a close relative. Patients who do not want to be told their diagnosis may change their minds. Physicians should regularly ask patients if they have questions or want to discuss anything else about their condition.

Physicians should never promise family members that the patient will not learn a serious diagnosis. A nurse, an x-ray technician, or an insurance company representative might disclose it inadvertently. It is usually counterproductive to devise elaborate schemes to keep patients from the diagnosis, instead of helping them cope with the bad news.

In some cases, excellent care can be provided without explicitly talking about the diagnosis with the patient. If the family in Case 6.1 provides care and emotional support and helps the patient reach closure in life, little may be gained from making the prognosis explicit. Such cases illustrate that ethical values taken for granted in the United States are not the only basis for good medicine.

DECEPTION TO THIRD PARTIES

Patients who seek benefits, such as insurance coverage, disability, and excuses from work, often need physicians to give information to third parties. Physicians may consider using deception about the patients' condition to help them gain such benefits. Although such deception may be motivated by a desire to help the patient, it is ethically problematical. Throughout this section, it is assumed that the patient has authorized disclosure to the third party.

Reasons for Deception

Physicians may believe that the ethical guideline of acting in the best interest of patients justifies deception. Physicians may regard themselves as patient advocates, helping their patients gain medical and social benefits. In some situations, the benefits of deception seem great, or the harm small.

Benefits of Deception Are Great

CASE 6.2. ACCESS TO NEEDED CARE. A man with severe hypertension has no health insurance and receives care at a public hospital. He is treated with an angiotensin-converting enzyme inhibitor because other medications have intolerable side effects. Because of budget cuts, the pharmacy has restricted this drug to patients with congestive heart failure. On the next visit, his blood pressure is 180/115. The patient says, "Doc, there's no way I can pay $70 a month for the pills." The physician considers saying that the patient has congestive heart failure to get him the medicine.

In Case 6.2, the benefits of deception about the patient's condition seem huge. Treatment for severe hypertension is effective, standard medical care. The patient apparently will not receive such highly beneficial care unless the physician bends the rules.

The physician may also believe that deception is justified by the unfairness of the health care system. About 43 million Americans lack health insurance, and public hospitals do not have the resources to provide them adequate care. The physician may believe that obtaining the drug for the patient is redressing a wrong, rather than breaking an ethical guideline.

Harms of Deception Are Small

CASE 6.3. EXCUSE FROM WORK. A patient asks a physician to sign a form excusing an absence from work. He says that he had a severe upper respiratory infection but has now recovered. The physician did not see the patient while he was ill.

In Case 6.3, the physician may sign the form, even though she does not know whether the patient was actually sick or not, because she believes that any resulting harm would be trivial.

The doctor may consider the harm—inappropriate absenteeism—minor and better handled directly by the employer (16). It would not be cost effective for patients to visit physicians for all self-limited illnesses that keep them from work. Nor would it be desirable to medicalize such conditions by encouraging patients to consult physicians. Even if the worker was not sick, perhaps he had a good reason to stay home, for example, to care for a sick child. For these reasons, physicians commonly certify work absences even when they have not examined the patient during the illness.

Reasons Not to Deceive

Physicians Should Avoid Lying

CASE 6.4. CERTIFICATION FOR DISABILITY. A patient with chronic back pain asks the physician to certify that he is disabled. He has no neurological symptoms of numbness or weakness in his legs, which are criteria for disability. Disability is the patient's only financial support. In addition, the patient finds a disabled parking card to be convenient.

In Case 6.4, the physician is asked to lie. The physician may believe that the patient deserves income support, but physicians, like all people, have a moral obligation not to lie, as previously discussed.

Physicians Should Avoid Deception

Some physicians believe that although it would be wrong to lie to third parties about a patient's condition, it is permissible to provide information that is deceptive but literally true. In one survey, between 32% and 58% of physicians said they would deceive an insurance company to obtain coverage for screening mammography and coronary bypass surgery (17).

CASE 6.5. INSURANCE COVERAGE. A 42-year-old accountant asks her physician for a screening mammogram. Her mother, grandmother, and aunt all had breast cancer diagnosed in their 40s. Her health insurance policy will not cover mammography for women under 50, but will pay for mammograms ordered to evaluate masses. The physician attempts to call the plan to obtain authorization for the test. Three times the line is busy. On the fourth call, the clerk says that he will mail the physician an authorization form to fill out.

It may seem unfair for the insurance company to deny coverage for care that is beneficial, or to require physicians to assume heavy bureaucratic burdens. Although it is controversial whether mammograms are generally indicated under age 50, this woman's family history justifies the test. In Case 6.5, rather than fight the bureaucracy, the physician may be tempted to write "breast mass" on the insurance form. The physician may argue that this statement is literally true; most women have fibrocystic disease.

Physicians have an obligation to avoid misrepresentation to patients, because of the fiduciary nature of the doctor–patient relationship (see Chapter 4). Physicians have similar obligations to avoid deception to third parties, but for different reasons. The relationship between physicians and third parties is contractual rather than fiduciary. In contracts, both parties are required to avoid deception and deal fairly but generally need not disclose information that the other side could readily obtain by its own efforts or that is not essential to the transaction (18). However, insurers commonly require physicians to affirm that the information provided is accurate and complete. In Case 6.5, insurers consider such deception to be fraud and might bring legal charges.

The Harms of Deception Outweigh the Benefits

When indirect and long-term harms are taken into account, the overall harms of deception outweigh the benefits (19).

Deception Undermines Trust in the Profession

If physicians use deception in one situation, patients and the public may question whether they also use deception in other situations, perhaps to patients' disadvantage.

It is unrealistic to expect that such deception will not be discovered. Computers help insurers to identify questionable claims. Similarly, claims for disability from Social Security and worker's compensation are reviewed according to published criteria (20). Once misled, third parties will mistrust other information from physicians. They may require additional documentation. Physicians, who already complain of bureaucratic intrusions on the practice of medicine, may then face additional paperwork.

Deception Harms Other Persons

Deception about a patient's condition indirectly harms other people. Giving disability parking cards to patients like the one in Case 6.4 makes it more difficult for persons who are truly disabled to park. Deceptive claims for disability or insurance coverage force the public, workers, and employers to pay higher taxes or insurance premiums.

Resolving Dilemmas About Deception to Third Parties

The following suggestions may help physicians deal with patients' requests to use deception in order to gain benefits (Table 6-2).

Consider Whether an Important Health Benefit is at Stake

Physicians need to ask in what sense they are helping the patient. In some cases, health care is not the issue.

CASE 6.6. CANCELLATION OF TRAVEL PLANS. A healthy patient who has bought a vacation tour wishes to change his plans. He asks his physician to write a note saying that he is ill, so that he can obtain a refund.

In Case 6.6, the patient simply wants to break a business deal with the travel agency and avoid a financial penalty. Although physicians have a duty to provide beneficial medical care, they have no obligation to help patients gain business advantages.

Other cases involve social benefits that promote health. In Case 6.4, the patient needs disability payments to obtain food, clothing, and shelter. Such necessities are essential for good health. Physicians have an obligation to provide truthful information that will help patients get social benefits to which they are entitled, but it is not at all clear that physicians should use de-

---

TABLE 6-2. *Resolving dilemmas about deception to third parties*

Consider whether an important health benefit is at stake.
Deception may not be necessary.
Exhaust other alternatives.
Involve patients who request deception.

ception to help patients get social benefits for which they do not qualify. Even if physicians believe that the current social system is unjust, deception in selective cases seems an inadequate way to address the problem.

Case 6.2, involving medications for hypertension, offers the most cogent case for deception because the patient apparently will not receive highly beneficial health care unless the physician bends the rules. It is permissible for the physician to do so if other alternatives for the patient to obtain the drug have been exhausted.

Deception May Not Be Necessary

The Literal Truth May Resolve the Dilemma

The strategy of using the literal truth is unethical if it is deceptive, as in saying that the patient has a breast mass in Case 6.5. However, the literal truth is appropriate if it is not deceptive and prevents harm to the patient (21). In Case 6.3, the physician was asked to certify an absence from work without having examined the patient during the illness. The physician does not know whether the patient was ill but does not want to deny justified sick leave. Some physicians write, "The patient reports that he was sick and unable to work" (16). This statement, which is true, puts the dilemma back onto the patient and employer. Furthermore, this strategy obviates physician visits simply to obtain work excuses for self-limited illnesses. The physician should also explain to the patient the substance of his note and the reasons for it.

The Third Party May Have No Right to the Information

Physicians should not disclose information that the third party has no right to receive, as in the following case.

CASE 6.7. PREEMPLOYMENT PHYSICAL EXAMINATION. A man with asymptomatic human immunodeficiency virus (HIV) infection applies for an office job. A preemployment physical examination form asks if the patient has any serious medical problems. The physician is reluctant to tell the employer about the HIV infection, fearing that the patient will not be offered the job, even though he can perform the work satisfactorily.

Under the Americans with Disabilities Act, employers have no legal right to information that is not relevant to the patient's ability to perform the job and may not require a medical examination until a job offer has been made (22). The physician has no duty to tell the employer about the patient's HIV infection, because it is not relevant to his ability to perform the job. For this reason, it would be appropriate to simply write that the patient has "no medical conditions that impair the patient's ability to perform the job." This is the literal truth. To avoid signaling to employers that patients have an unrelated illness, physicians should write this response even for patients who have no illness.

Exhaust Other Alternatives

Often physicians can achieve the goal of benefiting patients without using deception. In Case 6.2, the physician may have several options for obtaining the drug for the patient with hypertension. The physician should appeal to the hospital pharmacy committee or to the chief of service for an exception to the formulary restrictions. Also it may be possible to get the drug free from the manufacturer. Furthermore, the physician should protest the budget of the public hospital to appropriate governmental officials. Deception for individual patients does not change the system; it only redirects scarce resources from one underserved patient to another. To be sure, pursuing these alternatives requires time and effort by the physician, but exhausting these alternatives gives physicians a stronger ethical justification for using deception as a last resort.

Involve Patients who Request Deception

Physicians often believe that they alone must decide how to respond to requests for deception. In fact, patients who make such requests have ethical responsibilities as well. If patients request physicians to use deception on a disability application or an insurance bill, physicians can frankly say that they feel caught between two ethical duties, to help the patient and to be truthful. Physicians can reflect the dilemma back to patients, saying, "If I mislead your insurer, how would my patients trust me not to mislead them in other situations?" Furthermore, the physician can point out the problems that will occur later if documentation is requested by the insurer.

In summary, there are strong ethical reasons for physicians to avoid deception and nondisclosure with patients. In addition, physicians should avoid deception about the patient's condition to third parties who have a right to such information. Physicians should keep in mind how deception could undermine the doctor–patient relationship and should seek constructive ways to resolve such dilemmas.

APPENDIX: BREAKING BAD NEWS

Plan the conversation. When ordering the test, the physician should also plan how to communicate the results. Most patients prefer to hear bad news in person rather than by telephone. In the inpatient setting, it is important to determine who will talk to the patient: the house officer, the attending physician, or the consultant.

Provide a calm setting. The physician should hold the discussion in a quiet, private place, sit down, and have a colleague answer pages. Before going to see the patient, the doctor can take a few moments to collect himself.

Warn the patient that bad news is coming. "Mr. Jones, I'm afraid I have some bad news. Do you feel like talking now?" Such a warning allows patients to prepare for what is coming. A few patients will say that they are not ready to hear bad news.

Avoid euphemisms and jargon. Say "cancer," rather than "tumor," "growth," or "malignancy," which patients are likely to misinterpret.

Allow the patient to react. The patient may respond with "stunned silence, anger, disbelief, acute distress, or guilt" (10). Many physicians are uncomfortable with silence and fill it by talking, often with confusing medical jargon. It is better to give patients time to absorb the information, sort out their reactions, or cry.

Keep the first discussion brief. Patients generally comprehend little else after hearing they have a serious diagnosis. Doctors need to recognize "the glazed look that means the patient is no longer listening" (12). Detailed information about tests and treatments can often wait for subsequent visits.

Elicit the patient's reactions and concerns. Otherwise physicians may make incorrect inferences about how the patient is feeling. Open-ended questions are helpful. "Most people are overwhelmed in this situation. How are you feeling?"

Provide realistic hope. Physicians need to emphasize that they will provide the best care they can and that they will be with the patient. If effective treatments are available, this should be stressed.

Show your concern. A detached demeanor may be interpreted as lack of concern. Physicians can say that they are sorry, in the sense of communicating regret. It is often helpful to reflect back the patient's underlying emotions. "This must be very hard for you." Gestures such as touching the patient on the forearm or hand may convey empathy more effectively than words. Another way to show concern is to help with immediate details, such as calling a family member. Expressions such as "I know what you're going through" may be counterproductive; the patient may feel that a healthy person could not imagine having a fatal diagnosis.

Repeat the discussion at subsequent visits to ensure that the patient has understood. Providing information is a process, not a single conversation. At each visit, asking how the patient is doing can allow him to raise issues.

Share uncertainty with the patient. When patients ask how much longer they have to live, physicians usually do not give straightforward responses (8). In the spirit of respecting patient autonomy, physicians need to give patients the best information possible. When physicians cite an average prognosis, they need to make clear that an individual may have a longer or shorter survival than the mean. In addition to answering questions about prognosis literally, physicians also need to address the patient's psychosocial concerns, such as fears of losing control, suffering unrelieved pain, and dying alone.

REFERENCES

1. Reiser SJ. Words as scalpels: transmitting evidence in the clinical dialogue. Ann Intern Med 1980;92:837–842.
2. Novack DH, Plumer R, Smith RL, et al. Changes in physicians' attitudes toward telling the cancer patient. JAMA 1979;241:897–900.
3. Appelbaum PS, Roth LH. Patients who refuse treatment in medical hospitals. JAMA 1983;250:1296–1301.
4. Blackhall LJ, Murphy ST, Frank G, et al. Ethnicity and attitudes toward patient autonomy. JAMA 1995;274:820–825.
5. Gordon DB, Paci E. Disclosure practices and cultural narratives: understanding concealment and silence around cancer in Tuscany, Italy. Soc Sci Med 1997;46:1433–1452.
6. Surbone A. Truth telling to the patient. JAMA 1992;268:1661–1662.
7. Bok S. Secrets. New York: Pantheon Books, 1982.
8. President's Commission for the Study of Ethical Problems in Medicine and Biomedical and Behavioral Research. Making health care decisions. Washington: U.S. Government Printing Office, 1982.
9. Schreiber MH, Leonard M, Rieniets CY. Disclosure of imaging findings to patients directly by radiologists: survey of patients' preferences. AJR 1995;165:467–946.
10. Fallowfield L. Giving sad and bad news. Lancet 1993;341:476–478.
11. Miranda J, Brody RV. Communicating bad news. West J Med 1992;156:83–85.
12. Brewin TB. Three ways of giving bad news. Lancet 1991;337:1207–1209.
13. Quill TE, Townsend P. Bad news: delivery, dialogue, and dilemma. Arch Intern Med 1991;151:463–470.
14. McLauchlan CAJ. Handling distressed relatives and breaking bad news. BMJ 1990;301:1145–1149.
15. Ptacek JT, Eberthardt TL. Breaking bad news: a review of the literature. JAMA 1996;276:496–502.
16. Holleman WL, Holleman MC. School and work release evalutions. JAMA 1988;260:3629–3634.
17. Freeman VG, Rathore SS, Weinfurt KP, et al. Lying for patients: physician deception of third-party payers. Arch Intern Med 1999;159:2263–2270.
18. Farnsworth EA. Contracts, 2nd ed. Boston: Little, Brown, 1990:249–272.
19. Bok S. Lying: moral choices in public and private life. New York: Pantheon Books, 1978.
20. Carey TS, Hadler NM. The role of the primary physician in disability determination for Social Security and worker's compensation. Ann Intern Med 1986;104:706–710.
21. Nyberg D. The varnished truth. Chicago: University of Chicago Press, 1993.
22. Americans with Disabilities Act of 1990, 42 USC §§12181,12182.

ANNOTATED BIBLIOGRAPHY

1. Bok S. Lying: moral choices in public and private life. New York: Pantheon Books, 1978.
   Comprehensive discussion of lies, stressing that people who are lied to feel betrayed and consider lying more serious than the liar does.
2. Blackhall LJ, Murphy ST, Frank G, et al. Ethnicity and attitudes toward patient autonomy. JAMA 1995;274:820–825.
   Fewer Mexican-American and Korean-American patients want to be told a serious diagnosis or grave prognosis, compared with European-Americans and African-Americans.
3. Surbone A. Truth telling to the patient. JAMA 1992;268:1661–1662.
   In most other cultures, it is customary for families and physicians to shield patients from disturbing information about their diagnosis or prognosis.

7

Keeping Promises

Physicians, like all people, make promises and are sometimes tempted to break them. Once made, promises take on moral force and are generally regarded as binding. In retrospect, however, some promises may seem imprudent or mistaken. The following cases dramatize that some promises can be kept only if important ethical guidelines are violated.

CASE 7.1. PROMISE NOT TO TELL THE PATIENT THAT SHE HAS CANCER. *A 61-year-old Mexican-American widow undergoes a needle aspiration of a breast mass. Her daughter and son ask the physician not to tell the patient if the mass is cancer, because they fear she would not be able to handle the bad news. They point out that it is not customary for women of her age in Mexico to be told they have cancer. After breast cancer is diagnosed, the patient is referred to a surgeon. The surgeon believes that patients need to be involved in decisions regarding mastectomy or lumpectomy. In addition, the patient asks a Spanish-speaking nurse, "Why do I need surgery?" The surgeon and nurse feel constrained by the primary physician's promise not to tell the patient her diagnosis.*

CASE 7.2. PROMISE TO SCHEDULE TESTS. *A 54-year-old man, a heavy smoker, is hospitalized for hemoptysis, weight loss, and angina pectoris. A chest x-ray shows a 2-cm proximal lung mass, with hilar adenopathy. A bronchoscopy is scheduled to obtain a biopsy. When the intern walks by his room, the patient shouts, "This is outrageous. I haven't had breakfast, I haven't had lunch. Now they say they don't know when the test will be done and that I may have to go through all this again tomorrow. If this is how the hospital is run, I'm leaving." The intern, eager to appease the patient and continue with his other work, promises the patient that the test will get done that afternoon. He tells the nurse to call the bronchoscopy suite to say that the test needs to be done that afternoon.*

THE ETHICAL SIGNIFICANCE OF PROMISES

A promise is a commitment to act a certain way in the future, either to do something or to refrain from doing it. Promises generate expectations in other people, who in turn modify their plans and actions on the assumption that promises will be kept (1). In everyday social interactions, people commonly make promises and expect others to keep the promises they make. Promises may be exchanged for other promises, as in a business contract. For example, a merchant may promise to deliver goods in exchange for the promise of payment on delivery.

Keeping promises is desirable for several reasons. It results in beneficial consequences by making the future more predictable, relieving anxiety, and promoting trust. Indeed, another definition of "promise" is "that which causes hope, expectation, or assurance" (2). Keeping promises is also important even if there are no short-term beneficial consequences. Promise-keeping is essential for harmonious social interactions. If promises were widely broken, people could not rely on others. People would be reluctant to make commitments for the future if they could not trust others to honor their promises.

If promises are broken, the person to whom the promise is made often suffers a detriment (3). Tangible harms resulting from broken promises might include inconvenience and monetary losses. Moreover, it seems unfair to allow people to break promises simply because it would be to their advantage to do so, when the other person may have altered her plans in reliance on the promise. The very concept of promises is negated if people feel free to break them. It is manipulative to expect others to honor their promises, even to their detriment, but to break your own promises when it is in your self-interest (3). The promise-breaker is in a sense trying to get something for nothing.

Promise-keeping is especially important for physicians. Because the doctor–patient relationship is based on trust, patients may feel betrayed if physicians break promises. Once betrayed, patients may be less likely to trust the individual physician or the medical profession. Promises by physicians help patients cope with the uncertainty and fears inherent in being sick. In addition, promises establish mutual expectations that benefit both physicians and patients. For example, physicians promise confidentiality of medical information; in return, patients are more candid about discussing sensitive issues pertaining to their health. Ultimately the patient's well-being is enhanced, and the physician's work is facilitated.

EXCEPTIONS TO KEEPING PROMISES

No one wants to keep all promises he or she makes. Some promises are made on the spur of the moment, under emotional stress, with inadequate information, or without proper deliberation (3). Foolish promises that put one at a great disadvantage are often retracted, particularly if they confer a gratuitous boon on the other person. People may excuse breaking such promises because the other person is no worse off than if the promise had never been made in the first place. With many retracted promises, no promise has been made in return, and the promisee has taken no action in reliance on the promise.

Clinical dilemmas occur when keeping promises would require actions that violate other ethical guidelines. In Case 7.1, the surgeon and nurse believe the initial promise not to tell the patient violates the guideline of respecting patient autonomy. In Case 7.2, the intern's promise was misleading, because he could not guarantee that the test would take place that afternoon.

While keeping promises is important, it is not an absolute ethical duty. In exceptional situations, it may be justified to break a promise. The strongest case for overriding the promise-keeping would occur when the following conditions are met:

- Keeping the promise would violate another important ethical guideline. In the most disturbing cases, keeping the promise would require deception by the physician, compromise the patient's autonomy, or seriously harm the patient.
- The countervailing ethical considerations were not taken into account when the promise was made.
- The clinical and ethical situation has changed significantly since the promise was made. In Case 7.1, the promise not to tell the patient was made before she asked explicitly about her diagnosis.
- The promise was made by someone else. While a person's promise can bind his own future actions, he has no authority to bind other people, such as the surgeon in Case 7.1 or the consultant performing the bronchoscopy in Case 7.2.
- The promise was implicit rather than explicitly stated.

SUGGESTIONS FOR PHYSICIANS

Do Not Make Promises Lightly

A statement that the physician regards as kindly reassurance may be interpreted by the patient or family as a promise. Even if the physician does not think a promise is important, the patient is likely to. Patients typically are more upset when physicians break promises than are the physicians.

Address the Concerns Underlying the Request for a Promise

If someone asks the physician to make an unrealistic promise, the physician can elicit the underlying concerns and try to address them in other ways. Thus, in Case 7.1, the physician needs to understand the concerns underlying the family's request not to tell the patient her diagnosis. Chapter 6 suggests how to do this. In Case 7.2, the physician needs to listen to and empathize with the patient's feelings of frustration and anger.

Don't Promise Outcomes That Are Out of Your Control

Physicians should avoid making promises that are beyond their control to keep. Because clinical outcomes are inherently uncertain, it is unrealistic to make a promise that guarantees a good outcome or the absence of complications after a procedure. Given the complex organization of modern medicine, it is misleading to make promises about the actions of other members of the health care team. After all, other physicians and nurses are autonomous agents who have free will and their own moral and professional values. Thus, in Case 7.1, even if the physician agrees not to disclose the diagnosis to the patient, she cannot promise that no other health care worker will disclose it. Furthermore, the physician should be clear that she will tell the patient she has cancer if the patient asks directly.

In Case 7.2, physicians should not make promises about future care that they do not personally control, such as the scheduling of bronchoscopy. In the short run it may seem easier to promise that the test will be done, rather than to listen to the patient complain about problems. However, making a promise that may not be kept is likely to cause more problems in the long run. It may be better simply to listen and acknowledge that the patient has every right to be angry. Realistically, all the doctor can promise is to look into the matter and to do her best to make sure that such delays and inconvenience don't happen again. If the doctor makes such promises, she needs to follow up on them appropriately. For instance, calling the patient ombudsman or filing an incident report with the charge nurse are appropriate institutional mechanisms to ensure follow-up.

Don't Violate Ethical Guidelines Because of an Ill-Considered Promise

While promise-keeping is important, it is not an absolute duty. Other ethical guidelines are also important and may take priority in some situations. In some cases, breaking the promise may be the lesser of two evils. Trying to keep an ethically questionable promise may only make matters worse. In Case 7.1, suppose the patient asks the physician directly whether she has cancer, so that there is a conflict between keeping the promise and not deceiving the patient. In this situation, respect for patient autonomy and avoiding deception should prevail over keeping a promise. It is usually better to admit that the promise was a mistake and to deal with the consequences as directly and compassionately as possible.

In summary, promises can allay patients' fears and uncertainty. It is important to keep promises because other people rely on them. Breaking promises undermines trust in the individual physician and in the medical profession, yet keeping promises is not an absolute ethical duty. Sometimes respecting a promise may require the physician to violate other important ethical guidelines. In exceptional situations, breaking a promise may be justified as the lesser of two evils.

REFERENCES

1. Farnsworth EA. *Contracts*, 2nd ed. Boston: Little, Brown, 1990:39–110.
2. *Webster's revised unabridged dictionary*. http://www.dictionary.com
3. Fuller LL, Eisenberg MA. *Basic contract law*, 4th ed. St. Paul, MN: West Publishing, 1981:1–8.

SECTION II

Shared Decision-Making

8

An Approach to Decisions About Clinical Interventions

Medical interventions may allow accurate diagnosis and effective treatment, but they may also be applied when their benefit is questionable or when patients would not want them. Physicians therefore must try to avoid two types of errors: withholding potentially beneficial tests and therapies that the patient would want and imposing interventions that are not beneficial or not wanted.

This brief chapter presents an approach to decisions about clinical interventions. The general approach to ethical issues in Chapter 1 can be adapted to such decisions (Fig. 8.1). The key questions are as follows:

Is the intervention futile in a strict sense? Sound ethical judgments require accurate medical information. Physicians are under no obligation to provide interventions that are futile in a strict sense (*see* Chapter 9).

Does the patient have adequate decision-making capacity? This is a crucial branch point in decision-making. Chapter 10 discusses how to determine whether a patient lacks decision-making capacity.

If the patient is competent, what is her informed decision? Competent, informed patients may refuse medical interventions (*see* Chapter 11). Patients frequently lack decision-making capacity when decisions about medical interventions must be made. If the patient lacks decision-making capacity, two additional questions need to be posed.

If the patient is not competent, has she given advance directives? Clear and convincing advance directives should be respected (*see* Chapter 12). In the absence of such advance directives, decisions should be based on what the patient would want or what is in her best interests (*see* Chapter 12).

If the patient has not clearly indicated what she would want done in the situation, who should serve as surrogate? Generally the surrogate should be a person designated by the patient or a close family member (*see* Chapter 13).

The book then considers disagreements between doctors and patients over medical interventions. Chapter 14 discusses conclusions about life-sustaining interventions that are commonly drawn, but that prove misleading on closer analysis. Chapter 15 analyzes insistence by patients or surrogates on interventions that physicians regard as inappropriate. Chapter 16 discusses the opposite situation: the physician insists on interventions that the patient considers unwarranted. Chapter 17 discusses how ethics committees or ethics consultants can help physicians resolve ethical dilemmas.

Next the book analyzes life-sustaining interventions in specific situations. Chapter 18 discusses Do Not Resuscitate (DNR) orders. Often discussions about DNR orders are the first step

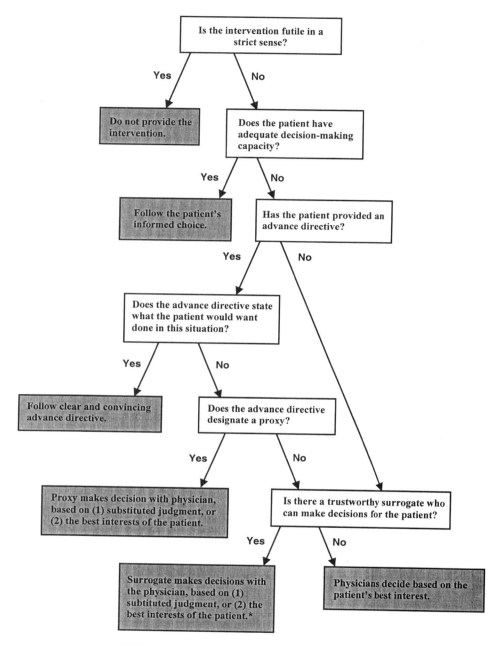

FIGURE 8-1. Flow chart for clinical decisions.

in a comprehensive evaluation of the goals and plans for care. Chapter 19 analyzes the controversial topics of assisted suicide and active euthanasia for terminally ill patients. Subsequent chapters discuss tube feedings, the persistent vegetative state, and the determination of death.

Legal issues are then presented. Chapter 23 analyzes landmark legal cases that have dramatized dilemmas about regarding life-sustaining interventions. Chapter 24 discusses myths about the law regarding clinical interventions.

REFERENCES

1. Lo B, Schroeder SA. Frequency of ethical dilemmas on a medical inpatient service. *Arch Intern Med* 1981;141:1062–1064.
2. LaPuma J, Stocking CB, Silverstein MD, et al. An ethics consulation service in a teaching hospital. *JAMA* 1988;260:808–811.
3. LaPuma J, Stocking CB, Darling CM, et al. Community hospital ethics consulation: evaluation and comparison with a university hospital service. *Am J Med* 1992;92:346–351.
4. Council on Ethical and Judicial Affairs, AMA. Guidelines for the appropriate use of do-not-resuscitate orders. *JAMA* 1991;265:1868–1871.

9

Futile Interventions

Patients or surrogates sometimes request medical interventions that physicians consider irrational or pointless. The concept of futility seems an appealing way to resolve such disagreements. The term "futility" comes from a Latin word meaning "leaky" (1). In classical mythology, the gods condemned the daughters of Danaus to carry water in leaky buckets (1). No matter how hard they tried, they could never achieve their goal of transporting water. By analogy, futile medical interventions would serve no meaningful purpose, no matter how often they are repeated.

Physicians do not need to provide futile interventions, even if patients or surrogates request them. Physicians claim that the judgment of futility is a matter of professional expertise. In this view, decisions to forego futile interventions may be made unilaterally by physicians rather than shared with patients or surrogates. Because the term futility gives decision-making power to physicians, it must be used with caution. The term is fraught with confusion, inconsistency, and controversy.

LEGAL CASES INVOLVING FUTILITY

Several publicized court rulings illustrate how physicians use the concept of futility to reject requests for interventions in patients who have an extremely poor prognosis.

The Gilguun Case

CASE 9.1. CPR AND MECHANICAL VENTILATION IN A PATIENT WITH MULTISYSTEM ORGAN FAILURE. *Catherine Gilguun was a 72-year-old woman with diabetes mellitus, leg ulcers, breast cancer, stroke, and Parkinson's disease. After hip surgery for a hip fracture, she developed status epilepticus and became unresponsive. After a temporary improvement, she developed a bowel obstruction, gastrointestinal bleeding, disseminated intravascular coagulation, and unresponsiveness. Her physicians believed that cardiopulmonary resuscitation (CPR) would be futile. One daughter refused a Do Not Resuscitate (DNR) order, saying that she would want everything done. The physicians wrote a unilateral DNR order, with the concurrence of the hospital ethics committee. The attending physician weaned the patient from the ventilator with the understanding that she would not be reintubated. After the patient died, the daughter sued the physicians and hospital for malpractice. A jury decided in favor of the physicians and hospital.*

The Gilguun case illustrates how physicians may use the concept of futility to respond to intractable disagreements with family members of incompetent patients who have a very poor prognosis.

72

The Baby K Case

CASE 9.2. MECHANICAL VENTILATION IN A CHILD WITH ANENCEPHALY. *Baby K had anencephaly (absence of the cerebral cortex). Infants with anencephaly generally survive less than a few weeks (2). After birth, Baby K's mother rejected the physicians' recommendations to withhold mechanical ventilation and allow her to die. The infant was weaned and discharged home. She developed many episodes of respiratory failure, which were treated with intubation and mechanical ventilation. The hospital sought court permission to withhold these interventions in the future, because they were futile. The mother disagreed, stating that "all human life has value" and that "God will work a miracle if that is His will. God and not other humans should decide the moment of her death." The appellate court ruled that mechanical ventilation was "emergency treatment" that was required under the federal Emergency Medical Treatment and Labor Act, which ensures access to necessary emergency care. The court rejected the argument that her quality of life was so poor that unilateral decisions by physicians to withhold interventions were justified.*

The Baby K case illustrates disagreements over the goals of care. Mechanical ventilation achieved the goal of allowing Baby K to recover from episodes of ventilatory failure, although it would not achieve the goal of improving her cerebral functioning. This case also illustrates how physicians' estimates of prognosis may be incorrect: Baby K lived for much longer than expected, dying of cardiac arrest at 2½ years of age.

STRICT DEFINITIONS OF FUTILITY

Physicians use the term in several different ways (3–5). In three strictly defined senses, medical futility justifies unilateral decisions by physicians to withhold or withdraw interventions (Table 9-1).

Intervention Has No Pathophysiologic Rationale

CASE 9.3. PATIENT WITH PROGRESSIVE SEPTIC SHOCK. *A 74-year-old woman has progressive septic shock with Staphylococcus infection, despite treatment with appropriate antibiotics. The patient's family requests an antibiotic that they learned about on the Internet. The antibiotic is active only against gram-negative bacteria.*

In this case, there is no pathophysiological rationale for the antibiotic, because it is not effective against the gram-positive bacteria causing this patient's illness. The antibiotic would provide no physiological benefit in terms of raising the patient's blood pressure. Even if the family insists on the drug, there is no medical reason to administer it.

Cardiac Arrest Occurs Despite Maximal Treatment

CASE 9.4. THE PATIENT WITH SEPTIC SHOCK HAS DETERIORATED DESPITE OPTIMAL THERAPY. *She is comatose, on renal dialysis, and on a ventilator. On increasing doses of vasopressors,*

TABLE 9-1. *When is an intervention futile in a strict sense?*

Intervention has no pathophysiologic rationale.
Cardiac arrest occurs despite maximal treatment.
The intervention has already failed in the patient.

her mean arterial pressure falls to 60 mmHg. Her physicians want to write an order not to resuscitate in case of a cardiopulmonary arrest.

Effective circulation cannot be sustained in this patient, despite appropriate therapy. If her hypotension results in cardiopulmonary arrest, CPR could not restore effective circulation. Even if cardiac rhythm were restored, she would be back in the situation of having refractory hypotension, which would again result in cardiopulmonary arrest. Thus a DNR order would be appropriate.

The Intervention Has Already Failed in the Patient

CASE 9.5. NO RESPONSE TO CPR. *A 54-year-old man suffers a cardiac arrest in the emergency room. CPR and advanced cardiac support are promptly initiated. After 30 minutes, all measures recommended in the American Heart Association guidelines have been attempted. He remains in asystole. His family insists that resuscitation be continued.*

An adequate clinical attempt of CPR has failed to achieve the fundamental goal of restoring effective circulation and breathing. It is pointless to continue or repeat interventions that have already failed.

These three strict senses of "futility" are as plain as the root metaphor of carrying water in leaky buckets. To be sure, a miraculous recovery might occur if such a futile intervention is attempted, but clinical decisions should not be based on the possibility of miracles. The determination that an intervention is futile in these strict senses is based on objective data or judgments within the expertise of physicians. Physicians have no ethical duty to provide interventions that are futile in these strict senses; indeed, they generally have an ethical obligation *not* to provide them.

LOOSE DEFINITIONS OF FUTILITY

The term "futility" is also used in several looser senses that are confusing, involve value judgments, and do not justify unilateral decisions by physicians to withhold interventions (5,6).

No Worthwhile Goals of Care Can Be Achieved

Futility can be defined only in terms of the goals of care. Some ethicists contend that the proper goal of medicine is not simply to correct physiological derangements. For these writers, it is inappropriate to prolong life if the patient will not regain consciousness or leave the intensive care unit (ICU) alive (1,7).

However, individual patients or the public may view the goals of care differently than physicians. Some people regard life as precious even if the patient will not leave the ICU alive. Indeed, certain states have established public policies that favor prolonging life in patients who will not regain consciousness (8). On a practical level, patients and surrogates may not agree with physicians about the goals of care or accept physicians' definition of goals. At a minimum, physicians need to discuss goals with patients, rather than attempting to define them unilaterally.

The Likelihood of Success Is Very Small

Some physicians contend that an intervention should be considered futile if the likelihood of success in a given situation is extremely small, for example, no success in the last 100 attempts or a less than 1% chance of success (7). However, there are conceptual problems with this quantitative, probabilistic concept of futility. Why set the threshold at 0/100 or at 1%? Some patients or families might consider a likelihood of success of 1% worth pursuing in some circumstances. On the other hand, some physicians might desire to make unilateral decisions to forego interventions whose likelihood of success is 2% or even 5%. Indeed, studies show that physicians commonly describe interventions as futile when the likelihood of success is far greater than 1% (9,10). Hence, even if agreement could be forged on a quantitative threshold for futility, in practice a much broader range of cases is characterized as futile.

The Patient's Quality of Life Is Unacceptable

In some situations, physicians may declare an intervention futile because they believe that the patient's quality of life is unacceptable. For example, some ethicists consider interventions futile for patients in a persistent vegetative state (PVS), who will never regain consciousness or interact with other people (1). They argue that sustaining biological life is not an appropriate goal when the patient has no likelihood of regaining consciousness. However, public policies may explicitly reject such quality-of-life determinations by physicians (8). In less extreme cases than PVS, it is problematic for physicians to make quality-of-life judgments that are not based on the patient's own values (*see* Chapter 4). Again, discussions with patients or surrogates are essential, and unilateral decisions by physicians may be counterproductive.

Prospective Benefit Is Not Worth the Resources Required

An intervention might be termed futile because the expected outcomes are not considered worth the effort and resources required. Allocating resources requires tragic choices, which may seem less divisive if not explicit (11). Terming an intervention futile may allow people to deny that tradeoffs are being made, or that the cost of saving some lives is too high (12), but trying to deny or hide value judgments by using the term "futile" may be counterproductive, leading patients or surrogates to assert a right to insist on whatever treatment they want. It may be preferable to reframe the question: are the benefits of the intervention worth the costs, including the loss of opportunity to treat patients who would have better medical outcomes? This question needs to be decided by society as a whole, not by physicians acting unilaterally at the bedside (*see* Chapter 32). Asserting that such interventions are futile closes off this difficult but essential debate (13).

PRACTICAL PROBLEMS WITH THE CONCEPT OF FUTILITY

Several problems occur in practice when physicians make unilateral decisions to withhold "futile" interventions.

Judgments of Futility Are Often Mistaken or Problematic

Physicians often make serious errors when they claim that an intervention has a very low probability of success. One study analyzed cases in which residents had written DNR orders on the basis of a probabilistic definition of futility (10). In 32% of such cases, residents estimated the probability of survival after CPR to be 5% or higher. In fully 20% of cases, the estimated probability of survival after CPR was 10% or greater. Thus the term "futility" was applied inappropriately to interventions whose probability of success far exceeds the 1% threshold for futility proposed in the literature. There are several reasons for such mistakes. Frequently, there are no reliable outcomes data on which to base determinations about the futility of an intervention in a specific situation. Physicians may misinterpret the medical literature.

Problems also occur when determinations of futility are based on quality of life. In the same study, residents determined that CPR would be futile in this sense for 40 competent patients. Physicians discussed quality of life with only 65% of these patients, even though such discussions were feasible (10). It is ethically problematical for physicians to make judgments about a competent patient's quality of life without talking to the patient directly. Many studies find that physicians underestimate the extent to which patients believe their lives are worth living (14,15).

Futility Applies to Few Patients

Patients for whom interventions can be reliably predicted to be futile, even in a loose sense, are rare (16). In the SUPPORT study, 0.2% of all hospitalized patients were predicted to have a less than 1% prospect of surviving for 2 months. In actuality, only 10% of this subgroup survived longer than 1 week. Thus, fewer than 2 of 10,000 hospitalized patients would be affected if life-sustaining interventions were limited a week after the patient was admitted. A tighter definition of futility would cover even fewer patients.

Unilateral Decisions by Physicians Polarize Disagreements

Attempts by physicians to resolve disputes by claiming the power to act unilaterally are likely to antagonize patients and surrogates. Furthermore, declaring an intervention futile may not settle other important issues in a case. For instance, CPR may be futile in a strict sense in a patient with multisystem failure in the ICU. However, a unilateral decision by physicians to withhold CPR would probably worsen disagreements regarding mechanical ventilation, vasopressor support, and antibiotics for infection.

Value Judgments May Be Masked as Scientific Expertise

When physicians term interventions futile, they claim total decision-making power, instead of sharing it with patients or surrogates (17). Unilateral decisions by physicians, based on futility, may therefore compromise patient autonomy. Assumptions and value judgments about the goals of the intervention and the acceptability of risk may be masked as scientific judgments. By suggesting that the decision is objective, the term "futile" may hide the fact that power and control are at stake.

Physicians Confuse Futility and Best Interests

Physicians need to distinguish futility and best interests as a basis for their decisions. Even if an intervention cannot be termed futile in a strict sense, physicians are not obligated to recommend it or provide it. Doctors need to explain why they believe that the burdens of an intervention outweigh the benefits and to recommend against interventions that they believe are not in the patient's best interests. However, physicians should try to persuade the patient or surrogate not to make a unilateral decision. Chapter 4 discusses the concept of best interests in detail.

SAFEGUARDS WHEN INTERVENTIONS ARE CONSIDERED FUTILE

Procedural safeguards are necessary to ensure that physicians' unilateral decisions to withhold "futile" interventions are appropriate (Table 9-2). Open discussions of medical futility help

TABLE 9-2. *Safeguards when physicians unilaterally decide that an intervention is futile*

Establish explicit guidelines on futility.
Obtain a second opinion.
Discuss the intervention with the patient or surrogate.

guard against errors and abuses. In the original meaning of "futile," there is no controversy that a leaky bucket will not hold water. Similarly, it should not be difficult for a physician to persuade colleagues, the patient or surrogate, or the public that a particular intervention is futile.

Establish Explicit Guidelines on Futility

Health care organizations should develop written guidelines regarding futile interventions (18). Written institutional guidelines demonstrate that unilateral decisions to forego futile interventions are made on the basis of carefully considered standards, not on *ad hoc* reasoning in particular cases. Several cities have developed policies and procedures for futility for a group of hospitals in a community (19–21). These policies have established procedures for managing intractable disputes between physicians and patients or surrogates. These policies reject unilateral decisions by the physician, instead requiring ongoing communication with patients or surrogates, a second opinion, and consultation with the hospital ethics committee.

Obtain a Second Opinion

The physician who is considering a unilateral decision to forego a "futile" treatment should obtain a second opinion from a colleague or from the institutional ethics committee. Such second opinions are important because judgments about futility are often flawed. Furthermore, second opinions help ensure that hidden value assumptions are made explicit and that all pertinent ethical considerations and management alternatives are considered.

Discuss the Intervention with the Patient or Surrogate

Some physicians believe that they need not discuss futile interventions with the patient or surrogate. For example, in Case 9.3, a vast array of interventions would be futile in a strict sense, such as cancer chemotherapy. It would be pointless to tell patients or surrogates of interventions that are irrelevant to the illness at hand. Indeed, discussing futile interventions with patients or surrogates may invite trouble by appearing to offer them a choice when actually there is none. In some cases, however, physicians may not discuss interventions because they fear that the patient or surrogate will disagree with their assessment that an intervention is futile. Physicians may use the idea of unilateral decisions about futility to avoid unpleasant discussions (18). However, the best approach to such situations is more discussion, not less.

Generally, discussing "futile" treatments with patients or surrogates is beneficial. It shows respect for patients and surrogates. It clarifies their expectations, goals, concerns, and needs. Chapter 4 gives specific suggestions for such discussions. Rather than trying to convince patients or surrogates to forego interventions, physicians may be better able to forge an acceptable plan for care by exploring the patient's and surrogate's perspective through open-ended questions and empathic comments (22). The physician might say, "I wonder if you feel sad and frustrated to see your mother so sick." Physicians should also be willing express their own feelings. "I'm also sad and frustrated that she hasn't improved. I wish we had a drug that would make her better." Moreover, such discussions help safeguard against improper uses of the term futility. Almost all patients or surrogates will eventually agree with physicians' judgments that interventions are futile (23). If patients or surrogates do not agree, physicians may need to reconsider whether the intervention is truly futile in a strict sense.

MEDICAL INDICATIONS FOR INTERVENTIONS

Physicians often use the term "not medically indicated" to justify unilateral decisions to withhold interventions that are admittedly not futile. The Wanglie case is an example (24).

CASE 9.6. MECHANICAL VENTILATION FOR A PATIENT IN A PERSISTENT VEGETATIVE STATE. *Helga Wanglie was an 87-year-old retired teacher who developed pneumonia and ventilatory failure after surgery for a hip fracture. Over the next 5 months, she was conscious but could not be weaned from the ventilator. She suffered a cardiac arrest and was resuscitated but never regained consciousness.*

A month later, the physicians suggested that the ventilator be discontinued because Mrs. Wanglie was in a PVS and could not be weaned from the respirator. Being in a PVS, Mrs. Wanglie had no awareness of her surroundings and no capacity to enjoy life. Her physicians conceded that mechanical ventilation could not be termed futile, because it would prolong her life. In their view, however, there were no medical indications for mechanical ventilation.

The family wanted the ventilator continued but agreed to a DNR order. Mr. Wanglie, a retired lawyer, said that during their 53-year marriage his wife had told him many times that she did not want "her life snuffed out," even if she was in a coma. Mr. Wanglie also argued, "Only He who gave life has the right to take life. The bills are being paid, so what are they complaining about?" Regarding the physicians' judgment that she would not improve, Mr. Wanglie said, "That may be true, but we hope for the best." The daughter and son agreed with their father. No other facility in the area would accept the patient in transfer.

Nine months after her cardiopulmonary arrest, the hospital went to court to discontinue the ventilator. The court rejected the hospital's request to appoint a guardian who would discontinue the ventilator. Mrs. Wanglie died, still on the ventilator, several days after the decision was handed down.

The physicians contended that mechanical ventilation has specific indications: to allow healing of underlying pulmonary disease, to palliate suffering in cases of terminal illness, and to enable disabled persons to enjoy life (24). The physicians believed that none of these indications was present in this case. Providing interventions that had no indications would compromise their professional judgment and moral integrity.

The concept of "no medical indications" suffers from the same problems as the concept of "medical futility." In a strict sense, the concept is compelling. No physician would provide mechanical ventilation to a patient whose condition was not caused by ventilatory failure or could be treated effectively by less invasive means. Used in looser senses, however, "no medical indications" is problematic. In the Wanglie case, the physicians made a value judgment that her quality of life was too poor to prolong with mechanical ventilation. Mr. Wanglie, on the other hand, claimed that his wife would want her life prolonged even in such a condition.

In conclusion, the concepts of futility and "not medically indicated" are intuitively appealing but need to be used extremely carefully. When futility is strictly defined, physicians may, and indeed should, make unilateral decisions to withhold interventions. However, it is problematic for physicians to use these concepts in looser ways to resolve disagreements with patients or families.

REFERENCES

1. Schneiderman LJ, Jecker NS, Jonsen AR. Medical futility: its meaning and ethical implications. *Ann Intern Med* 1990;112:949–954.
2. Peabody JL, Emery JR, Ashwal S. Experience with anencephalic infants as prospective organ donors. *N Engl J Med* 1989;321:344–350.
3. Youngner SJ. Who defines futility? *JAMA* 1988;260:2094–2095.
4. Lo B. Unanswered questions about DNR orders. *JAMA* 1991;265:1874–1875.
5. Truog RD, Brett AS, Frader J. The problem with futility. *N Engl J Med* 1992;326:1560–1564.
6. Lantos JD, Singer PA, Walker RM, et al. The illusion of futility in clinical practice. *Am J Med* 1989;87:81–84.
7. Schneiderman LJ, Jecker NS, Jonsen AR. Medical futility: response to critiques. *Ann Intern Med* 1996; 125:669–674.
8. Cruzan *v.* Harmon, 760 S.W.2d 408.
9. Prendergast TJ, Luce JM. Increasing incidence of withholding and withdrawal of life support from the critically ill. *Am Rev Respir Dis Crit Care Med* 1997;155:15–20.
10. Curtis JR, Park DR, Krone MR, et al. The use of the medical futility rationale in do not attempt resuscitation orders. *JAMA* 1995;273:124–128.
11. Calabresi G, Bobbitt P. *Tragic choices.* New York: WW Norton, 1978.
12. Miles SH. Medical futility. *Law Med Health Care* 1992;20:310–315.
13. Alpers A, Lo B. Futility: not just a medical issue. *Law Med Health Care* 1992;20:327–329.
14. Pearlman RA, Uhlmann RF. Quality of life in chronic diseases: perceptions of elderly patients. *J Gerontol* 1988;43:M25–30.
15. Danis M, Patrick DL, Southerland LI, N, et al. Patients' and families' preferences for medical intensive care. *JAMA* 1988;260:797–802.
16. Teno J, Murphy D, Lynn J, et al. Prognosis-based futility guidelines: does anyone win? *J Am Geriatr Soc* 1994;42:1202–1207.
17. Wolf SM. Conflict between doctor and patient. *Law Med Health Care* 1988;16:197–203.
18. Council on Ethical and Judicial Affairs, AMA. Medical futility in end-of-life care. *JAMA* 1999;281:937–941.
19. Bay Area Network of Ethics Committees (BANEC) Nonbeneficial Treatment Working Group. Nonbeneficial or futile medical treatment: conflict resolution guidelines for the San Francisco Bay Area. *West J Med* 1999; 170:287–290.
20. Halevy A, Brody B. A multi-institutional collaborative policy on medical futility. *JAMA* 1996;276:571–574.
21. Murphy DJ, Barbour E. GUIDe (Guidelines for the Use of Intensive Care in Denver): a community effort to define futile and inappropriate care. *New Horizons* 1994;2:326–331.
22. Lo B, Snyder L, Sox H. Care at the end of life: guiding practice where there are no easy answers. *Ann Intern Med* 1999;130:772–774.
23. Smedira NG, Evans BH, Grais LS, et al. Withholding and withdrawing of life support from the critically ill. *N Engl J Med* 1990;322:309–315.
24. Miles SH. Informed demand for "non-beneficial" medical treatment. *N Engl J Med* 1991;325:511–515.

ANNOTATED BIBLIOGRAPHY

1. Truog RD, Brett AS, Frader J. The problem with futility. *N Engl J Med* 1992;326:1560–1564.
   Contends that the concept of futility is riddled with ambiguities and hidden assumptions and should be banished from discussions of medical ethics.
2. Curtis JR, Park DR, Krone MR, et al. The use of the medical futility rationale in do not attempt resuscitation orders. *JAMA* 1995;273:124–128.
   Empirical study documenting problems and mistakes that occur when physicians claim that CPR would be futile.
3. Alpers A, Lo B. When is CPR futile? *JAMA* 1995;273:156–158.
   Suggests safeguards when unilaterial decisions are made based on futility.

10

Decision-Making Capacity

Physicians must respect the autonomous choices of patients. However, illness or medications may impair the capacity of patients to make decisions about their health care. Such patients may be unable to make any decisions, or they may make decisions that contradict their best interests and cause them serious, irreparable harm. Decision-making ability falls along a continuum, with no natural threshold for adequate decision-making capacity, yet for any proposed intervention, a binary decision needs to be made: either patients have adequate decision-making capacity and their choices should be respected, or they do not and their preferences can be set aside (1). The following case illustrates how it may be difficult to decide whether decision-making power should be taken away from a patient.

CASE 10.1. REFUSAL TO EXPLAIN A DECISION. *Mrs. C., a 74-year-old widow with mild dementia, is admitted for congestive heart failure and angina pectoris that has progressed despite maximal medical therapy (2). In the past 3 years, she has suffered two myocardial infarctions. Her physician recommends coronary angiography and, if possible, angioplasty.*

Mrs. C. recognizes her primary care physician, but seldom knows the date or the name of the clinic. She has forgotten to come to several clinic appointments. Her mental functioning gets worse when she is hospitalized. A nephew, her only relative, pays a woman to shop, cook, and clean house for her. He reports that Mrs. C. enjoys watching television, attending the senior center, and sitting in the park.

When asked about her wishes for care, Mrs. C. says that she wants to go home. After many discussions, the cardiology team convinces her to have the angiogram. On the morning of the procedure, however, she changes her mind, saying that she doesn't want anyone to put a tube into her heart and that she has been in the hospital long enough. Her nephew believes that angioplasty would be best for her but is reluctant to contradict her wishes because she has always been independent and stubborn. Mrs. C. is generally adverse to medical interventions. She refused mammography, even though she has a family history of breast cancer. She also refused treatment for a cholesterol level of 318 mg/dL.

The team asks a psychiatrist to see her. On a mental status examination, she does not know the date, the name of the hospital, or the city. She recalls only one of three objects and cannot perform serial subtraction. She refuses to talk further with the psychiatrist, saying that she is not crazy.

In this case, Mrs. C.'s mental functioning is obviously impaired. Is it so impaired that her nephew should assume the authority to make medical decisions for her? Her refusal did not seem so unreasonable to some physicians and nurses. Furthermore, some nurses asked why her consent to angiography was not questioned, only her refusal.

This chapter analyzes how physicians should assess whether patients like Mrs. C. have the capacity to make decisions about their care. This book uses the term *competent* to refer to patients who have the capacity to make informed decisions about medical interventions. Strictly speaking, all adults are considered competent to make such decisions unless a court has declared them *incompetent*. In everyday practice, however, physicians usually make *de facto* determinations that patients lack decision-making capacity and arrange for surrogates to make decisions, without involving the courts (3–6). This clinical approach has been defended because routine judicial intervention imposes unacceptable delays and generally involves only superficial hearings. Because legal competency hearings are far less common than informal determinations by physicians, this book does not use the legal term incompetent. Instead, we say that a patient *lacks decision-making capacity* if a physician rather than a court determines that the patient is unable to make informed decisions about health care (3).

ETHICAL IMPLICATIONS OF DECISION-MAKING CAPACITY

Caring for patients whose decision-making capacity is questionable involves two conflicting ethical guidelines. On the one hand, physicians must respect the authority of competent patients to make decisions that others might regard as foolish, unwise, or harmful (*see* Chapter 11). On the other hand, physicians should act in their patients' best interests (*see* Chapter 4). Patients who lack decision-making capacity are vulnerable and may be seriously harmed by decisions that are contrary to their best interests. Such persons need to be protected from harm (6,7). The patient's decision-making capacity is therefore crucial. If it is intact, the patient's decisions will be respected. If it is seriously impaired, decision-making power is taken from the patient and given to a surrogate.

Generally, a patient's decision-making capacity is not challenged if she agrees with the physician. On its face, this practice suggests that patients are only incapacitated when they disagree with physicians. However, it makes sense to raise more questions about decision-making capacity when a patient refuses a beneficial intervention than when she consents to it. When Mrs. C. accepts angiography, her care would be the same whether or not she has decision-making capacity. If she has adequate decision-making capacity, her consent to angioplasty would be valid. If she lacks it, the physician and her surrogate agree that angiography was necessary, because it was in her best interests. Now consider Mrs. C.'s refusal of angiography (assuming that she had not previously given an informed refusal). If she has decision-making capacity, her refusal would have to be respected. If she lacks it, a surrogate would assume decision-making power. The physician and her nephew agree that angiography is in her best interests. Hence, if she refuses, her management hinges on whether her decision-making capacity is considered impaired. Thus it is appropriate that Mrs. C.'s refusal of recommended interventions triggers questions about her capacity to make medical decisions. Such a refusal, however, does not by itself prove that she lacks such capacity.

LEGAL STANDARDS FOR COMPETENCE

The courts have not enunciated clear standards of competency to make medical decisions (4,8). A comprehensive legal treatise concludes that "the meanings of competence and incompetence are usually taken for granted or dealt with only in a cursory way by courts" (8). Many older legal cases viewed incompetence in general or global terms. Either the patient was competent in all aspects of life, or she was not competent in any sphere. The courts inferred incompetence from a person's overall ability to function in life, medical diagnoses, general mental functioning, and personal appearance.

However, a person may be capable of performing some tasks adequately, but not others (6). For example, she may be capable of making informed medical decisions, but not informed decisions about finances. Thus it would be more appropriate to consider a person competent or incompetent for specific tasks, rather than in all aspects of her life (5). The modern legal consensus is that a person should be considered competent to make medical decisions if she is capable of giving informed consent (5). More specifically, a patient is considered competent if she appreciates her diagnosis and prognosis, the nature of the tests or treatments proposed, the alternatives, the risks and benefits of each, and the probable consequences. Chapter 3 discusses informed consent in detail.

CLINICAL STANDARDS FOR DECISION-MAKING CAPACITY

A patient's decision-making capacity should be subjected to scrutiny in several situations. As in Case 10.1, the patient may refuse a treatment that the physician strongly recommends, or vacillate in her decision. In other cases, patients may have conditions that commonly impair decision-making capacity, such as dementia, schizophrenia, or depression. Although these conditions justify closer scrutiny of the patient's decision-making capacity, they are not tantamount to impaired decision-making capacity. Physicians need to test directly the patient's ability to give informed consent for the proposed intervention (3,6,9). Decision-making capacity requires a cluster of abilities (Table 10-1), as outlined below.

The Patient Makes and Communicates a Choice

The patient must appreciate that she—and not the physician or family members—has ultimate decision-making power. In addition, the patient must be willing to choose among the alternative courses of care. A patient who vacillates repeatedly between consent and refusal is incapable of making a decision, let alone an informed one. Such profound indecision must be distinguished from changing her mind as the situation changes, as she receives more information or advice, or after she deliberates.

The patient must communicate her choice. Persons who are unable to speak, for example, because they are on a ventilator, do not necessarily lack decision-making capacity. They may be able to communicate through writing messages, using an alphabet board, or blinking or nodding in response to questions.

The Patient Understands Information that Is Pertinent to the Decision and Appreciates its Relevance to Her Own Situation

The patient needs to understand her medical situation and prognosis, the nature of the proposed intervention, the alternatives, the risks and benefits, and the likely consequences of each alter-

TABLE 10-1. *Clinical standards for decision-making capacity*

The patient makes and communicates a choice.
The patient appreciates the following information:
- the medical situation and prognosis
- the nature of the recommended care
- alternative courses of care
- the risks, benefits, and consequences of each alternative.

Decisions are consistent with the patient's values and goals.
Decisions do not result from delusions.
The patient uses reasoning to make a choice.

native. Patients need this information to make an informed decision. In addition to comprehending this information, the patient needs to appreciate that she has the disorder and what consequences of treatment would be for her. She needs to accept that the information that the physician discussed is relevant to her own situation. In Case 10.1, the health care team could not determine whether Mrs. C. understood that angioplasty usually relieves chest pain but has certain risks.

Decisions Are Consistent With the Patient's Values and Goals

Choices should be consistent with the patient's character and core values. If Mrs. C. wants to be more active without pain, refusing surgery or angioplasty would be inconsistent with her goals. However, many patients do not have well-articulated values and goals, or may have multiple, conflicting goals. Mrs. C. may want to return home, but also to be more active and pain free. A choice may be consistent with some goals but not with others. People do not necessarily have a fixed hierarchy of goals and values. Mrs. C. might define her goals or set priorities only by making a decision about angiography. Thus physicians should not regard a patient as lacking decision-making capacity merely because she cannot articulate a set of general values or goals.

Decisions Do Not Result from Delusions or Distorted Views of Reality

Some patients have delusions that preclude informed decision-making. For instance, Mary Northern was an elderly woman who refused amputation of her gangrenous legs, denying that gangrene had caused her feet to be "dead, black, shriveled, rotting and stinking" (10). Instead, she believed that they were merely blackened by soot or dust. The court declared her incompetent, because she was "incapable of recognizing facts which would be obvious to a person of normal perception" (10). The court said that if she had acknowledged that her legs were gangrenous but refused amputation because she preferred death to the loss of her feet, she would have been considered competent to refuse the surgery.

The Patient Uses Reasoning to Make a Choice

Processing information logically is another element of the capacity to make medical decisions. Patients should compare and weigh the various options for care (9). This requirement does not require the patient to choose what most people consider reasonable in the situation. Unconventional decisions do not necessarily imply lack of decision-making capacity. Expectations for reasoning must take into account that many people do not deliberate but instead rely on emotional or intuitive factors in making important decisions.

Assessments of Decision-Making Capacity Should Take into Account the Clinical Context

Assessments must consider the patient's functional abilities, the demands of the specific clinical situation, and the possible harm that may result from her choice. Some writers have suggested that a patient who chooses an option that has great risk and little prospect of benefit should meet higher standards for decision-making capacity than a patient who chooses an option that has great prospect of benefit and little risk (6,9,11). The benefits and risks of alternatives should also be taken into account; a patient who chooses an option that is has less benefit and greater risk than the alternatives should be held to a stricter standard of decision-making capacity. Also, the nature of the intervention may be important. A patient may be given more leeway to refuse disfiguring surgery, such as amputation, than treatments with less drastic side effects. Such a sliding scale offers more protection to patients when the potential harm resulting from their decisions is greater. According to this view, it seems plausible in Case 10.1 to apply a more rigorous standard of capacity when Mrs. C. refuses treatment for symptomatic, life-threatening cardiac disease than when she refuses screening tests or treatment for cardiac risk factors. Although such a sliding scale is intuitively appealing, it may be problematic in practice. People are likely to disagree over what risks are serious and over what standard should be required for a particular decision. A sliding scale might allow physicians to exercise inappropriate control over patients with whom they disagree. To guard against such problems, physicians need to define explicitly the criteria they are using in assessing a patient's decision-making capacity.

ASSESSING THE CAPACITY TO MAKE DECISIONS

Many helpful and practical suggestions for determining decision-making capacity have been offered (9,12). The assessment presupposes that the patient has received adequate information about her condition and the interventions. If there is any doubt, the physician needs to repeat the information.

Does the Patient Understand the Disclosed Information?

Helpful questions include:

- "Tell me what you believe is wrong with your health now."
- "What is angiography likely to do for you?"

Does the Patient Appreciate the Consequences of Her Choices?

The physician can ask:

- "What do you believe will happen if you do not have angiography?"
- "I've described the possible benefits and risks of angiography. If these benefits or risks occurred, how would your everyday activities be affected?"

Does the Patient Use Reasoning to Make a Choice?

The doctor can use such questions as:

- "Tell me how you reached your decision. . . ."
- "Help me understand how you decided to refuse the angiogram."
- "Tell me what makes angiography seem worse than the alternatives."

In addition, it is helpful to talk to family and friends, nurses, and other physicians caring for the patient, particularly when the physician does not know the patient well. These persons can clarify whether the patient's mental function or choices have changed over time.

The Role of Mental Status Testing

Clinicians often use mental status tests to assess whether a patient has the capacity to make medical decisions. Such tests evaluate orientation of the subject to person, place, and time, attention span, immediate recall, short-term and long-term memory, ability to perform simple calculations, and language skills (13).

However, mental status tests are less useful than directly assessing whether the patient understands the nature of the intervention, the risks and benefits, the alternatives, and the consequences (9). For example, Mrs. C. scored poorly on standard mental status tests, but if she appreciates that angioplasty would probably improve her chest pain and shortness of breath, she has the capacity to make an informed refusal.

In several court rulings, patients with abnormal mental status tests were found competent to make decisions about health care. For example, a 72-year-old man who withdrew his consent for amputation of his gangrenous legs was found competent even though one psychiatrist found that he was disoriented to place and to the people around him and had visual hallucinations. The probate judge found that "his conversation did wander occasionally but to no greater extent than would be expected of a 72-year-old man in his circumstances." The patient hoped "for a miracle" but realized that "there is no great likelihood of its occurrence."

In another case, a 77-year-old woman was found competent to refuse amputation of her leg for gangrene (14). Testimony indicated that she was "lucid on some matters and confused on others," that her "train of thought sometimes wanders," and that "her conception of time is distorted." One psychiatrist claimed that her refusal to discuss the amputation with him indicated that "she was unable to face up to the problem." The court found that she understood that in "rejecting the amputation she is, in effect, choosing death over life."

Consultation by Psychiatrists

Psychiatrists may be helpful in evaluating patients whose decision-making capacity is questionable (4,12,15). Psychiatrists are skilled at interviewing patients with mental impairment. Compared with nonspecialists, they may be more successful at engaging the patient in discussions and better able to evaluate a patient's understanding of the proposed intervention. In addition, psychiatrists specialize in diagnosing and treating mental illnesses that might impair a patient's decision-making capacity. Psychiatrists are also skilled at identifying and resolving interpersonal and intrapsychic conflicts that impair decision-making (15).

Attending physicians can readily acquire the skills to assess patients' decision-making capacity, and routine psychiatric consultation is not necessary (9). Ultimately, attending physicians are responsible for judging whether the patient lacks decision-making capacity.

Enhancing the Capacity of Patients to Make Decisions

Impairments in decision-making capacity may be reversible if underlying medical or psychiatric conditions are treated. In addition, physicians can enhance patient understanding of pertinent information by presenting information in simple language, in small chunks, slowly and repeatedly over time. Diagrams and videotapes may improve comprehension. Furthermore, the presence of family members or friends can help reduce anxiety, correct misunderstandings, and focus on the salient issues.

Engaging the Patient in Discussions

Patients like Mrs. C. may refuse to answer questions or explain their decisions. They need to understand that lack of cooperation may lead to a determination of impaired decision-making capacity and loss of the power to make health care decisions. However, repeated attempts to assess decision-making capacity or to persuade them may be counterproductive.

Patients may be angry at losing control or resent being badgered. In turn, health care workers may feel frustrated.

DECISION-MAKING CAPACITY IN SPECIFIC CLINICAL SITUATIONS

Mental Illness and Decision-Making Capacity

Many patients with mental illness are competent to make decisions about their medical care. However, lack of decision-making capacity is more common in certain psychiatric conditions. Patients with schizophrenia or depression commonly fail to appreciate the relevance of information to their situation. Among inpatients with schizophrenia, 35% did not acknowledge their symptoms and diagnosis (16). Furthermore, 13% to 14% of patients with schizophrenia or major depression denied the potential benefit of treatment.

Psychiatric illness may also impair decision-making capacity more subtly (17). Patients who are depressed may overemphasize the risks of treatment, underestimate the benefits, believe that treatment is less likely to be successful for them than for others, or feel unworthy of the intervention.

Psychiatric patients may be so gravely disabled or unable to care for themselves that they may be involuntarily committed (*see* Chapter 42). However, involuntary commitment does not empower physicians to give whatever medical treatment they consider advisable. If such a patient refuses treatment for medical problems, an appropriate surrogate or a separate court order is needed to authorize treatment.

Unconventional Decisions Based on Religious Beliefs

Patients may refuse effective medical treatments because of religious beliefs. Religious beliefs are matters of faith; empirical evidence and reasoning are not pertinent. In the United States, freedom of religion is deeply respected. Furthermore, it is troubling for physicians to label some religious beliefs as acceptable and others as not. Thus, refusals of treatment by competent adults based on religious grounds are accepted. (Parental refusals of effective treatment for children may be overridden, as is discussed in Chapter 39.) Religious beliefs need not be articulated as formal or orthodox doctrines. As one court ruling declared, beliefs that others consider "unwise, foolish, or ridiculous" do not render a person incompetent (18). Indeed, informed consent would be meaningless if such individualistic refusals were not respected, even though they conflict with medical or popular wisdom.

The physician's inquiry generally is limited to whether the religious beliefs are sincere in the sense that they antedate the illness and are consistent with prior actions (9) and whether other aspects of decision-making are problematic. Some patients have religious delusions or hallucinations. For example, a patient may believe that he is Christ, that the devil has caused his colon cancer, or that he should refuse surgery because it is God's will that he suffer. Because of his delusions, he is not capable of making informed decisions. It does not matter that his delusions are based on religious ideas.

Emergencies

A patient with questionable decision-making capacity may present with an emergency condition that requires immediate treatment. Rather than evaluating the patient's decision-making capacity, physicians should provide emergency care, unless it is known that the patient or surrogate would refuse such care. This approach is justified by implied consent to emergency care (*see* Chapter 3).

CARING FOR PATIENTS WHO LACK DECISION-MAKING CAPACITY

After physicians determine that a patient lacks decision-making capacity, further care should be guided by advance directives or surrogate decision-making (*see* Chapters 12 and 13).

Even if a patient lacks the capacity to make decisions, her stated preferences should be given substantial consideration. For instance, mentally incapacitated patients may balk at phlebotomy or x-rays, sometimes screaming their refusal. Even if the courts declared such a patient incompetent, it would be morally and emotionally repugnant to impose interventions on an unwilling patient. Health care workers may consider it inhumane to force a patient to undergo a highly invasive intervention when she cannot understand its purpose and benefits. Furthermore, future cooperation may be undermined. It is preferable if the patient assents to interventions decided on by a surrogate or court, even if she cannot give informed consent. Persuasion, cajoling, and asking family members and friends to talk to the patient are acceptable to try to gain the patient's cooperation. Often a patient will agree to treatment after caregivers have listened to her objections, modified the treatment plans, or changed the hospital routine.

In summary, physicians commonly decide that patients lack the capacity to make informed decisions about their care without resorting to the courts. Physicians need to understand the clinical standards for decision-making capacity and be able to apply these standards in specific cases. Good communication skills are crucial for assessing decision-making capacity.

REFERENCES

1. Brock DW. *Life and death*. New York: Cambridge University Press, 1993.
2. Lo B. Assessing decision-making capacity. *Law Med Health Care* 1990;18:193–201.
3. President's Commission for the Study of Ethical Problems in Medicine and Biomedical and Behavioral Research. *Making health care decisions*. Washington: US Government Printing Office, 1982.
4. Appelbaum PS, Lidz CW, Meisel A. *Informed consent: legal theory and clinical practice*. New York: Oxford University Press, 1987:266.
5. Meisel A. *The Right to Die*. New York: John Wiley & Sons, 1989.
6. Buchanan AE, Brock DW. *Deciding for others*. Cambridge: Cambridge University Press, 1989.
7. Beauchamp TL, Childress JF. *Principles of biomedical ethics*, 4th ed. New York: Oxford University Press, 1994.
8. Meisel A. *The right to die*, 2nd ed. New York: John Wiley & Sons, 1995.
9. Grisso T, Appelbaum P. *Assessing competence to consent to treatment: a guide for physicians and other health professionals*. New York: Oxford University Press, 1998:22–26,47–48,77–80,90–91.
10. State Department of Human Resources *v.* Northern. 563 S.W.2d 197 (Tenn. Ct. App. 1978).
11. Drane JF. Competency to give an informed consent. *JAMA* 1984;252:925–927.
12. Appelbaum PS, Grisso T. Assessing patient's capacities to consent to treatment. *N Engl J Med* 1988;319:1635–1638.
13. Kane RL, Ouslander JG, Ibrass IB. *Essentials of clinical geriatrics*. 2nd ed. New York: McGraw-Hill, 1989.
14. Lane *v.* Candura. 6 Mass. App. 377,376 N.E.2d 1232 (1978).
15. Perl M, Shelp EE. Psychiatric consultation masking moral dilemmas in medicine. *N Engl J Med* 1982;307:618–621.
16. Appelbaum PS, Grisso T. The MacArthur Treatment Competence Study, I: mental illness and competence to consent to treatment. *Law Hum Behav* 1995;19:105–126.
17. Bursztajn HJ, Gutheil TG, Brodsky A. Affective disorders, competence, and decision making. In: Gutheil TG, Bursztajn HJ, Brodsky A, Alexander V, ed. *Decision making in psychiatry and the law*. Baltimore: Williams & Wilkins, 1991:153–170.
18. In re Brooks. 32 Ill.2d 361, 205 N.E.2d 435 (1965).

ANNOTATED BIBLIOGRAPHY

1. Grisso T, Appelbaum P. *Assessing competence to consent to treatment: a guide for physicians and other health professionals.* New York: Oxford University Press, 1998.
   Lucid, practical, and comprehensive discussion of how to assess decision-making capacity.
2. Buchanan AE, Brock DW. *Deciding for others.* Cambridge: Cambridge University Press, 1989.
   Comprehensive discussion of different definitions and standards for decision-making capacity.

11

Refusal of Treatment by Competent, Informed Patients

Competent and informed patients may refuse interventions that their physicians recommend. In some cases, physicians may hesitate to accept refusals that jeopardize the patient's life or health. Although concern for a patient's well-being is commendable, as discussed in Chapter 4, it is important for physicians to understand the strong ethical and legal reasons for respecting refusals by informed, competent patients. This chapter discusses the reasons for respecting such refusals, the problems that result from refusals of transfusions by Jehovah's Witnesses, and restrictions on patient refusal.

REASONS FOR RESPECTING PATIENT REFUSALS

Respect for Patient Autonomy

Honoring refusal of treatment by competent, informed patients respects their self-determination and individuality. Ethically, physicians should respect the autonomy of persons to make decisions about their care (1–4). Patients should be free of unwanted medical interventions. The option of declining treatment is fundamental to the concept of informed consent. If patients must give consent for treatment, then logically they have the right to decline treatment. The U.S. Supreme Court has suggested that the Constitution protects a competent patient's refusal of life-sustaining treatment (5). A large body of case law supports the right of competent, informed patients to refuse unwanted treatment (6).

Imposing Medical Interventions Would Be Unacceptable

On a practical level, it is difficult to imagine imposing unwanted medical interventions on a competent patient. Sedating or restraining patients to impose treatment over their objections seems intrusive and inhumane. Most people would find such means repugnant, even if the original refusal of treatment was unwise.

SCOPE OF REFUSAL

Competent patients are permitted to refuse virtually any treatments, even highly beneficial ones with few side effects. The range of interventions includes surgery, mechanical ventilation, renal dialysis, antibiotics, cardiopulmonary resuscitation, and tube feedings (6). Competent patients have the right to refuse treatment even if such refusal might shorten their lives or lead to their deaths. They are not required to have a terminal illness as a condition of refusing treatment.

Competent patients may refuse treatment even if their family, friends, or physicians disagree with them. As one court ruling declared, even decisions that are "unwise, foolish, or ridiculous" (7) may need to be respected. Indeed, informed consent would be meaningless unless patients could refuse interventions for highly personal reasons or make decisions that conflict with medical or popular wisdom.

JEHOVAH'S WITNESS CASES

Jehovah's Witnesses do not accept blood transfusions, basing their refusal on an interpretation of the Bible (8). They believe that although a blood transfusion might save their corporeal life, it will deprive them of everlasting salvation. Their refusals are clearly articulated, are usually steadfast over time, and are supported by their family and friends. Refusals of blood transfusions by Jehovah's Witnesses may be distressing to physicians because, from a purely clinical perspective, the benefits of transfusion are great and the risks trivial. Many patients are young, previously healthy, and could be restored to perfect health.

Reactions of Health Care Providers

Jehovah's Witnesses generally consent to other interventions, including surgery, provided that transfusions are not used. Physicians may feel that Jehovah's Witnesses, by refusing transfusions but agreeing to other care, unnecessarily compromise medical outcomes, make their job more difficult, and require them to provide substandard care. Physicians may believe that they are being asked to accomplish the goal of saving the patient's life without using the best available means. Some surgeons complain that operating on a Jehovah's Witness without transfusions is like having to operate with one hand tied behind their back. They have less margin for error or complications. On a psychological level, some physicians resent the loss of control over the patient's care. Some health care workers may also blame the patient for making their job more complicated. Many surgeons and anesthesiologists prefer not to care for Jehovah's Witnesses. Often, however, transferring such patients to another institution or physician is impractical.

Frustrated health care workers may develop imaginative plans for administering blood to Jehovah's Witnesses. Some physicians suggest waiting until such patients are unconscious and then asking if they object to a transfusion. Because patients are then no longer able to refuse, these physicians would administer blood. Other physicians advocate simply giving transfusions after patients are under anesthesia, and not telling them about it. Both such actions, however, are unacceptable because they are deceptive and undermine trust in physicians.

Health care workers need to appreciate that without transfusions medical outcomes for Jehovah's Witness are often quite good, even though care is more difficult. For example, operative mortality for open-heart surgery on Jehovah's Witnesses has been reported as acceptably low, using intraoperative cell salvage and other blood conservation techniques (9).

Legal Issues

The courts have consistently upheld refusals of blood transfusions by competent adult Jehovah's Witnesses (6,10–12). Recent controversies have involved incompetent Jehovah's Witnesses. Some physicians object that wallet cards signed by Jehovah's Witnesses are not sufficient evidence that the patient made an informed decision (13).

Practical Suggestions

Physicians caring for Jehovah's Witnesses can take several steps to ensure that the patient's refusal of transfusions is informed and steadfast. First, the physician should ask the adult patient about transfusions when no family members, friends, or religious advisors are present. This lessens the chance that the patient feels coerced into refusing. When alone, some Jehovah's Witnesses will agree to transfusions. Second, the physician should ask patients whether they would accept transfusions if they are ordered by a court. Some Jehovah's Witnesses will accept a transfusion as long as they do not personally give consent for it. Under these circumstances, many judges are willing to order that transfusions be given. Third, some Jehovah's Witnesses will refuse all blood products, whereas others will accept various blood components. Most will accept erythropoietin and fluorinated blood substitutes. Fourth, physicians should ask whether the patient has any other concerns about receiving blood, such as the risk of HIV infection or hepatitis. If the underlying reason for refusal is really a fear of infection, this concern should be addressed directly.

Having ensured that the refusal is steadfast and informed, health care workers should respect the patient's decision. From the point of view of a Jehovah's Witness, the decision to refuse transfusions is simple. They would be pleased to survive the hospitalization, but as one patient put it, "What good is a few years of life compared to everlasting damnation?" (14). Even if health care workers do not agree with this belief, they need to respect it. Continuing to try to convince a Jehovah's Witness shows disrespect. Furthermore, using deception to administer blood cannot be condoned.

When an adult Jehovah's Witness who requires a transfusion lacks decision-making capacity, the situation is more complicated. Advance directives that reflect informed decisions should be respected, as Chapter 12 discusses. Many Jehovah's Witnesses have completed wallet-sized "blood cards" declaring they would refuse transfusions. The ethical validity of these cards has been questioned because completion of the cards may have been coerced by peer pressure and because the patient may not have been informed about the risks and benefits of transfusions (13).

Physicians should respond differently if the patient is a minor and the parents are refusing a medically indicated transfusion (*see* Chapter 39). In this situation, physicians should ask a court to approve the transfusion. As one court declared, parents are "not free to make martyrs of their children" (15).

RESTRICTIONS ON REFUSAL

The right of competent, informed patients to refuse medical treatment may be limited in certain situations.

Communicable Diseases

In certain circumstances, competent patients may be required to undergo treatment against their wishes in order to prevent harms to third parties. The clearest examples are infectious diseases that can be transmitted by casual contact, such as tuberculosis (16,17). To reduce the risk of transmitting a serious disease to other persons, infected individuals may be required to be treated, or else be quarantined until they no longer pose a risk to others.

Compelled Treatment of Pregnant Women

In several cases, pregnant women were ordered by the courts to undergo cesarean sections or blood transfusions over their objections, allegedly to protect the health of the fetus. These rulings, however, have been sharply criticized for violating the woman's bodily integrity and right of self-determination. Recent court rulings that strongly rejected this practice will probably set a strong legal precedent (18–20).

Trying to prevent harm to the fetus who will be carried to term is praiseworthy (*see* Chapter 41). However, compelled treatment is not feasible in most situations in pregnancy. In diabetes or drug addiction, interventions must be continued over an extended period, the cooperation of the pregnant woman is needed, and the infringement of her autonomy caused by ongoing forced treatment is substantial.

Treating Competent Patients for Their Own Benefit

Providing interventions over the objections of a competent patient in order to prevent harm to third parties needs to be clearly distinguished from providing treatment in order to prevent harm to the patient herself. The physician's duty to prevent harm to competent patients is considered weaker than the duty to prevent harm to unsuspecting third parties. Physicians should try to persuade patients and to negotiate a mutually acceptable plan of care (*see* Chapter 4). They may not, however, override the informed decisions of a competent patient because they believe it would be better for her.

In some situations, physicians may be tempted to administer treatment to prevent serious harm to patients. Jonsen et al. discuss the perplexing case of a young man with bacterial meningitis who refused antibiotics (21). The patient shows no indication of impaired decision-making capacity, other than his "enigmatic refusal" of treatment. As they present the case, there is no time for prolonged discussions. Rather than allow the patient to die from such a readily treatable infection, these authors advocate administering antibiotics, because they believe that "something essential is missing in the case." Indeed, the authors later disclose that earlier the patient's cousin had died from an anaphylactic reaction to penicillin and that this incident had led to his refusal.

This is admittedly a difficult case, and difficult cases often lead to bad generalizations. Although it is troubling to allow a patient to die from a easily treated infection, it is also troubling to override the refusal of a patient when the only evidence of impaired decision-making capacity is the patient's refusal of treatment. Without hindsight, it is problematical to establish a rule that such patients can be considered to have impaired decision-making capacity. Any such rule would give physicians virtually unlimited power to override patients who cannot provide satisfactory reasons for refusing treatment.

In summary, there are cogent ethical and legal reasons to accept refusals of treatment by competent and informed patients. Subsequent chapters discuss how physicians can try to persuade patients to accept beneficial interventions while respecting their right to refuse.

REFERENCES

1. Lo B, Jonsen AR. Clinical decisions to limit treatment. *Ann Intern Med* 1980;93:764–768.
2. President's Commission for the Study of Ethical Problems in Medicine and Biomedical and Behavioral Research. *Making health care decisions.* Washington: US Government Printing Office, 1982.
3. President's Commission for the Study of Ethical Problems in Medicine and Biomedical and Behavioral Research. *Deciding to forego life-sustaining treatment.* Washington: US Government Printing Office, 1983.
4. American College of Physicians. American College of Physicians ethics manual. *Ann Intern Med* 1998; 128:576–594.
5. Lo B, Steinbrook R. Beyond the Cruzan case: the U.S. Supreme Court and medical practice. *Ann Intern Med* 1991;114:895–901.
6. Meisel A. *The right to die*, 2nd ed. New York: John Wiley & Sons, 1995;538–542.
7. In re Brooks. 32 Ill.2d 361, 205 N.E.2d 435 (1965).

8. Sheldon M. Ethical issues in the forced transfusion of Jehovah's Witness children [see comments]. *J Emerg Med* 1996;14:251–257.

9. Rosengart TK, Helm RE, DeBois WJ, et al. Open heart operations without transfusion using a multimodality blood conservation strategy in 50 Jehovah's Witness patients: implications for a "bloodless" surgical technique. *J Am Coll Surg* 1997;184:618–629.

10. Furrow BR, Johnson SH, Jost TS, et al. *Health law: cases, materials and problems.* St. Paul, MN.: West Publishing, 1991.

11. Fosmire *v.* Nicoleau, 552 N.E.2d 77 (N.Y. 1990).

12. Norwood Hosp. *v.* Munoz, 564 N.E.2d 1017 (Mass. 1991).

13. Migden DR, Braen GR. The Jehovah's Witness blood refusal card: ethical and medicolegal considerations for emergency physicians. *Acad Emerg Med* 1998;5:815–824.

14. In re Osborne, 294 A. 2d 372 (D.C. 1972).

15. Prince *v.* Massachusetts, 321 U.S. 158 (1944).

16. Oscherwitz T, Tulsky JP, Roger S, et al. Detention of persistently nonadherent patients with tuberculosis. *JAMA* 1997;278:843–846.

17. Gasner MR, Maw KL, Feldman GE, et al. The use of legal action in New York City to ensure treatment of tuberculosis. *N Engl J Med* 1999;340:359–366.

18. Curran W. Court-ordered cesarean sections receive judicial defeat. *N Engl J Med* 1990;323:489–492.

19. Levy JK. Jehovah's Witnesses, pregnancy, and blood transfusions: a paradigm for the autonomy of all pregnant women. *J Law Med Ethics* 1999;27:171–189.

20. Goldblatt AD. Commentary: no more jurisdiction over Jehovah. *J Law Med Ethics* 1999;27:190–193.

21. Jonsen A, Siegler M, Winslade W. *Clinical ethics,* 3rd ed. New York: Macmillan, 1991:61–63.

ANNOTATED BIBLIOGRAPHY

1. President's Commission for the Study of Ethical Problems in Medicine and Biomedical and Behavioral Research. *Deciding to forego life-sustaining treatment.* Washington: US Government Printing Office, 1983.
Lucid and thoughtful exposition of refusal of treatment by patients.

2. Meisel A. *The right to die,* 2nd ed. New York: John Wiley & Sons, 1995.
Comprehensive legal treatise that describes court rulings permitting competent patients to refuse treatment.

12

Standards for Decisions When Patients Lack Decision-Making Capacity

Decisions for patients who lack decision-making capacity may be more difficult than decisions for patients who can give informed consent or refusal. For such patients, physicians must address two questions:

- What standards should be used when informed consent or refusal from the patient is not possible?
- Who should act as surrogate for patients who cannot decide for themselves?

Chapter 13 addresses the latter question. This chapter addresses the first question, discussing advance directives, substituted judgments, and the best interests of the patient. These should be viewed as a hierarchy: decisions based on advance directives generally should take priority over those grounded in substituted judgments, which in turn should supersede decisions based on best interests (Table 12-1).

ADVANCE DIRECTIVES

Many patients fear that they will lose control over care if their decision-making capacity is impaired and that medical interventions will be imposed on them against their wishes. Advance directives are statements by competent patients that indicate *who* should act as surrogate or *what* interventions they would accept or refuse in case they should lose decision-making capacity. Advance directives respect patients as persons by allowing their preferences and values to guide care even when they can no longer make informed decisions. While patients are still competent, they give informed consent or refusal. In addition, advance directives allow patients to relieve stress on family members who must make decisions for them (1).

The following case illustrates the usefulness and limitations of advance directives.

CASE 12.1. ORAL ADVANCE DIRECTIVES. *Mrs. A., a 76-year-old widow with Alzheimer's disease, resides in a nursing home. Often she does not recognize relatives and friends or respond when asked questions. She requires assistance with dressing, bathing, and eating. When still lucid, she told her children and her friends many times that she wanted "no heroics" if she became senile. After visiting a neighbor who was in intensive care, unconscious after a severe stroke, she told her son, "That is not living. I don't want to die plugged into a machine, unable to recognize my family and having to depend on others to take care of me. If I'm like that, just let me die in peace."*

Mrs. A. develops pneumonia and sepsis. Her son and daughter remind the physician of these conversations and ask him not to administer antibiotics for the infection or transfer her to an

94

TABLE 12-1. *Standards for making decisions when patients lack decision-making capacity*

Advance directives
Substituted judgments
Best interests of the patient

acute care hospital. However, her brother strongly believes that life-sustaining treatment should be provided regardless of her previous statements or the expected quality of life. He asserts, "Life is sacred; you can't just let her die." The brother adds, "She's a totally different person. She was so afraid of being senile. But look at her now. She's not suffering. Even though she usually doesn't recognize us, she smiles when I hold her hand or when I play music on the radio."

Types of Advance Directives

Oral Statements to Family Members or Friends

Conversations with relatives or friends about what interventions they would want or not want in future situations are the most common advance directives (2,3). Such discussions are frequently used in everyday clinical practice to guide decisions for patients who have lost decision-making capacity.

Limitations of Oral Directives

People may comment about the care of other people without intending to direct their own future care. They also may state preferences without thinking deeply about them. In addition, observers may not accurately recall a patient's statements or may disagree over what the patient said.

Legal Status of Oral Directives

Although oral directives are commonly used in decisions to provide or forego an intervention, a few states severely restrict their use. Courts have ruled that advance directives must be "clear and convincing," which requires stronger evidence than a "preponderance of the evidence" but less evidence than "beyond a reasonable doubt." Applying this standard strictly, New York and Missouri have rejected typical oral advance directives to guide decisions about which interventions are appropriate (4). In these states, oral directives must mention the specific intervention and clinical situation at hand, for example, a feeding tube in severe dementia (4). Courts in other states, however, have interpreted the clear and convincing standard for oral advance directives less stringently, accepting oral statements similar to those by Mrs. A. in Case 12.1 as clear and convincing (4).

Evaluating the Trustworthiness of Oral Directives

Certain characteristics make oral advance directives more trustworthy guides to whether the patient wanted an intervention (Table 12-2).

- The patient's preferences are *informed*. Patients who have experienced serious illness or who have had relatives or friends with serious illness are more likely to be informed.

TABLE 12-2. *Characteristics of trustworthy advance directives*

The patient's preferences are informed.
The directive discusses specific treatments and clinical situations.
The directive is repeated over time, in different situations, to various individuals.

- The directive indicates what *specific treatments* the patient would want or not want *in various clinical situations*, rather than simply expressing general preference or values.
- The directive is *repeated* over time, in different situations, to various individuals. Such consistency makes it more likely that the choices are carefully considered and based on deeply held values.

Oral Statements to Physicians

Discussions with physicians are more common and less problematical than written advance directives (2,3,5). Unlike oral statements to relatives or friends, directives to physicians are not casual comments. Moreover, physicians can check whether directives are informed. For instance, a physician can discuss with Mrs. A. how most patients with moderate dementia appear to enjoy many activities.

Written Advance Directives

Almost all states have enacted laws authorizing living wills or the appointment of health care proxies (6,7). Patients complete a formal legal document that must be witnessed or notarized. A lawyer is not needed to complete these documents. Because state statutes vary, caregivers and patients need to be familiar with their state laws.

The courts consider written advance directives more reliable evidence of patient choices than oral statements. Courts presume that patients are more likely to think about the issues and to appreciate the consequences of their actions if they complete a formal legal document. However, in many reports, only about 5% of patients have given written advance directives (8–11).

Living Wills

In living wills, patients direct their physicians to withhold or withdraw life-sustaining treatment if they develop a terminal condition or, in some states, enter a persistent vegetative state. Various states define "terminal condition" differently, usually only in very general terms. In most states, conditions such as dementia of Alzheimer's type would not be covered by living wills. Patients typically may refuse only interventions that "merely prolong the process of dying." People may disagree whether this phrase includes antibiotics for pneumonia in Case 12.1. Some states do not allow patients to decline artificial nutrition and hydration through living wills. Caregivers who follow living wills in good faith are given immunity from civil and criminal liability and professional disciplinary actions.

Because of these limitations, living wills are less flexible and comprehensive than the health care proxy (12–14).

Health Care Proxy

Competent patients may appoint a health care proxy or agent to make medical decisions if they were to lose decision-making capacity. In some states, this process is called "executing a durable power of attorney for health care." As long as patients remain competent, they continue to make their own health care decisions. This proxy, typically a relative or close friend, has decision-making priority over other potential surrogates. In Case 12.1, if Mrs. A. had appointed her sister as health care proxy, her brother would have no authority to make health decisions. The health care proxy applies to all situations in which the patient is incapable of making decisions, not just terminal illness. Proxy decisions must be consistent with the patient's previously expressed choices or best interests. Appointing a health care proxy, supplemented with statements of what life-sustaining the patient would want or refuse in various scenarios, is the best way to provide advance directives.

Physicians need to be familiar with the relevant laws in their state. Laws usually authorize standard forms, which must be witnessed or notarized. A typical statutory form for appointing a health care proxy is reproduced in the Appendix. The language in the forms may be difficult to comprehend, and forms are typically several pages long. Many states honor forms from other states. Certain people may not serve as surrogates because of potential conflicts of interest. In California, the surrogate may not be the treating physician or employees of the treating physician or institution, unless they are relatives of the patient. Caregivers who in good faith follow the directives of duly appointed health care proxies are given legal immunity from civil suits, criminal prosecution, and professional disciplinary action.

Limitations of Advance Directives

Advance directives have several significant limitations (15).

Advance Directives May Not Be Informed

Even after discussions with physicians, only 33% of patients know that patients on a ventilator cannot talk, and about one-half believe that ventilators are oxygen tanks or that ventilated people are always comatose (16). Similarly, patients have serious misunderstandings about cardiopulmonary resuscitation (CPR). Over one-fourth cannot identify any basic characteristics of CPR, such as chest compressions or assisted breathing (16). Only one-third know that even if CPR succeeds in restarting the heart, a breathing machine is usually needed. The authors found it "disconcerting" that "patients expressed strong preferences about treatments that they did not understand" (16).

Patients also overestimate the chance of survival after CPR is attempted (16,17). Patients generally overestimate their prognosis. In one study of patients with a 50% chance of surviving 2 years, 27% of patients think they would be cured, and only 10% judge their life expectancy to be less than 2 years (18). In a cohort of patients with metastatic lung or colon cancer, who had a 6-month survival of 45%, most patients were decidedly overoptimistic: 59% believed that their chance of surviving 6 months was greater than 90% (19).

With competent patients, physicians can have further discussions and correct misunderstandings. After patients lose decision-making capacity, however, such discussions are no longer feasible.

Interpretations of Advance Directives May Be Problematical

Because advance directives seldom address the exact decision at hand, the patient's previous statements usually need to be interpreted.

Vague Terms

Advance directives often use vague terms such as "heroic" or "extraordinary" care. Directives commonly refuse interventions when "the burdens outweigh the benefits of care." In Case

12.1, such vague terms provide little guidance. Did Mrs. A. decline antibiotics for infection, or only more invasive interventions such as CPR and intensive care? Mrs. A. said that she did not want life-sustaining treatment if she became "senile," but when does "senility" commence: when she can no longer pursue favorite activities, when she sometimes does not recognize family members, or only when she no longer responds at all? Studies show that patients' choices in specific scenarios cannot be accurately predicted from their general preferences and goals (9,20).

Application to Similar Situations

A patient may give advance directives regarding one situation but develop a different condition. For example, a patient may give directives regarding dementia but develop a major stroke. Patients differ in how much leeway they want surrogates to take to apply the patient's directive to other circumstances or interventions (21). In one study, 39% of patients wanted their directives to be followed literally, while 31% of patients wanted their surrogates to override their advance directives if their surrogates believed it was best for them (21).

Advance Directives May Conflict With the Patient's Best Interests

Following the patient's advance directives may not be in her current best interests. Surrogates and physicians therefore might wish to override prior refusal of care, for example, if a brief intervention is virtually certain to restore the patient to previous health (22).

When providing advance directives, patients make implicit assumptions about their prognosis or family situation, but promising new therapies might become available, other serious medical conditions might develop, a treatment might prove unsuccessful, or a spouse might die. Such developments might make prior directives less pertinent to the current situation.

More fundamentally, the incompetent may be a different person from when she gave the directives (23,24). In this view, advance directives therefore are not binding. Mrs. A.'s brother questions whether her previous statements are still relevant because she has changed so dramatically. On the other hand, many people believe that although Mrs. A. is only a shadow of her former self, she is in essence still the same person and that her directives should be respected.

Patients May Change Their Minds

After patients indicate that they would decline interventions, in 21% to 28% of cases they subsequently decide that they would accept the interventions, or at least try them (25,26). Acceptance of life-sustaining interventions is less stable. After patients indicate that they would accept life-sustaining interventions, from 43% to 50% indicate in later interviews that they would decline the intervention. Furthermore, 68% of patients who say they would accept a trial of treatment subsequently say they would decline the intervention (25).

Despite these limitations, advance directives should be encouraged. They promote respect for patients as individuals with unique characters and values. They also encourage discussions of life-sustaining interventions among patients, family members, and physicians.

Rationale for Discussing Advance Directives With Patients

Most patients—between 59% and 85% of outpatients—want to talk with their physicians about life-sustaining interventions before a clinical crisis occurs (2,3,5), yet fewer than 6% have done so. When thinking or talking about life-sustaining interventions, most patients feel in control, relieved, or cared for (2). Even patients who feel sad or anxious when thinking about life-sustaining treatment still want to have such conversations (2,5). Among hospitalized patients, between 42% and 81% want to discuss end-of-life decisions with their physicians (27,28). Most patients want physicians to take the initiative in discussing advance directives (2,29).

The Federal Patient Self-Determination Act is intended to promote discussions about advance directives (30). Hospitals, nursing homes, and health maintenance organizations that participate in Medicaid and Medicare must inform patients about their rights to provide advance directives at the time of admission or enrollment. Institutions must also carry out advance directives and educate their staffs about them. Patients are not required to complete an advance directive.

Problems with Discussions About Advance Directives

Currently, discussions about advance directives are problematical. In one study, only 11% of patients who had executed advance directives had discussed them with their physician. Almost all discussions concerned general attitudes and feelings rather than specific interventions (31).

A detailed analysis of doctor–patient conversations about advance directives found serious problems (32). Almost all physicians posed hypothetical scenarios to patients. However, physicians discussed scenarios in which there was little variation in patient preferences. In 91% of cases, the physicians discussed dire scenarios, in which patients were permanently unconscious, in an intensive care unit indefinitely, or about to die. No patients wanted interventions in such a dire scenario. In about one-half of cases, physicians discussed reversible scenarios in which patients were expected to regain their previous health. Almost all patients accepted even "heroic" interventions in a reversible scenario. Thus, discussions of theses scenarios provided little guidance. Physicians less frequently discussed more difficult situations, such as when recovery is unpredictable or the patient has chronic disability after treatment.

Typically, physicians used vague language, asking patients what they would want if they were "very, very sick" or "had something that was very serious." Doctors rarely tried to define such terms or ascertain how patients interpreted them. In almost all cases, physicians also discussed specific interventions, most commonly CPR or mechanical ventilation. However, in only 16% of conversations did physicians attempt to learn what patients knew about these interventions. In discussing outcomes, only 11% of physicians gave numerical probabilities of success, and only 13% mentioned outcomes other than death and complete recovery. Hence patients did not receive sufficient information to make informed decisions.

Physicians explicitly elicited patients' values, goals for care, and reasons for choices in only 34% of cases. Most commonly, physicians merely determined whether patients wanted specific interventions in scenarios without exploring the reasons for those preferences. Even when reasons were discussed, physicians rarely asked patients to define a poor quality of life or being a burden to their family, which were frequent reasons for refusing interventions.

Improving Discussions About Advance Directives

When Should Discussions About Advance Directives Be Initiated?

Physicians should discuss advance directives when it would not be surprising if the patient were to lose decision-making capacity or to die (33). Hence physicians should target not only patients who are "terminal" or in a progressively downhill course, but also those with serious chronic illness like congestive heart failure, whose course is not so predictable. Patients want discussions to occur earlier than physicians do: earlier in the natural history of disease, and earlier in the patient–physician relationship (29). If the physician waits until clinical deterioration has already occurred, the patient is often too sick to make informed decisions (34).

In some cultures, advance directives are undesirable. For example, many traditional Chinese patients believe that talking about future illness will anger the ghosts, who then will make the illness occur or cause bad luck. Such reluctance to discuss future plans needs to be respected.

Physicians can resolve many problems with advance directives by explicitly addressing the following issues (Table 12-3).

Who Should Serve as Surrogate?

Most patients find it easier to discuss the choice of surrogate than preferences regarding care. Straightforward questions may broach the topic: "I ask all my patients with heart disease how they want decisions to be made. Who would you want to make decisions for you in case you are too sick to talk with me directly?" Those who do not wish to discuss these topics can easily demur. Physicians should urge patients to discuss with surrogates their choices regarding life-sustaining treatment and help to do so.

What Are the Patient's General Preferences and Values?

Many physicians focus discussions on specific medical decisions, such as Do Not Resuscitate (DNR) orders. However, it is premature to discuss particular decisions before understanding patient's concerns and expectations. Often specific decisions can more easily be made after the patient expresses her general values and preferences. Open-ended questions help to elicit the patient's perspective (35):

- "When you think of serious illness, what concerns you the most?" Alternatively, "When you think of serious illness, what is most important to you?"
- "Sometimes your family may need to make decisions about your medical care. What things would you want them to take into account?" These questions elicit how the patient defines her best interests or an acceptable quality of life.
- "Are there conditions under which you would not want life-prolonging interventions?"

What Are the Patient's Preferences in Specific Clinical Situations?

It is unrealistic to try to discuss all future medical situations. The goal of discussions is not to be exhaustive, but to elicit informed choices about likely scenarios and to understand what considerations are important to the patient.

Discuss Scenarios That are Likely to Occur

Although the persistent vegetative state has captured public attention, it is uncommon. Rather than discussing hopeless or completely reversible situations, physicians should dis-

TABLE 12-3. *Topics to discuss regarding advance directives*

Who should serve as surrogate?
What are the patient's general preferences and values?
What are the patient's preferences in specific clinical situations?
How should advance directives be interpreted?

cuss common scenarios (36) in which the outcome is uncertain and the interventions are burdensome (16).

Physicians need to describe interventions and their likely outcomes. For CPR, patients need to know about chest compressions, artificial respirations, electroshock, the low likelihood of survival after CPR, and the possibility of neurological compromise (*see* Chapter 18). For mechanical ventilation, patients need to understand that they will have a tube in their throat, will not be able to speak, and will probably need sedation.

For patients with coronary artery disease, cardiopulmonary arrest, cardiogenic shock, and respiratory failure from pulmonary edema should be discussed. What limits would the patient place on life-prolonging interventions if prolonged ventilatory or multisystem failure develops?

For patients with cancer, the physician should discuss altered mental status and sepsis in advanced disease. What types of intervention would the patient be willing to accept? For what likelihood, magnitude, and duration of improvement?

With elderly patients, physicians should discuss severe dementia and stroke. In these situations, would the patient want infections treated with antibiotics or intensive care? Would she want a feeding tube if she was unable to swallow food? How would the patient define severe dementia or severe stroke?

Correct Unrealistic Expectations

Patients may have unrealistic expectations. For example, a woman with lung cancer metastatic to liver and bone may indicate that she wants everything done. In such cases, physicians should elicit expectations, concerns, and emotions, using open-ended questions. The physician could say, "What do you think happens to patients whose cancer spreads like that?" In some cases, physicians may need to explain that the patient's goals are impossible. "I wish that were the case. Unfortunately when cancer has spread that much, even breathing machines don't help patients live much longer."

Use of Specific Checklists

The Medical Directive is a checklist of 12 interventions in each of four clinical scenarios: terminal illness, dementia, persistent vegetative state, and coma (37). Such specific directives are useful when the patient and physician have discussed these situations and the patient has made truly informed decisions, but specific directives may be misleading if the patient expresses choices without fully appreciating the issues and deliberating about them.

How Should Advance Directives Be Interpreted?

Because advance directives cannot cover all contingencies, it is important to understand how the patient would want the surrogate and physician to interpret her preferences.

Clarify Ambiguous Terms

Physicians need to ask patients to clarify vague statements: "Can you tell me what you mean by 'No heroic treatment'?"

Clarify Discretion by Surrogates

Physicians should ask patients how much leeway they would allow surrogates to interpret their directives, extrapolate them to unforeseen situations, or override their directives if it seemed in their best interests (21). Following such preferences respects the values of the individual patient.

Continue Discussions Over Time

Physicians should not expect to understand the patient's preferences after a single conversation. In addition, patients' choices and values may change as their illness, their life situation, or their appraisal of their situation changes. If patients change their mind, they should tell both the surrogate and the physician, destroy all copies of written advance directives, and complete a new advance directive.

How Do Patients Want to Be Treated Near the End of Life?

A recent advance directive form enables patients to indicate that they want their family to know that "I love them," "I wish to be forgiven for the times I may have hurt them," and "I forgive them for what they have have done to me" (38). In addition, patients can fill out what they would like their family to say if anyone asks how they want to be remembered (38). By shifting the focus from decisions about medical care, these parts of the directive may help patients find closure at the end of life.

Recommend Written Directives

Physicians should tell patients about the advantages of written advance directives and encourage patients to complete them. This is particularly important in states like New York and Missouri, whose courts have rejected most oral directives (39).

Document Discussions in the Medical Record

The physician's note should describe the patient's decision-making capacity, appreciation of the consequences of their choices, and her specific preferences regarding interventions in various situations. It is not necessary for the patient to sign the record.

SUBSTITUTED JUDGMENT

Clear and specific advance directives should be respected, as previously discussed, but often patients have given only general directives or no indication of their preferences. How should physicians and surrogates make decisions in such situations?

CASE 12.2. DISAGREEMENTS OVER SUBSTITUTED JUDGMENT. *Mr. S., a 76-year-old widower, suffers a massive stroke and aphasia. Two weeks later, he still has paralysis of his right arm and leg. He does not respond consistently to simple requests or questions but sometimes smiles when his hand is held. He develops pneumonia.*

Throughout his life, he had been reluctant to see physicians and did not take prescribed medications to lower his cholesterol regularly. He loved to take walks and work in his garden. When his wife died of a sudden heart attack, he said, "Death isn't the enemy. She wanted to be active and healthy to the end, and the good Lord granted her wish." He was a proud and independent man who was reluctant to accept help from others. He has given no oral or written advance directives. His son and daughter believe Mr. S. would refuse antibiotics. "He disliked being dependent on others and would hate being in a nursing home. In his condition, he can't do any of the things he loved in life."

In the absence of clear and specific advance directives, surrogates should try to construct the decision that the patient would make under the circumstances, taking into account all that is known about the patient. The surrogate might imagine that the patient miraculously regains decision-making capacity. What care would the patient choose under the circumstances?

Reconstructing patients' choices is ethically justified because it respects their individuality to the extent that this is possible. Even if patients are no longer able to make informed decisions, it is respectful to treat them as unique individuals and to make decisions for them that are consistent with their self-conception and life story (24). Patients trust a family member or other surrogate to make the best decision possible under circumstances that were not foreseen (1). Several problems, however, may occur with substituted judgments.

Problems with Substituted Judgment

Inconsistency

Reasonable people acting in good faith may disagree over what the patient would want. For example, his sister might believe that Mr. S. would want antibiotics. "He's been a fighter all his life and never gave up." She recalled that as a young man, Mr. S. had overcome tremendous odds to come to America and get a college education.

Inaccuracy

Neither family members nor physicians can accurately state a competent patient's choices regarding future life-sustaining treatment (18,40–42). In one study, only 68% of family members correctly stated a competent patient's preferences for CPR if he developed dementia, and only 59% of physicians were able to do so (40). This level of agreement between proxies and patients would be expected by chance alone. The accuracy of substituted judgments could probably be improved. Surrogates' predictions of patients' preferences are more accurate when surrogate and patient had discussed end-of-life issues (18,42).

Based on Questionable Considerations

Competent patients may not want to be a burden or may want to spare the family the expenses and stress of terminal care (43). It seems reasonable for surrogates to consider these factors when the patient himself has already done so, but it may be self-serving for surrogates to consider such factors when patients have not stated their importance (44). Family members may confound what they would want with what the patient would want.

Hypothetical and Unavoidably Speculative

Substituted judgments are inherently less certain than advance directives (45–47). Even though Mr. S. could no longer take walks and read, he might adapt to his illness and find life worthwhile. His comments regarding his wife do not necessarily express his own desires for medical care. Furthermore, many independent people learn to accept disabilities and assistance from others. In Case 12.2, the children's reasoning is unconvincing when applied to the converse situation. If a patient had seen physicians regularly, taken medications faithfully, and pursued no hobbies, it would be illogical to infer that he wanted all life-sustaining interventions in this situation.

Conflicting with the Patient's Best Interests

In unusual cases, substituted judgments may lead to decisions that contradict the patient's current best interests. For example, family members may say that a mildly demented patient would not want life-prolonging interventions, even though he still enjoys activities such as listening to music or playing with grandchildren. Although it would be appropriate to withhold treatment in this situation on the basis of a clear and specific advance directive, it is problematic to do so as a substituted judgment.

Despite the potential pitfalls of substituted judgments, they are desirable because they respect the patient's individuality as a person with unique values and preferences (24).

BEST INTERESTS

In many cases, a substituted judgment would be so speculative that it is more honest for the surrogate and physician to base decisions on what they believe is best for the patient (48). A consensus of medical ethicists and clinicians supports decisions based on the patient's best interests (6,45,49). Such decisions are justified by the ethical guideline of beneficence: physicians must act for the patient's well being and need to weigh the benefits and burdens of interventions for the patient.

Some scholars advocate a best-interests standard because statements previously made by an incapacitated patient in a vastly different situation may not be relevant (23,45,48). For example, these writers believe that preferences expressed by a young, healthy person should not carry much weight years later when he is severely demented. Indeed some writers have suggested that the patient with severe dementia should be considered a different person from the one who provided the advance directives, with different values and preferences. In this view, previous directives are irrelevant to current decisions.

Problems with Best Interests

Different people may disagree over what is best for a patient. Disagreements may involve the goals of care, the assessment of the benefits and burdens of an interventions, or the evaluation of the patient's quality of life. Judgments about quality of life are particularly controversial if made by a surrogate rather than by the patient, because other people underestimate patients' quality of life. Chapter 4 discusses these issues in more detail.

Some interpretations by surrogates of the patient's best interests are ethically problematic. Surrogates may assert that the patient wanted to spare the family the emotional or financial burdens of a protracted terminal illness. If there is compelling evidence that this is the patient's own view, it should be respected. In the absence of such evidence, however, the surrogate may be projecting his own wishes or acting out of self-interest.

Some surrogates request painful interventions that will only prolong the patient's life a few days. Surrogates may believe that suffering serves a spiritual purpose or that biological life should be prolonged even if the interventions required are very burdensome. Decisions based on such beliefs need to be scrutinized carefully (50). Did the patient hold such views, as opposed to the surrogate? Did the patient say that he or she would accept painful interventions or decline palliative relief? Many patients who believe their illness serves a spiritual purpose will still decline burdensome interventions. Caregivers may believe that they are causing the patient to suffer if they do not provide standard palliative care or if they carry out interventions that provide little prospect of benefit but cause considerable discomfort (50,51). The ethical guideline of nonmaleficence allows health care workers to refrain from interventions that cause significant suffering and prolong the patient's life for only a few hours or days (50).

Despite problems with best interests, it is important to recognize that acting for the benefit of patients is a fundamental ethical guideline for physicians. All medical interventions have both benefits and burdens, and physicians must assess whether the benefits of interventions outweigh the burdens for the particular patient in the given clinical situation. Some doctors believe all life-sustaining interventions should be provided to patients who lack decision-making capacity, unless they are futile. This approach, however, may impose interventions that are burdensome but provide little benefit. The guideline of acting in the patient's best interests provides a strong reason to forego such interventions.

In summary, advance directives are the preferred way to make decisions for patients who lack decision-making capacity. Advance directives may be oral statements or documents such as living wills or durable powers of attorney for health care. The most comprehensive and flexible advance directives both appoint a surrogate and express choices regarding treatments. In discussions with patients, physicians can ensure that advance directives are informed, specific, and up-to-date. In the absence of clear advance directives, surrogates should try to make substituted judgments. If the patient's values and preferences are not known, decisions need to be based on the patient's best interests.

REFERENCES

1. Singer PA, Martin DK, Lavery JV, et al. Reconceptualizing advance care planning from the patient's perspective. *Arch Intern Med* 1998;158:879–884.
2. Lo B, McLeod G, Saika G. Patient attitudes towards discussing life-sustaining treatment. *Arch Intern Med* 1986;146:1613–1615.
3. Emanuel LL, Barry MJ, Stoeckle JD, et al. Advance directives for medical care—a case for greater use. *N Engl J Med* 1991;324:889–895.
4. Lo B, Rouse F, Dornbrand L. Family decision-making on trial: who decides for incompetent patients? *N Engl J Med* 1990;322:1228–1231.
5. Steinbrook R, Lo B, Moulton J, et al. Preferences of homosexual men with AIDS for life-sustaining treatment. *N Engl J Med* 1986;314:457–460.
6. Meisel A. *The right to die*, 2nd ed. New York: John Wiley & Sons, 1995.
7. Sabatino CS. The legal and functional status of the medical proxy: suggestions for statutory reform. *J Law Med Ethics* 1999;27:46–51.
8. Rubin SM, Strull WM, Fialkow MF, et al. Increasing completion of the durable power of attorney for health care: a randomized controlled trial. *JAMA* 1994;271:209–212.
9. Schneiderman LJ, Kronick R, Kaplan RM, et al. Effects of offering advance directives on medical treatments and costs. *Ann Intern Med* 1992;117:599–606.
10. Sulmasy DP, Song KY, Marx ES, et al. Strategies to promote the use of advance directives in a residency outpatient practice. *J Gen Intern Med* 1996;11:657–663.
11. Meier DE, Fuss BR, O'Rourke D, et al. Marked improvement in recognition and completion of health care proxies. *Arch Intern Med* 1996;156:1227–1232.
12. Orentlicher D. Advance medical directives. *JAMA* 1991;263:2365–2367.
13. Annas GJ. The health care proxy and the living will. *N Engl J Med* 1991;324:1210–1213.
14. Steinbrook R, Lo B. Decision making for incompetent patients by designated proxy. *N Engl J Med* 1984;310:1598–1601.
15. Wolf SM, Boyle P, Callahan D, et al. Sources of concern about the Patient Self-Determination Act. *N Engl J Med* 1991;325:1666–1671.
16. Fischer GS, Tulsky JA, Rose MR, et al. Patient knowledge and physician predications of treatment preferences after discussions of advance directives. *J Gen Intern Med* 1998;13:447–454.
17. Murphy DJ, Burrows D, Santilli S, et al. The influence of the probability of survival on patients' preferences regarding cardiopulmonary resuscitation. *N Engl J Med* 1994;330:545–549.
18. Sulmasy DP, Terry PB, Weisman CS, et al. The accuracy of substituted judgments in patients with terminal diagnoses. *Ann Intern Med* 1998;128:621–629.
19. Weeks JC, Cook EF, O'Day SJ, et al. Relationship between cancer patients' predictions of prognosis and their treatment preferences. *JAMA* 1998;279:1709–1714.
20. Fischer GS, Alpert HR, Stoeckle JD, et al. Can goals of care be used to predict intervention preferences in an advance directive? *Arch Intern Med* 1997;157:801–807.
21. Sehgal A, Galbraith A, Chesney M, et al. How strictly do dialysis patients want their advance directives followed? *JAMA* 1992;267:59–63.

22. Danis M, Southerland LI, Garrett JM, et al. A prospective study of advance directives for life-sustaining care. *N Engl J Med* 1991;324:882–888.
23. Dresser RS, Robertson JA. Quality of life and non-treatment decisions for incompetent patients: a critique of the orthodox approach. *Law Med Health Care* 1989;17:234–244.
24. Blustein J. Choosing for others as continuing a life story: the problem of personal identity revisited. *J Law Med Ethics* 1999;27:13–19.
25. Emanuel LL, Emanuel EJ, Stoeckle JD, et al. Advance directives. Stability of patients' treatment choices. *Arch Intern Med* 1994;154:209–217.
26. Danis M, Garrett J, Harris R, Patrick DL. Stability of choices about life-sustaining treatments. *Ann Intern Med* 1994;120:567–573.
27. Reilly BM, Magnussen CR, Ross J, et al. Can we talk? Inpatient discussions about advance directives in a community hospital. Attending physicians' attitudes, their inpatients' wishes, and reported experience. *Arch Intern Med* 1994;154:2299–2308.
28. Hoffman JC, Wenger NS, Davis RH, et al. Patient preferences for communication with physicians about end-of-life decisions. *Ann Intern Med* 1997;127:1–12.
29. Johnston SC, Pfeifer MP, McNutt R. The discussion about advance directives. Patient and physician opinions regarding when and how it should be conducted. End of Life Study Group. *Arch Intern Med* 1995;155:1025–1030.
30. Omnibus Budget Reconciliation Act of 1990, Pub. L. No. 101–508 §§4206,4751.
31. Virmani J, Schneiderman LJ, Kaplan RM. Relationship of advance directives to physician-patient communication. *Arch Intern Med* 1994;154:909–913.
32. Tulsky JA, Fischer GS, Rose MR, et al. Opening the black box: how do physicians communicate about advance directives? *Ann Intern Med* 1998;129:441–449.
33. Lynn J, Schuster JL. *Improving care for the end of life: a sourcebook for health care managers and clinicians.* New York: Oxford University Press, 1999.
34. Council on Ethical and Judicial Affairs, AMA. Guidelines for the appropriate use of do-not-resuscitate orders. *JAMA* 1991;265:1868–1871.
35. Lo B, Snyder L, Sox H. Care at the end of life: guiding practice where there are no easy answers. *Ann Intern Med* 1999;130:772–774.
36. Singer PA. Disease-specific advance directives. *Lancet* 1994;344:594–596.
37. Emanuel LL, Emanuel EJ. The medical directive. *JAMA* 1989;261:3288–3293.
38. *Acting with dignity. Five wishes.* Available at www.agingwithdignity.org.
39. Lo B, Steinbrook R. Beyond the Cruzan case: the U.S. Supreme Court and medical practice. *Ann Intern Med* 1991;114:895–901.
40. Seckler AB, Meier DB, Mulvihill M, et al. Substituted judgment: how accurate are proxy predictions? *Ann Intern Med* 1991;115:92–98.
41. Emanuel EJ, Emanuel LL. Proxy decision making for incompetent patients: an ethical and empirical analysis. *JAMA* 1992;267:2067–2071.
42. Suhl J, Simons P, Reedy T, et al. Myth of substituted judgment: surrogate decisionmaking regarding life support is unreliable. *Arch Intern Med* 1994;154:90–96.
43. Hare J, Pratt C, Nelson C. Agreement between patients and their self-seleted surrogates on difficult medical decisions. *Arch Intern Med* 1992;152:1049–1054.
44. Lo B. Caring for the incompetent patient: is there a doctor in the house? *Law Med Health Care* 1990;17:214–220.
45. Buchanan AE, Brock DW. *Deciding for others.* Cambridge: Cambridge University Press, 1989.
46. Annas GJ. Quality of life in the courts: Earle Spring in fantasyland. *Hastings Center Rep* 1980;10:9–10.
47. Annas GJ. The case of Mary Hier: when substituted judgment becomes sleight of hand. *Hastings Center Rep* 1984;14:23–25.
48. Rhoden N. How should we view the incompetent? *Law Med Health Care* 1989;17:264–268.
49. President's Commission for the Study of Ethical Problems in Medicine and Biomedical and Behavioral Research. *Deciding to forego life-sustaining treatment.* Washington: US Government Printing Office, 1983.
50. Alpers A, Lo B. Avoiding family feuds: responding to surrogates' demands for life-sustaining treatment. *J Law Med Ethics* 1999;27:74–80.
51. Braithwaite S, Thomasma DC. New guidelines on foregoing life-sustaining treatment in incompetent patients: an anti-cruelty policy. *Ann Intern Med* 1986;104:711–715.

ANNOTATED BIBLIOGRAPHY

1. Buchanan AE, Brock DW. *Deciding for others.* Cambridge: Cambridge University Press, 1989.
   Thoughtful book on making decisions for patients who lack the capacity to make informed decisions.
2. Tulsky JA, Fischer GS, Rose MR, et al. Opening the black box: how do physicians communicate about advance directives? *Ann Intern Med* 1998;129:441–449.
   Well-designed study elucidating problems that occur when physicians discuss advance directives with patients.
3. Wolf SM, Boyle P, Callahan D, et al. Sources of concern about the Patient Self-Determination Act. *N Engl J Med* 1991;325:1666–1671.
   Thoughtful discussion of some common objections to advance directives.

4. Sehgal A, Galbraith A, Chesney M, et al. How strictly do dialysis patients want their advance directives followed? *JAMA* 1992;267:59–63.
   Patients vary regarding how much leeway they would grant surrogates to override their directives, if the surrogate believed it would be in the patient's best interests to do so.
5. Dresser RS, Robertson JA. Quality of life and non-treatment decisions for incompetent patients: a critique of the orthodox approach. *Law Med Health Care* 1989;17:234–244.
   Best interests may be a more realistic and honest standard than substituted judgment for patients who have not provided advance directives.
6. Blustein J. Choosing for others as continuing a life story: the problem of personal identity revisited. *J Law Med Ethics* 1999;27:13–19.
   Argues that surrogate decision-making is justified as a way of continuing the life stories of those who have lost the capacity to make their own decisions.
7. Emanuel EJ, Emanuel LL. Proxy decision making for incompetent patients: an ethical and empirical analysis. *JAMA* 1992;267:2067–2071.
   Summarizes data showing how families and physicians may not be able to state patients' preferences accurately.

Appendix: California statutory form for durable power attorney for health care

(health care proxy)

Appendix

Excerpts from California statutory form for

Durable Power of Attorney for Health Care

(California Probate Code Section 4771)

Creation of Durable Power of Attorney for Health Care

By this document I intent to create a durable power of attorney for health care by appointing the person designated below to make health care decisions for me, as allowed by the California Probate Code 4600-4806. This power of attorney will remain valid even if I become incapacitated and am unable to communicate my health care wishes...

Appointment of Health Care Agent

I, _____, hereby appoint:

Name: _____   ...
as my agent to make health care decisions for me as authorized in this document.

Authority of Health Care Agent

I grant my agent full power and authority to make health care decisions for me if I become incapable of giving informed consent for these health care decisions. This power is subject to the limitations set forth below. Unless I have limited my agent's authority in this document, that authority shall include the right to consent, refuse consent, or withdraw consent to any medical care, treatment, service, or procedure; to receive and to consent to the release of medical information... I understand that, by law, my agent may not consent to the following: commitment to a mental health treatment facility, convulsive treatment, psychosurgery, sterilization or abortion.

Medical Treatment Preferences and Limitations

Your agent must make health care decisions that are consistent with your known preferences. You may, but are not required to, state your wishes about the kinds of medical care you do or do not want, including your wishes concerning life-sustaining treatment, in the space provided below. If your preferences are unknown, your agent has the duty to act in your best interests.

_____

_____

_____

_____

Duration

I understand that this durable power of attorney for health care will be effective from the date I sign this document and will exist indefinitely, unless I specify a shorter time. However, I can revoke this documents at any time by telling my health care agent and my doctor that I no longer want it to be effective.

Date and signature

I sign my name to this durable power of Attorney for Health Care on

____(date)____ at _____(city)_____, _____(state)_____

_____(signature)_____

Statement of Witness

I declare under penalty of perjury under the laws of California that the person who signed or acknowledged this document is personally known to me to be the principal, or that the identity of the principal was proved to me by convincing evidence, that the principal signed or acknowledged this Durable Power of Attorney for Health Care in my presence, that the principal appears to be of sound mind and under no duress, fraud, or undue influence, that I am not the person appointed as attorney in fact (agent) by this document, and that I am not the principal's health care provider, an operator of a community care facility or residential care facility for the elderly, nor an employee of the principal's health care provider, or an employee of a community care facility or residential care facility for the elderly.

Signature: _____
Print name: _____
Date: _____
Residence address: _____

_____

Signature:_____
Print name: _____
Date: _____
Residence address: _____

_____

At least one of the above witnesses must also sign the following declaration.

I further declare under penalty of perjury that I am not related to the principal by blood, marriage, or adoption, and, to the best of my knowledge, I am not entitled to any part of the estate of the principal upon the death of the principal under a will now existing or by operation of law.

Signature: _____

If the patient residents in a skilled nursing facility, one of the witnesses must be a patient advocate or ombudsman.

The patient may have the form notarized by a Notary Public instead of witnessed by two witnesses.

13

Surrogate Decision-Making

When patients lack decision-making capacity, physicians turn to surrogates to make decisions on their behalf. Traditionally, family members serve as surrogate decision-makers for patients who lack decision-making capacity. This practice, however, may break down in cases like the following. Note that this book uses the term *surrogate* for anyone who makes decisions for a patient who lacks decision-making capacity and reserves the term *proxy* for a surrogate appointed by the patient. Chapter 12 discusses the related issue of what standards should be used in making decisions for patients who lack decision-making capacity.

   CASE 13.1. DISAGREEMENT BETWEEN FAMILY MEMBERS. *Mrs. R. is a 72-year-old widow with severe Alzheimer's disease. She does not recognize her family but often smiles when someone holds her hand or gives her a hug. She lives with her sister, who provides help with all activities of daily living together with an attendant. Mrs. R. develops pneumonia. She had never indicated what she would want in such a situation or whom she would want to make decisions for her. Her sister believes that Mrs. R. would not want her life prolonged in this condition because she prized her independence and asks the physician to withhold antibiotics. Mrs. R.'s only child is a son who visits once or twice a year. He is outraged at this request. He asserts, "Life is sacred; it's God's gift. We can't just snuff it out."*

   Because Mrs. R. had given no advance directives, decisions about care need to be made by a surrogate. Both the sister and the son desire to act as Mrs. R.'s surrogate. The sister asserts priority because she cared for Mrs. R. and has been close to her sister most of her life, yet the son has closer ties of kinship. What justifies selecting one surrogate over the other? How can decisions be made in the face of family disagreements?

WHO SHOULD SERVE AS SURROGATE?

Among potential surrogates, there is a hierarchy that physicians should keep in mind. However, often decisions are best made by consensus, rather than giving one potential surrogate priority over others.

Court-Appointed Guardians

The courts have legal authority to declare a patient incompetent and to appoint a guardian to make medical decisions for the patient. The legal system offers procedural safeguards, such as notice to all parties, the right to call and cross-examine witnesses, impartial judges, explicit justification for decisions, and an appeals process. However, involving the courts routinely in decisions has serious drawbacks (1,2). First, the courts intrude on highly personal and private issues. The adversarial judicial system may polarize families and physicians, rather than fostering a mutually acceptable decision. Second, guardianship hearings usually are superficial, and courts do not monitor guardians' decisions (3). Finally, intolerable delays would occur if the courts were involved more frequently in decisions about life-sustaining treatment. As one court decision declared, "Courts are not the proper place to resolve the agonizing personal problems that underlie these cases. Our legal system cannot replace the more intimate struggle that must be borne by the patient, those caring for the patient, and those who care about the patient" (4). Court-appointed guardians have legal priority over other potential surrogates. However, physicians and hospitals should involve the courts only as a last resort, when disputes cannot be resolved in the clinical setting.

Surrogates Selected by Patients

As discussed in Chapter 12, almost all states have legal procedures for competent patients to appoint a health care proxy (5). Generally, the patient must complete a form and have it witnessed or notarized. Many patients find it easier to select who should act as proxy, rather than anticipate what they would want in future scenarios. Appointing a proxy may prevent disputes in the future. For example, many homosexual men with human immunodeficiency virus (HIV) infection want their friends or partners to act as proxy decision-makers, rather than biological relatives, who may be estranged. Similarly, patients who anticipate disagreements among family members may select one person to be proxy.

   In some cases, the patient indicates the selection of a surrogate informally but does not complete a legal document appointing the person. If the surrogate and close relatives disagree over plans for care, the physician may then face a conflict between what is ethically appropriate and what is legally protected. Ethically speaking, the person whom the patient wanted to serve as surrogate should have priority. Legally, however, persons may have no standing to make decisions. The physician should try to persuade the family to respect the patient's choice of proxy.

Family Members

Decisions by families of patients who lack decision-making capacity are standard medical practice (6,7). There are compelling ethical justifications for family decision-making.

Most People Want Family Members to Serve as Surrogates

In a public opinion poll, 30% of respondents wanted their families to make medical decisions for them if they became incapacitated. An additional 53% wanted their family to make decisions together with their physicians (8). Only 3% of respondents wanted the courts to decide.

Family Members Often Know What the Patient Would Want

Because family members generally have close relationships with patients, they are more likely than other people to have discussed life-sustaining interventions with patients.

Families Members are Presumed to Act in the Patient's Best Interests

Ties of kinship and affection generally lead family members to do what is best for the patient, rather than what is best for themselves. Strong social, cultural, and religious norms encourage family members to subordinate their own interests for the sake of relatives in need.

The term "family" should be interpreted in light of demographic facts, such as the large number of unmarried couples living together. Ethically, the crucial issue is not the legal status of the relationship, but whether it is reasonable to presume that the partner will act in the best interests of the patient.

Decision-Making by the Family as a Group

For many families, the idea of singling out one person as a surrogate may seem to disrespect the family as a whole. Family connections have both ethical and practical significance. Proponents of an ethics of care (*see* Chapter 1) have argued that more attention should be paid to how decisions affect various relationships and that families should have a greater voice in health care decisions (9,10). In this view, relationships among family members will survive after the patient's death. These relationships deserve respect, and physicians should support attempts to maintain family harmony. From a pragmatic point of view, many proxies are reluctant to contradict the views of close relatives. They may feel torn between what they think is best for the patient and what other family members want to do (11).

No Family Members Available

Decisions are most difficult when patients with impaired decision-making capacity have no advance directives and no family members. In some cases, a friend may be an appropriate surrogate. If the friend has an emotional bond to patients, it is plausible to presume that he or she will act in the patient's best interests (12).

If no one is available as surrogate, it is appropriate for physicians to make decisions, based on what they believe is in the patient's best interests. Physicians do not need to administer life-sustaining interventions simply because there is no surrogate to decline them on behalf of the patient. In this situation, physicians may forego interventions that they do not consider to be in the patient's best interests. When there is no surrogate, it is advisable for physicians to consult with the hospital ethics committee or a physician not involved in the case. Simply explaining one's reasoning to another person can clarify thinking, identify unwarranted assumptions and unconvincing arguments, and suggest new options for care.

LEGAL ISSUES REGARDING SURROGATE DECISION-MAKING

Many states allow relatives to refuse interventions on behalf of such patients, even in the absence of advance directives (5,7). The highest courts in New York State and Missouri, however, have rejected family decision-making when patients have not given clear and convincing advance directives. In these states, physicians face a dilemma because the law does not permit actions that are recommended by medical ethics and sound clinical practice.

In several states, legislation specifies which relatives have priority to act as surrogates for incapacitated patients (13). Generally, the patient's spouse takes priority over adult children, followed by parents and more distant relatives. Such laws, however, may lead to ethically troubling results, such as favoring the distant son in Case 13.1 over the sister who is apparently closer to the patient. These laws may also be problematical when a spouse is estranged but not legally divorced.

PROBLEMS WITH SURROGATE DECISION-MAKING

The physician should serve as the patient's advocate if the surrogate's decision conflicts with the patient's previous statements or best interests.

Emotional Barriers to Decisions

Surrogates commonly find it difficult to make decisions because of the emotional stress of the patient's illness. Sadness or denial may complicate decisions. Surrogates may also feel guilty over not doing everything for the patient or "pulling the plug."

Unacceptable Reasons for Decisions

Surrogates are given less leeway than competent patients concerning the basis for their decisions. For example, patients may forego interventions in order to spare family members emotional distress or to preserve an inheritance for children. Such refusals are heeded in order to respect patient autonomy. However, as Chapter 12 discusses, claims by surrogates that the patient would refuse interventions for these reasons may be self-serving and need to be scrutinized (14).

Decisions Inconsistent with the Patient's Preferences or Values

Some surrogate decisions are not consistent with the patient's preferences or values. Surrogates may impose their own values on the patient, rather than respecting her choices and values. In Case 13.1, the son is basing decisions on religious beliefs about the sanctity of life. When patients themselves hold such views, they are followed out of respect for patient autonomy (*see* Chapter 4). However, it is inappropriate for surrogates to impose their own views onto the patient. Thus, the physician needs to inquire whether the patient herself held such religious views.

Conflicts of Interest

Caring for a relative with serious chronic illness may cause emotional distress, fatigue, financial burdens, or conflicts with other responsibilities (15). Consciously or unconsciously, it might be a relief in Case 13.1 for Mrs. R.'s sister to be freed from the burdens of care. In some cases, relatives may promote their own interests, not the interests of the patient. Unscrupulous family members may try to gain control of an inheritance or a pension. In other cases, long-standing family tensions and disputes may flare in the context of a terminal illness. However, physicians should not be overly suspicious about surrogates. Most family members subordinate their interests to those of the patient and make considerable sacrifices (16). Simply making sacrifices to care for a relative or being mentioned in a will is not a conflict of interests.

Disagreements Among Potential Surrogates

Case 13.1 illustrates how family members may disagree over decisions. Some physicians withhold interventions only when all family members agree. However, giving every relative a veto may impose interventions that are not in the patient's best interests. Furthermore, it is problematical to give distant or estranged relatives a voice equal to that of those closest to the patient. Realistically, physicians often make decisions with family consensus rather than unanimity. Some relatives may be willing to accept a decision made by the rest of the family, even though they would have decided differently themselves.

Despite problems with surrogate decision-making, physicians should try to make joint decisions with surrogates of patients who lack decision-making capacity. Patients want family members or other surrogates to make decisions for them and trust them to do their best under circumstances that might not be foreseen (17).

Common Misconceptions About Surrogate Decision-Making

Physicians may have misconceptions about decisions for patients who lack decision-making capacity.

Unrealistic Standards for Advance Directives

Patients cannot predict the clinical situations that they will face. It is unrealistic to expect patients to have given directives about the specific intervention and situation at hand, as Chapter 12 discusses.

Undue Suspicion of Surrogates

Some doctors fear that the burdens of caregiving or the possibility of an inheritance may create a conflict of interest for surrogates. However, physicians should not be overly distrustful or cynical. Most family members make substantial commitments to care for relatives with serious illness. Respecting close family relationships is an important social value, and physicians should support families who are trying to deal with difficult situations as best they can.

Unrealistic Expectations of Certainty

In every aspect of clinical medicine, physicians need to work under uncertainty. Physicians seldom know with certainty what a patient would want in a particular situation. However, it is problematical to insist on life-sustaining interventions because it is not certain that the patient would not want them. Imposing burdensome interventions on patients makes them "prisoners of technology" (18).

IMPROVING SURROGATE DECISION-MAKING

After sufficient discussions, physicians and surrogates agree on decisions about life-sustaining interventions in almost all cases (19). Physicians can take steps to improve surrogate decision-making (Table 13-1). Chapter 15 also gives additional detailed suggestions for reaching agreement.

Elicit and Respond to Surrogates' Concerns

In Case 13.1, open-ended questions may help the son articulate his concerns (20). "As you think about your mother's condition, what concerns you the most? . . . What do you hope for?" In Case 13.1, the physician might also give the son time to understand and accept the situation.

Discuss the Decision-Making Process

Physicians should acknowledge that decisions are difficult and that people with good intentions may disagree. Families find it helpful when physicians clarify their role and accom-

TABLE 13-1. *Suggestions for improving surrogate decision-making*

Elicit and respond to surrogates' concerns.
Discuss the decision-making process.
Give a recommendation.
Get help from other health care workers.

modate their grief (21). Physicians should remind everybody that decisions should be based on the patient's preferences and values, not on what surrogates or doctors would choose for themselves.

The physician should also discuss the relationship between the patient and surrogates. Acknowledging emotional reactions is helpful. In Case 13.1, the physician might say to the son, "For many relatives who live far away, it is difficult to make decisions. I wonder how you are feeling about making decisions for your mother."

Give a Recommendation

Physicians should not merely list options and leave it to family members to decide. Doctors should make a recommendation based on what is known about the patient's preferences and values. Recommendations are particularly important when family members disagree or are overwhelmed by guilt or grief.

Get Help from Other Health Care Workers

Often a nurse, social worker, or chaplain can help the family work through past antagonisms with the patient or among themselves. Furthermore, such persons may provide valuable emotional support to family members. The hospital ethics committee may be able to facilitate such discussions.

In summary, surrogates should know the incapacitated patient's preferences, be willing to respect them, and act in the best interests of the patient. The patient's own choice of surrogate should be respected. In most cases, the standard clinical practice of family decision-making is ethically appropriate. When family members disagree, physicians should make efforts to resolve conflicts and achieve consensus.

REFERENCES

1. Meisel A. *The right to die.* New York: John Wiley & Sons, 1989:145–169.
2. Lo B, Rouse F, Dornbrand L. Family decision-making on trial: who decides for incompetent patients? *N Engl J Med* 1990;322:1228–1231.
3. Bulcroft K, Kielkopf MR, Tripp K. Elderly wards and their legal guardians: analysis of county probate records in Ohio and Washington. *Gerontologist* 1991;31:156–164.
4. In re Jobes, 529 A. 2d 434 (N.J. 1987).
5. Sabatino CS. The legal and functional status of the medical proxy: suggestions for statutory reform. *J Law Med Ethics* 1999;27:46–51.
6. President's Commission for the Study of Ethical Problems in Medicine and Biomedical and Behavioral Research. *Deciding to forego life-sustaining treatment.* Washington: US Government Printing Office, 1983.
7. Meisel A. *The right to die,* 2nd ed. New York: John Wiley & Sons, 1995.
8. Blendon RJ, Szalay US, Knox RA. Should physicians aid their patients in dying? The public perspective. *JAMA* 1992;267:2658–2662.
9. Jecker N. The role of intimate others in medical decision making. *Gerontologist* 1990;30:65–71.
10. Hardwig J. What about the family? *Hastings Center Rep* 1990;20:5–10.
11. Alpers A, Lo B. Avoiding family feuds: responding to surrogates' demands for life-sustaining treatment. *J Law Med Ethics* 1999;27:74–80.
12. Veatch RM. An ethical framework for terminal care decisions. *J Am Geriatr Soc* 1984;32:665–669.
13. Menikoff JA, Sachs GA, Siegler M. Beyond advance directives: health care surrogate laws. *N Engl J Med* 1992;322:1165–1169.
14. Lo B. Caring for the incompetent patient: is there a doctor in the house? *Law Med Health Care* 1989;17:214–220.
15. Covinsky KE, Landefeld CS, Teno J, et al. Is economic hardship on the families of the seriously ill associated with patient and surrogate care preferences? *Arch Intern Med* 1996;156:1737–1741.
16. Covinsky KE, Goldman L, Cook FS, et al. The impact of serious illness on patients' families. *JAMA* 1994;272:1839–1844.
17. Singer PA, Martin DK, Lavery JV, et al. Reconceptualizing advance care planning from the patient's perspective. *Arch Int Med* 1998;158:879–884.

18. Angell M. Prisoners of technology: the case of Nancy Cruzan. *N Engl J Med* 1990;322:1226–1228.
19. Prendergast TJ, Luce JM. Increasing incidence of withholding and withdrawal of life support from the critically ill. *Am Rev Respir Dis Crit Care Med* 1997;155:15–20.
20. Lo B, Quill T, Tulsky J. Discussing palliative care with patients. *Ann Intern Med* 1999;130:744–749.
21. Tilden VP, Tolle SW, Garland MJ, et al. Decisions about life-sustaining treatment: impact of physicians' behaviors on the family. *Arch Intern Med* 1995;155:633–638.

ANNOTATED BIBLIOGRAPHY

1. Lo B, Rouse F, Dornbrand L. Family decision-making on trial: who decides for incompetent patients? *N Engl J Med* 1990;322:1228–1231.
   Argues that families should be presumed to be appropriate decision-makers for patients who lack decision-making capacity.
2. Buchanan AE, Brock DW. *Deciding for others*. Cambridge: Cambridge University Press, 1989.
   Detailed ethical analysis of surrogate decision-making.
3. Sabatino CS. The legal and functional status of the medical proxy: suggestions for statutory reform. *J Law Med Ethics* 1999;27:46–51.
   Recent analysis of state laws regarding surrogate decision-making.

Decisions About Life-Sustaining Interventions

14

Confusing Ethical Distinctions

In discussions about life-sustaining interventions, physicians often draw distinctions that seem intuitively plausible but prove problematical on closer analysis. Examples are distinctions between withdrawing and withholding interventions and between extraordinary (or heroic) and ordinary care. On the other hand, some ethical distinctions, although less intuitive, are nonetheless ethically valid. In particular, physicians may not understand the important distinction between providing very high doses of opioids to relieve symptoms and intentionally administering opioids to kill the patient (1). Physicians need to appreciate which distinctions are ethically meaningful and which are not, because failure to do so often leads to confusion and poor care.

CASE 14.1. WITHDRAWAL OF MECHANICAL VENTILATION. *Mr. C., a 68-year-old man with severe chronic obstructive lung disease, developed respiratory failure after an episode of bronchitis. He had told his outpatient physician repeatedly that he was willing to be on a ventilator in the intensive care unit, but only for a brief period. If he did not recover, he wanted the physicians to let him to die in peace. After 2 weeks on antibiotics, bronchodilators, and mechanical ventilation, Mr. C. showed little improvement and was still in respiratory failure. He asked his physicians to discontinue the ventilator and to keep him comfortable while he died. His family and primary physician believed that his decision was informed.*

Some health care workers objected to discontinuing the ventilator. They argued that although the patient can refuse life-sustaining interventions in the first place, removing them would be tantamount to murder. Other health care workers believed that it would be appropriate to discontinue heroic treatments such as the mechanical ventilation but that ordinary treatments like antibiotics and intravenous fluids needed to be continued. Still others objected to the use of sedating doses of opioids for the relief of dyspnea after the ventilator was withdrawn because they would hasten death.

WITHDRAWING AND WITHHOLDING INTERVENTIONS

Many physicians and nurses are willing to withhold interventions but reluctant to withdraw them once they have been started. In one survey, 82% of attending physicians were willing to withhold mechanical ventilation from a patient with severe chronic obstructive lung disease who refused it, whereas only 59% were willing to withdraw the ventilator in such a situation (2). In another survey, 57% of attending physicians and 73% of nurses said there is an ethical difference between not starting life support and stopping it once it has been started (3).

This distinction seems plausible because discontinuing the ventilator is frequently characterized as a positive action, whereas not starting the ventilator may seem more passive and therefore less reprehensible. In everyday life, people generally are held more responsible for their actions than for their omissions. This distinction between acting and refraining from action, however, is not tenable in clinical medicine. Philosophers have devised ingenious examples to illustrate how the distinction between acting and refraining from acting cannot, by itself, be decisive (4). Suppose that the ventilator is accidentally disconnected from the patient. A physician might argue that it was permissible to refrain from reconnecting the ventilator but not to take action to disconnect it. This position is problematical because the physician has an ethical obligation to respect the patient's preferences and act in the patient's best interests. If the patient wishes the ventilator continued and the physician does not reconnect it, it is morally wrong, even though the physician may be said to withhold the ventilator or refrain from acting. On the other hand, if a patient connected to a ventilator wishes to cease interventions, as in Case 14.1, respecting the patient's wishes requires the physician to withdraw the ventilator. Hence the physician may be ethically obligated to perform an act or refrain from acting, depending on the patient's preferences. The distinction between withdrawing and withholding is not decisive.

In many cases, justifications for withdrawing treatment are more powerful than reasons to not initiate it. Additional information may become known after treatment has started, for example, that the patient did not want treatment or has end-stage disease. Furthermore, a hoped-for benefit may not materialize, as in Case 14.1 (5). Typically decisions about life-sustaining treatment must be made when the patient's prognosis is still uncertain. A time-limited trial of intensive therapy may be appropriate in this situation (6). If a treatment proves ineffective, there is no point in continuing it. However, if people were not able to discontinue a treatment once it was started, they might not even try interventions that might prove beneficial (7).

More generally, there is no ethical difference between stopping and not starting a medical intervention. In either case, the physician is responsible for a decision. The considerations that justify not initiating a treatment—in Case 14.1 informed refusal by a competent patient—also justify discontinuing it. In addition, the courts have consistently ruled that there is no distinction between discontinuing medical interventions and not initiating them (8,9). In this book, we use the term "forego" to include both withholding and withdrawing interventions (5).

EXTRAORDINARY OR HEROIC CARE

People may intuitively distinguish between extraordinary and ordinary care. Interventions that are highly technological, invasive, complicated, expensive, or unusual are sometimes regarded as "heroic" or "extraordinary." Examples include mechanical ventilation and renal dialysis. In contrast, antibiotics, intravenous fluids, and tube feedings are typically considered "ordinary" care. Some ordinary measures are commonly considered basic care or a standard nursing measure, such as a warm, dry bed. Often it is argued that extraordinary treatments may be withheld or withdrawn, but not ordinary ones. In one survey, 74% of doctors and nurses found this distinction helpful in making decisions (3).

This distinction, however, is not a reliable guide to decisions (5). It is indeed appropriate to withdraw mechanical ventilation from Mr. C. in Case 14.1. However, the reason is not that the ventilator can be characterized as extraordinary or heroic, but rather that it provides little benefit and the patient does not want it. Instead of focusing on whether the technology may be considered extraordinary or ordinary, physicians should examine the benefits and burdens of the intervention in the situation, as well as the patient's preferences. In other clinical settings, such as during general anesthesia for surgery, mechanical ventilation is highly effective, desired by patients, and universally used. The courts have rejected distinctions between ordinary and extraordinary interventions (8,9). Numerous rulings have declared that interventions ranging from ventilators to tube feedings may be withheld or withdrawn in appropriate circumstances. Chapter 20 discusses tube feedings in more detail.

RELIEVING SYMPTOMS WITH HIGH DOSES OF OPIOIDS AND SEDATIVES

Relief of pain and other symptoms in terminal illness, such as shortness of breath, is often inadequate. In the SUPPORT study of seriously ill patients, 50% of patients who died experienced moderate to severe pain in their last 3 days of life (10). Doctors may be reluctant to prescribe opioids in sufficient doses to relieve symptoms, or nurses may be reluctant to administer them (11). Some health care workers withhold opioids because they fear patients will become addicted. However, addiction rarely develops in terminal illness and should not be a primary consideration under these circumstances. Another concern is that the dose of opioids required to relieve symptoms might hasten the patient's death by suppressing respiration or causing hypotension. The doctrine of double effect, long-standing in moral philosophy, addresses this concern.

The Doctrine of Double Effect

Like all interventions, opioids and sedatives have both intended effects and unintended "side" effects. The doctrine of double effect distinguishes effects that are intended from those that are foreseen but unintended (12–15). In this view, intentionally causing death is wrong. However, physicians may provide high doses of opioids and sedatives to relieve suffering, provided that they do not intend the patient's death. Such high doses are permitted even if the risk of hastening death is foreseen. The double effect doctrine also requires that the bad effect (the patient's death) not be the means to accomplish the good effect (relief of suffering). In addition, the unintended but foreseen bad effect must be proportional to the intended good effects. For example, it would be inappropriate to begin treatment of mild pain with very large doses of opioids. However, if the patient's suffering is greater, the physician can justify a greater risk of potentially contributing to the patient's death.

Problems With the Double Effect Doctrine

The doctrine of double effect is widely accepted in this context of high doses of opioids and sedatives to relieve pain. In a survey, almost 90% of physicians and nurses agreed that it is appropriate to administer medication to relieve pain even if it hastens a patient's death (3). The U.S. Supreme Court has accepted it (*see* Chapter 23).

However, the doctrine presents several problems (16). First, the doctrine of double effect presents a questionable account of intention (12,17). Physicians may have multiple intentions (18). In one study, physicians who ordered sedatives and analgesics while withholding life-sustaining interventions said they intended both to decrease pain and to hasten death in about a third of cases (19). Second, the doctrine of double effect seems to focus on how physicians articulates their intentions. The doctrine of double effect seems to imply that physicians are more justified in administering large doses of opioids if they can put out of mind the possibility that death may be hastened. Third, people generally are held accountable for consequences they foresee or should have foreseen, not merely for those consequences that they intended (5). Thus the doctrine of double effect may be inconsistent with widely held ideas regarding responsibility for actions.

The issue of intention is further clouded because refusal of medical interventions by a competent patient may involve the intention to hasten death in some cases. Many competent patients who forego life-sustaining interventions do not want to continue a particular treatment, but hope nevertheless that they can live without it. However, some patients who refuse life support intend to bring about their death. There is broad agreement that physicians should respect patient refusals of interventions, even when the patient's intention is to die. Thus, although intention is central to the doctrine of double effect, it should not be the only criterion for judging an action right or wrong.

Despite problems with the doctrine of double effect, it is well established that it is acceptable to use opioids to relieve pain and other symptoms, even if it hastens the patient's death. Because of controversies surrounding the doctrine of double effect, it may be helpful to give an alternative justification for high doses of opioids and sedatives to relieve refractory symptoms. When terminally ill patients experience refractory symptoms, the physician is caught between two duties: to relieve suffering and not to cause the patient's death. In balancing these conflicting duties, proportionality is important. The risk of hastening death is warranted if lower doses have failed to relieve the symptoms (5). In this situation, it is more important to relieve refractory symptoms than to prolong a painful existence for a few hours or days.

Practical Aspects of Relieving Refractory Symptoms

Intention is judged by a person's actions, as well as by her statements. Physicians cannot simply say that they intended to relieve pain; their actions must also be consistent with their statements (20). What approach to the use of opioids and sedatives is consistent with an intent to relieve pain, but not to hasten death?

If the physician's intent is to palliate symptoms, her actions must allow the possibility for symptoms to be relieved without hastening death. The initial dose should not be expected to suppress respiration or cause hypotension. If a lethal dose is administered, there is no possibility that the patient would survive. Suffering is relieved only by the death of the patient. This action would constitute active euthanasia.

If the physician intends only to palliate suffering, there is no warrant for increasing the morphine dose when the patient is comfortable. In conscious patients, the dose can be increased if the patient reports unacceptable symptoms. If patients are unconscious or otherwise unable to report pain, physicians and nurses must assess whether patients are comfortable. The dosage should be increased if the patient is restless or grimaces, withdraws from stimuli, or has hypertension, tachycardia, tachypnea, or any other findings that could reasonably be interpreted as suffering. Increasing sedation in absence of signs of distress would imply that the physician intended to hasten death and would cross the line from palliative care to active euthanasia (20).

RESPONSES TO REFRACTORY SUFFERING

Some terminally ill patients may experience suffering that is not relieved even by excellent palliative care and high-dose opioids. Examples include uncontrollable pain, dyspnea, or bleeding and inability to swallow oral secretions. How should physicians respond in such dire situations? Other options include terminal sedation and voluntarily stopping of eating and drinking (12). Unlike physician-assisted suicide and active euthanasia, these practices are legal in all states.

Terminal Sedation

Terminal sedation goes beyond high-dose opioids in several ways. The patient is sedated to unconsciousness in order to control symptoms, usually through administration of barbiturates or benzodiazepines. In addition, all life-sustaining interventions are withheld. The patient then dies of dehydration, starvation, or some other intervening complication. Although death is inevitable, it is delayed for a few hours to over 7 days, depending on clinical circumstances.

Although widely accepted, terminal sedation is not free of controversy (12). Terminal sedation is sometimes done without the express agreement of patients or surrogates or without explicit discussion that other interventions will be withheld (21). Such cases are problematical. In withholding life-sustaining interventions while a patient is terminally sedated, doctors claim that they are not killing the patient but simply respecting the patient's or surrogate's refusal of interventions. This claim is ethically acceptable only if the patient or surrogate has consented to foregoing these interventions. In addition, there may be confusion regarding the physician's intention and responsibility. It seems implausible to claim that death is unintended when a patient who wants to die is sedated to unconsciousness, life-sustaining interventions and artificial nutrition are withheld, and death is certain. Although sedation is intended to relieve the patient's suffering, the additional step of withholding fluids and nutrition is not needed to relieve pain, but is done to hasten the patient's wished-for death. Furthermore, the notion that terminal sedation is merely "letting nature take its course" is unconvincing because often the patient dies from the withholding of nutrition and fluids, not of the underlying disease. Some writers argue that terminal sedation cannot be meaningfully distinguished from active euthanasia (22).

Terminal sedation also has limitations as a response to refractory suffering. First, some patients find terminal sedation unacceptable because prolonged unconsciousness before death violates their dignity or causes their families to suffer. Patients who wish to die in their own homes may not be able to arrange terminal sedation at home. Second, terminal sedation cannot relieve some symptoms, such as uncontrollable bleeding or inability to swallow secretions. Although patients are not conscious of these conditions once sedated, their death cannot be considered dignified or peaceful.

Despite these concerns, terminal sedation is both ethically and legally acceptable. Doctors can ensure that terminal sedation is appropriate. Physicians should check that the patient has received excellent palliative care, that the decision to carry out terminal sedation is informed and voluntary, and that the patient does not have major depression.

Voluntary Stopping of Eating and Drinking

When voluntarily stopping eating and drinking, the patient decides to discontinue oral intake and is "allowed to die," primarily of dehydration or some intervening complication (12). Ethically and legally, the right of competent, informed patients to refuse life-prolonging interventions is firmly established. Forcibly feeding a competent patient who refuses food and fluids would violate the patient's autonomy. Because stopping eating and drinking requires considerable patient resolve, the voluntary nature of the action is clear. Stopping eating and drinking may seem natural, because severe anorexia commonly occurs in the final stage of many illnesses.

The main disadvantage is that voluntary stopping of eating and drinking requires considerable resolve. The process may last for up to 2 weeks and therefore may seem inhumane. Initially the patient may experience thirst and hunger. Ice chips and mouth care usually relieve discomfort, and pain medication may also be needed. Subtle coercion may occur if patients are not regularly offered the opportunity to eat and drink, yet such offers may be viewed as undermining the patient's resolve. Patients are likely to lose mental clarity toward the end of this process, which may raise questions about voluntariness or seem unacceptable to some patients or families.

EMOTIONAL REACTIONS TO THESE DISTINCTIONS

Physicians need to appreciate that these topics raise emotional as well as philosophical issues. To many people, stopping a treatment is much more difficult emotionally than not starting it. Health care workers may feel that they are causing the patient's death by withdrawing a ventilator, discontinuing vasopressors, turning off a pacemaker or automatic implantable cardiac defibrillator, or administering large doses of opioids or sedatives. The shorter the time between the withdrawal of the intervention and the patient's death, the more responsible the health care worker may feel for killing the patient. Such feelings may be particularly strong in nurses who are asked to actually disconnect the ventilator or to turn down the settings (23).

Doctors should routinely elicit the concerns, feelings, and objections of other health care workers regarding these issues. Moreover, doctors need to acknowledge the depth and sincerity of such feelings. Team meetings are often helpful for this purpose. Similarly, physicians need to ascertain whether the patient or family has reservations about the plan of care.

Strong emotional reactions, such as a pang of conscience, may be a clue that more deliberation and discussion are needed. However, health care workers should articulate the reasons for their emotional reactions. The fact that something is emotionally difficult does not necessarily mean that it is unethical. In Case 14.1, the attending physician needs to explain that ethically and legally, the cause of Mr. C.'s death is considered his chronic obstructive pulmonary disease, not the discontinuation of mechanical ventilation. Supporting this ethical position, the law clearly states that discontinuing treatment is not murder or suicide (8,24).

The concerns of nurses and house staff should be accommodated if reasonably possible. Nurses who have strong personal objections to the plan of care should not be required to carry it out if other arrangements can be made to care for the patient. Generally other nurses will volunteer to care for the patient. The attending physician should closely monitor the administration of opioids and sedatives, rather than leaving it to the nurses and house staff. Nurses and house officers appreciate it when the attending physician is at the bedside when mechanical ventilation is withdrawn.

In summary, several commonly held distinctions regarding life-sustaining interventions are not logically tenable. Physicians should appreciate that it may be appropriate to withdraw interventions that have been started or that some persons consider ordinary care. In addition, administering high doses of opioids and sedatives is appropriate to relieve symptoms in patients who have terminal illness or who have refused mechanical ventilation.

REFERENCES

1. Emanuel EJ, Daniels ER, Fairclough DL, et al. The practice of euthanasia and physician-assisted suicide in the United States: adherence to proposed safeguards and effects on physicians. *JAMA* 1998;280:507–513.
2. Caralis PV, Hammond JS. Attitudes of medical students, house staff, and faculty physicians toward euthanasia and termination of life-sustaining treatment. *Crit Care Med* 1992;20:683–690.
3. Solomon MZ, O'Donnell LO, Jennings B, et al. Decisions near the end of life: professional views on life-sustaining treatments. *Am J Public Health* 1993;83:14–23.
4. Brock D. Forgoing life-sustaining food and water: is it killing? In: Lynn J, ed. *By no extraordinary means* (expanded edition.) Bloomington: Indiana University Press, 1989:117–131.
5. President's Commission for the Study of Ethical Problems in Medicine and Biomedical and Behavioral Research. *Deciding to forego life-sustaining treatment.* Washington: US Government Printing Office, 1983:73–89.
6. Ruark J, Raffin TA, Stanford University Medical Center Committee on Ethics. Initiating and withdrawing life support. *N Engl J Med* 1988;318:25–30.
7. Lo B, Rouse F, Dornbrand L. Family decision-making on trial: who decides for incompetent patients? *N Engl J Med* 1990;322:1228–1231.
8. Meisel A. Legal myths about terminating life support. *Arch Intern Med* 1991;1551:1497–1502.
9. Meisel A. *The right to die*, 2nd ed. New York: John Wiley & Sons, 1995.
10. The SUPPORT Investigators. A controlled trial to improve care for seriously ill hospitalized patients. *JAMA* 1995;274:1591–1598.
11. Edwards MJ, Tolle SW. Disconnecting the ventilator at the request of a patient who knows he will then die: the doctor's anguish. *Ann Intern Med* 1992;117:254–256.
12. Quill TE, Dresser R, Brock DW. The rule of double effect—a critique of its role in end-of-life decision making. *N Engl J Med* 1997;3337:1768–1771.
13. Quill TE, Lo B, Brock DW. Palliative options of last resort: a comparison of voluntarily stopping eating and drinking, terminal sedation, physician-assisted suicide, and voluntary active euthanasia. *JAMA* 1997;278:2099–2104.

14. Gillon R. Foreseeing is not necessarily the same thing as intending. *BMJ* 1999;318:1431–1432.
15. Sulmasy DP, Pellegrino ED. The rule of double effect: clearing up the double talk. *Arch Intern Med* 1999;159:545–550.
16. Warnock M. *An intelligent person's guide to ethics.* London: Duckworth, 1998:27–31.
17. Beauchamp TL, Childress JF. *Principles of biomedical ethics*, 4th ed. New York: Oxford University Press, 1994:206–211.
18. Quill TE. Doctor, I want to die. Will you help me? *JAMA* 1993;270:870–873.
19. Wilson WC, Smedira NG, Fink C, et al. Ordering and administration of sedatives and analgesics during the withholding and withdrawal of life support from critically ill patients. *JAMA* 1992;267:949–953.
20. Alpers A, Lo B. The Supreme Court addresses physician-assisted suicide: can its decisions improve palliative care. *Arch Fam Pract* 1999;8:200–205.
21. Billings JA. Slow euthanasia. *J Palliat Care* 1996;12:21–30.
22. Orentlicher D. The Supreme Court and physician-assisted suicide: rejecting physician-assisted suicide but embracing euthanasia. *N Engl J Med* 1997;337:1236–1239.
23. Asch DA. The role of critical care nurses in euthanasia and assisted suicide. *N Engl J Med* 1996;334:1374–1379.
24. Lo B. The death of Clarence Herbert: withdrawing care is not murder. *Ann Intern Med* 1984;101:248–251.

ANNOTATED BIBLIOGRAPHY

1. President's Commission for the Study of Ethical Problems in Medicine and Biomedical and Behavioral Research. *Deciding to forego life-sustaining treatment.* Washington: US Government Printing Office, 1983:60–90.
   Lucid discussion of the distinctions brought up in this chapter, showing how they are confusing and therefore best avoided.
2. Brock D. Forgoing life-sustaining food and water: is it killing? In: Lynn J, ed. *By no extraordinary means* (expanded edition) Bloomington: Indiana University Press, 1989:117–131.
   Thoughtful analysis of the distinctions discussed in this chapter.
3. Quill TE, Dresser R, Brock DW. The rule of double effect—a critique of its role in end-of-life decision making. *N Engl J Med* 1997;3337:1768–1771.
   Analysis of the doctrine of double effect and its application to decisions about life-sustaining interventions.
4. Quill TE, Lo B, Brock DW. Palliative options of last resort: a comparison of voluntarily stopping eating and drinking, terminal sedation, physician-assisted suicide, and voluntary active euthanasia. *JAMA* 1997;278:2099–2104.
   Analysis of different approaches to responding to refractory suffering at the end of life.

15

Patient or Surrogate Insistence on Life-Sustaining Interventions

In early cases that presented dilemmas involving life-sustaining interventions, patients or families wanted to forego such interventions, while the physicians wanted to continue them. Increasingly, however, physicians encounter the opposite situation: patients or their families insist on life-sustaining interventions that physicians believe are inappropriate (1–3). In some cases, physicians believe that the requested interventions are futile or not medically indicated; Chapter 9 discusses such situations. This chapter analyzes cases in which physicians believe that a hospice approach is appropriate, but the patient or family wants life-sustaining interventions continued or initiated.

CLINICAL CONSIDERATIONS

Many health care professionals believe that they should help patients achieve a peaceful, gentle death (4,5). Physicians are exhorted to give greater attention to palliative care near the end of life (6). The following case illustrates the conflicts that may arise when patients and surrogates want life-sustaining interventions that physicians believe are inappropriate (4,5).

CASE 15.1. DESIRE FOR CPR AND MECHANICAL VENTILATION IN END-STAGE LUNG DISEASE. *Mr. H. was a 29-year-old man with end-stage cystic fibrosis who was admitted to the hospital for antibiotics and respiratory therapy. He was emaciated, required home oxygen, and was dyspneic walking around his home. During conversations, he often paused to catch his breath or to cough up thick secretions. Lung transplantation was not an option for him because of a concomitant swallowing problem that resulted in aspiration and lung infections. Mr. H. understood that his shortness of breath would get worse. He appreciated that if he suffered a cardiac arrest, the doctors believed that he would not survive the hospitalization even if cardiopulmonary resuscitation (CPR) were attempted. He further realized that the physicians believed that if he required intubation and mechanical ventilation he could not be weaned off the ventilator. He responded, "My entire life has been a struggle. No one thought I would live this long. I've always beaten the odds. I've always been a fighter. I'll keep fighting until the man upstairs tells me it's time to stop."*

Mr. H. was willing to accept odds that physicians believed are unacceptable. His core values included overcoming situations that others believed were hopeless. Other patients want at least to try life-sustaining interventions that offer some hope of success, albeit a faint hope.

The SUPPORT study provides a rich description of care at the end of life. This study enrolled over 9000 hospitalized patients with an advanced stage of one of nine illnesses (7). For these patients, the hospital mortality was over 25%, and the 6-month mortality was almost 50%. In the latter part of this project, physicians were given computer-generated prognoses for each patient; thus they knew which patients were seriously ill. For many patients who died, their last days included "undesirable states": 38% spent at least 10 days in an intensive care unit, 46% received mechanical ventilation within 3 days of death, and 45% were unconscious during their last 3 days of life (7,8). Relatives reported that 50% of conscious dying patients experienced moderate or severe pain during their last 3 days of life (7). These findings were widely interpreted as evidence of inappropriately aggressive use of technology and failure to relieve suffering near the end of life (4,5,7).

However, like Mr. H., many patients with a poor prognosis want high-technology interventions attempted and agree to limit interventions only after therapeutic trials have failed. Although patients in SUPPORT had a bad prognosis, they were not moribund. Three-fourths of the patients survived the hospitalization, and almost one-half survived for 6 months. It was reasonable for such patients and families to seek a trial of aggressive care and decide to forego interventions only after they had proved unsuccessful.

The SUPPORT study found that patients who overestimate their prognosis desire interventions that have a low likelihood of success. Consider patients with metastatic cancer whose physicians predicted a 6-month survival of 10%. Thirty-six percent of such patients preferred life-extending therapy rather than relief of pain and discomfort as the primary goal of care (9). Among those patients who believed that they had a 90% chance or better of surviving for 6 months, 61% wanted life-extending therapy, compared with only 15% of patients who estimated their chance for surviving 6 months to be less than 90%. Thus patient misunderstanding of prognosis was significantly associated with wanting life-extending therapy that had a low prospect of success. Case 15.1 illustrates that when patients do not understand or accept their prognosis, they are unlikely to agree to the physician's recommendations to forego life-sustaining interventions. Providing more statistical information on prognosis is unlikely to persuade such patients. Later in the chapter, we discuss how to explore the patient's perspective on his illness in ways that may help him to accept a more realistic view of his condition.

ETHICAL CONSIDERATIONS

The ethical guideline of beneficence requires physicians to act in the patient's best interests (*see* Chapter 4). The physician's view of what is best for the patient may differ from what the patient or surrogate believes is best. The patient's values generally should be respected. However, physicians are not required to provide interventions requested by patients or surrogates when there is compelling evidence that the requested intervention would not improve survival and would cause serious medical harms. After physicians understand the patient's or surrogate's point of view, they should try to persuade him or negotiate an acceptable compromise.

In this section, we apply these general ethical considerations to three particularly difficult requests for interventions: requests that "everything" be done, requests for interventions based on religious beliefs, and requests for interventions that cause suffering with little prospect of medical benefit.

CASE 15.2. FAMILY INSISTENCE THAT EVERYTHING BE DONE (10). *Bishop P. is a 60-year-old African-American man with diabetes, quadriplegia, and persistent infections. One year ago, he developed* Staphylococcus aureus *meningitis, epidural abscess, and pneumonia. During his hospitalization, Bishop P. developed quadriplegia, respiratory failure, renal failure, and persistent fevers.*

Ten months later, Bishop P. was rehospitalized with urosepsis from Enterobacter cloacae. *His course was complicated by hypotension, respiratory failure, renal failure, stroke, and seizures. He required mechanical ventilation and dialysis. Despite multiple courses of antibiotics, his blood cultures remained positive for* E. cloacae, *resistant to all antibiotics. A drug reaction caused a total body rash, and his skin sheared away around his bandages and electrocardiographic leads. The physicians predicted that he would not survive the hospitalization and that attempts at CPR would be futile and disfigure his body.*

Bishop P.'s Pentecostalist church emphasizes faith healing. Bishop P. was obtunded and could not state his preferences for care. His family insisted that everything be done because he believed that all life was sacred.

Bishop P.'s family wanted to act in accordance with his lifelong values. Such substituted judgments by surrogates are a legitimate basis for decisions when patients lack decision-making capacity and have not given clear advance directives (*see* Chapter 12).

Requests That "Everything" Be Done

In Case 15.2, the family requested that "everything" be done. The physicians should first clarify what is meant by "everything" (10). Many patients or surrogates do not want literally everything done and acknowledge that in some situations, interventions may be far more likely to cause suffering or harm than benefit. For example, many patients or surrogates agree to DNR orders if their condition were to worsen. It is important for physicians to distinguish among these possible meanings of "everything." Such understanding is a necessary first step in reaching a mutually acceptable plan of care. It is also useful to elicit the values and concerns that animate such requests. Some patients or surrogates may be concerned that if they do not insist on interventions, beneficial treatments will be withheld. Such concerns can be addressed directly.

As in Case 15.2, some religiously based reasons for insisting on interventions present dilemmas. Some patients or surrogates may believe that a miraculous recovery will occur if their faith is strong enough; insisting on treatments may be a way of demonstrating their faith. Finally, some patients or surrogates may want any intervention that prolongs life, even for a very short time. They may have vitalist religious views that life is a good in itself, regardless of its quality, and that human beings must preserve and prolong life until God determines its end (11).

Religious-Based Insistence on Interventions

Deeply held religious beliefs reflect a person's core values and identity. Physicians should give special attention to religiously based reasons for patient or surrogate decisions because they may arise from integral aspects of the person's character. However, physicians need sufficient information about the patient's religious beliefs to make specific clinical decisions. Individuals may hold idiosyncratic beliefs, even if they belong to religions with extensive doctrines regarding medical care. For instance, some Jehovah's Witnesses will accept blood transfusions if a court orders the transfusions. Furthermore, people who share general beliefs, such as the sacredness of life, may differ in their preferences regarding specific medical technologies (12).

Physicians can disrespect patients' and families' religious beliefs in several ways. Some doctors do so by discounting such beliefs. However, physicians also fail to show respect if they accept decisions based on religion, without first trying to understand the patient's beliefs (10). It is possible for physicians to inquire how religion shapes decisions without denigrating the patient's or family's faith. For example, a physician might say to Bishop P.'s daughter, "I know that religion plays an important part in your father's life. I'd like to understand it better. Please help me learn more." Physicians need to understand details about the patient's religious beliefs, such as his attitude toward miracles, prayer, and divine intervention (13).

Request for Interventions That Cause the Patient Suffering

In Case 15.2, the family's requests for CPR troubled caregivers, who believed that attempts at CPR would cause disfiguration, without preventing death. The health care workers believed that they would be actively increasing the patient's suffering. Many caregivers believe that it is unethical for them to provide interventions that cause suffering without proportionate benefit (14). The ethical guideline of nonmaleficence, as well as professional integrity, allows health care workers to refrain from providing an intervention that causes significant suffering and would prolong the patient's life for only a very brief period (10). This rationale justifies overriding the family and withholding interventions in rare cases.

Some surrogates state that the patient believes suffering serves a spiritual purpose. Spiritual aspects of dying are important to patients and have not been well appreciated by physicians. However, caregivers should examine surrogates' claims about the redemptive nature of suffering. Many patients who believe their illness serves a spiritual purpose will accept medications for pain and decline burdensome interventions (10). Furthermore, many patients who believe that suffering caused by terminal illness serves some higher purpose choose to forego medical interventions that cause additional suffering but provide limited benefits. Statements by surrogates regarding the redemptive or spiritual value of suffering, even if stated as the belief of the patient, should be evaluated more carefully than such statements made directly by the patients themselves.

RECOMMENDATIONS

Physicians can respond to requests for life-sustaining interventions in several constructive ways (Table 15-1).

Understand the Patient's or Surrogate's Perspective, Using Open-Ended Questions and Empathic Comments

When patients or surrogates request life-sustaining interventions that the physician considers inadvisable, the doctor should first try to understand their perspective, rather than trying to persuade them to change their minds or discussing specific clinical decisions (6). In Case 15.1, after Mr. H.'s concerns and general goals are clarified, specific decisions, such as whether to write a Do Not Resuscitate order, may be easier to make. In contrast, many doctors begin by discussing specific management decisions and talk about general goals and the option of palliative care only after a decision has been made to limit life-prolonging interventions (15).

TABLE 15-1. *Recommendations for responding to requests for life-sustaining interventions*

Understand the patient's or surrogate's perspective.
Use time constructively.
Be sensitive to ethnic and cultural issues.
Use other resources in discussions with patients or surrogates.
Negotiate with patients or surrogates.

In Case 15.1, the physician can use open-ended questions to elicit and probe Mr. H.'s perspective (6):

- "What concerns you most about your illness?"
- "How is treatment going for you (your family)?"
- "As you think about your illness, what is the best and the worst that might happen?"
- "What has been most difficult about this illness for you?"
- "What are your hopes (your expectations, your fears) for the future?"
- "As you think about the future, what is most important to you (what matters the most to you)?"

Physicians can direct similar open-ended questions to surrogates if the patient lacks decision-making capacity.

Open-ended questions help elicit patient concerns and emotions (16,17). The above questions are open-ended in that they ask for an expansive answer and cannot be answered simply with a yes or no. However, they focus attention on frequently avoided, emotionally significant issues.

Additional communication skills can help physicians elicit the patient's or surrogate's perspective and show that they understand it. The patient's own words can guide the physician's follow-up responses and questions. Using the patient's words in further comments and questions lets him know that he is being carefully listened to and that his perspective is important. Patients who sense they are understood may feel more comfortable revealing additional concerns and emotions.

Empathic comments, which reflect back the speaker's emotions, can help patients or surrogates articulate emotions, explore emotions, and also encourage further discussion of difficult topics (6,18,19). In Case 15.1, when Mr. H. has difficulty completing sentences, the physician might ask, "Is it frightening when you can't get enough air?" Similarly, in Case 15.2, the physician might say, "Does it make you feel sad to see your father so sick and not be able to talk to him?" Some physicians may fear that exploring emotions may arouse in the patient and family feelings of hopelessness and despair that doctors are powerless to alleviate. However, patients and families will have these emotional responses whether or not physicians choose to probe them. At a minimum, once these emotions are discussed openly, the patient and family no longer must face them alone. Frequently, talking about emotional reactions to serious illness is therapeutic and helps patients and families accept a grave prognosis. Furthermore, fear, anxiety, and depression may be amenable to simple interventions once they are identified.

Use Time Constructively

Frequently patients or surrogates are given bad news in the context of being asked to limit life-sustaining interventions. If possible, they should be given time to absorb the new information before making a decision. Often a time-limited trial of interventions is useful (20). However, the passage of time alone may not persuade patients or surrogates to limit interventions. Physicians should use the time to direct attention to making the patient's death meaningful. Doctors might say, "Your father is so seriously ill that we would not be surprised if he died in the hospital. What would be left undone if he were to die suddenly?" Social workers or chaplains can also help the family reach closure.

Be Sensitive to Ethnic and Cultural Issues

Bishop P. and his family were African-Americans. Ethnic factors can be significant in end-of-life care. For example, African-Americans and Hispanic-Americans complete advance directives or wish to forego life support less frequently than other patients (21–23). African-Americans may mistrust physicians and hospitals because of a history of discrimination and limited access to medical care.

Once ethnic or cultural issues have been identified, physicians should address them. Rather than leave concerns and suspicions unspoken, physicians might ask, "Many African-Americans worry that they will not receive the care they need. How do you feel about that?" Physicians should not immediately try to reassure the family that all appropriate care will be provided (24). Premature reassurance may deter patients from disclosing their concerns and emotions in enough detail that they can be understood (17). Instead, doctors may first need to listen and express empathy. "Is it distressing to think that you may not get the care you need?" Addressing issues of mistrust directly may demonstrate to family members that the doctor understands their concerns.

Use Other Resources in Discussions with Patients or Surrogates

Physicians can draw on the hospital ethics committee, chaplains, or social workers in discussing patient or surrogate insistence on interventions that they consider inappropriate. Often third parties can help the physician, patient, and family understand each other's viewpoints or can suggest alternative approaches that all will find acceptable.

Negotiate with Patients or Surrogates

When patients insist on life-sustaining interventions, a common compromise involves not adding or increasing interventions but also not withdrawing them (25). Although law and ethics do not distinguish between withholding life support and withdrawing it, the emotional difference may be significant to families. Willingness to continue interventions also may allay suspicions about physicians' motives for recommending limits to care. The rapid spread of managed care has raised public concern that physicians may be more concerned with saving money than with benefiting the patient (26).

In most cases, physicians can reach an agreement with patients or surrogates on an acceptable plan of care (27,28). In rare instances, physicians may conclude after repeated discussions that they simply cannot agree with the patient's or surrogate's request. If the request is for interventions that are futile in a strict sense or that cause significant suffering to the patient, it is ethically acceptable for the physician to decline to provide them. The patient or surrogate should be notified of this decision and of their right to seek another provider. The physician should also facilitate transfer of the patient to another doctor or hospital. If physicians decide to forego requested interventions, they should be realistic about the possibility of adverse publicity or even a future lawsuit from disgruntled relatives.

REFERENCES

1. Paris JJ, Crone RK, Reardon F. Physicians' refusal of requested treatment: the case of Baby L. *N Engl J Med* 1990;322:1012–1014.
2. Miles SH. Informed demand for "non-beneficial" medical treatment. *N Engl J Med* 1991;325:511–515.
3. Annas GJ. Asking the courts to set the standard of emergency care—the case of Baby K. *N Engl J Med* 1994;330:1542–1545.
4. Lo B. End-of-life care after termination of SUPPORT. *Hastings Center Rep* 1995;25:S6–S8.
5. Lo B. Improving care near the end of life: why is it so hard? *JAMA* 1995;274:1634–1636.
6. Lo B, Snyder L, Sox H. Care at the end of life: guiding practice where there are no easy answers. *Ann Intern Med* 1999;130:772–774.
7. The SUPPORT Investigators. A controlled trial to improve care for seriously ill hospitalized patients. *JAMA* 1995;274:1591–1598.

8. Lynn J, Teno JM, Phillips RS, et al. Perceptions by family members of the dying experience of older and seriously ill patients. *Ann Intern Med* 1997;126:97–106.
9. Weeks JC, Cook EF, O'Day SJ, et al. Relationship between cancer patients' predictions of prognosis and their treatment preferences. *JAMA* 1998;279:1709–1714.
10. Alpers A, Lo B. Avoiding family feuds: responding to surrogates' demands for life-sustaining treatment. *J Law Med Ethics* 1999;27:74–80.
11. Boozang KM. An intimate passing: restoring the role of family and religion in dying. *University of Pittsburgh Law Rev* 1997;58:549–617.
12. Dworkin R. *Life's dominion*. New York: Alfred A. Knopf, 1993:328.
13. Orr RD, Genesen LB. Requests for "inappropriate" treatment based on religious beliefs. *J Med Ethics* 1997;23:142–147.
14. Braithwaite S, Thomasma DC. New guidelines on foregoing life-sustaining treatment in incompetent patients: an anti-cruelty policy. *Ann Intern Med* 1986;104:711–715.
15. Tulsky JA, Chesney MA, Lo B. How do medical residents discuss resuscitation with patients? *J Gen Intern Med* 1995;10:436–442.
16. Lipkin M, Frankel RM, Beckman HB, et al. Performing the interview. In: Lipkin M, Putnam SM, Lazare A, eds. *The medical interview*. New York: Springer-Verlag, 1995:65–82.
17. Maguire P, Faulkner A, Booth K, et al. Helping cancer patients disclose their concerns. *Eur J Cancer* 1996;32A:78–81.
18. Buckman R. *How to break bad news*. Baltimore: Johns Hopkins University Press, 1992:98–171.
19. Suchman AL, Markakis K, Beckman HB, Frankel R. A model of empathic communication in the medical interview. *JAMA* 1997;277:678–682.
20. Ruark J, Raffin TA, Stanford University Medical Center Committee on Ethics. Initiating and withdrawing life support. *N Engl J Med* 1988;318:25–30.
21. Rubin SM, Strull WM, Fialkow MF, et al. Increasing completion of the durable power of attorney for health care: a randomized controlled trial. *JAMA* 1994;271:209–212.
22. Blackhall LJ, Murphy ST, Frank G, et al. Ethnicity and attitudes toward patient autonomy. *JAMA* 1995;274:820–825.
23. McKinley ED, Garrett JM, Evans AT, et al. Differences in end-of-life decision making among black and white ambulatory care cancer patients. *J Gen Intern Med* 1996;11:651–656.
24. Lo B, Quill T, Tulsky J. Discussing palliative care with patients. *Ann Intern Med* 1999;130:744–749.
25. Christakis NA, Asch DA. Biases in how physicians choose to withdraw life support. *Lancet* 1993;342:642–646.
26. Sulmasy DP. Managed care and managed death. *Arch Intern Med* 1995;155:133–136.
27. Smedira NG, Evans BH, Grais LS, et al. Withholding and withdrawing of life support from the critically ill. *N Engl J Med* 1990;322:309–315.
28. Prendergast TJ, Luce JM. Increasing incidence of withholding and withdrawal of life support from the critically ill. *Am Rev Respir Dis Crit Care Med* 1997;155:15–20.

ANNOTATED BIBLIOGRAPHY

1. Alpers A, Lo B. Avoiding family feuds: responding to surrogates' demands for life-sustaining treatment. *J Law Med Ethics* 1999;27:74–80.
   Analyzes cases in which surrogates insisted on interventions that physicians believed were not indicated.
2. Lo B, Quill T, Tulsky J. Discussing palliative care with patients. *Ann Intern Med* 1999;130:744–749.
   In response to patient and family requests for interventions that are unlikely to be successful, the physician can use empathic comments and open-ended questions to understand their perceptions of illness, concerns, and emotions.
3. Orr RD, Genesen LB. Requests for "inappropriate" treatment based on religious beliefs. *J Med Ethics* 1997;23:142–147.
   Analyzes religious-based requests for interventions.

16

Physician Insistence on Life-Sustaining Interventions

Physicians and hospitals may insist on providing life-prolonging interventions to an unwilling patient, claiming that their conscience or religious beliefs would be violated if they allowed the patient to die. Such insistence by caregivers clashes with the patient's refusal of treatment.

CASE 16.1. WITHDRAWAL OF MECHANICAL VENTILATION. *William Bartling was a 70-year-old man with chronic obstructive lung disease, coronary artery disease, and depression (1,2). He was admitted to a hospital for depression and chronic back pain. His admission chest radiograph showed a new pulmonary nodule. A needle aspirate revealed adenocarcinoma. After the procedure, he suffered a pneumothorax and required a chest tube and mechanical ventilation. During the next 2 months, he could not be weaned from the respirator. Mr. Bartling requested that the respirator be disconnected and signed a living will, a durable power of attorney for health care, and a declaration of his wishes. His family also signed documents releasing the physicians and hospital from liability.*

The hospital and physicians refused Mr. Bartling's request, arguing that they had an ethical duty to preserve life and that withholding life-sustaining treatment was incompatible with their Christian and pro-life beliefs. Attempts to transfer the patient to another hospital that would comply with his wishes were unsuccessful. Mr. Bartling sued to have the ventilator discontined.

The Bartling case posed the question of whether the caregivers may insist on providing life-sustaining interventions over a patient's refusal. Such insistence may be common. In one survey, 60% of attending physicians said they would not withdraw a ventilator from a patient with severe chronic obstructive lung disease who wished it discontinued (3). This chapter will analyze the ethical arguments for and against such caregiver insistence on carrying out interventions. In addition, the chapter discusses the appropriateness of transferring patients to caregivers who will respect their refusal of interventions.

ARGUMENTS FOR INSISTENCE BY CAREGIVERS ON INTERVENTIONS

Health care professionals and institutions offer several reasons why their moral or religious beliefs should allow them to impose life-sustaining interventions on unwilling patients. This chapter excludes cases in which caregivers seek to provide life-sustaining interventions, not because of their own moral views, but because they believe that the patient's refusal is not informed or because the surrogate is contradicting the patient's wishes.

Respect the Autonomy of Caregivers

Health care professionals are moral agents with values, rights, and consciences. Just as patient autonomy must be respected, many physicians and nurses claim that their autonomy should also be respected. They do not regard themselves simply as agents of the patient, mere technicians who carry out the patient's plans and goals. In this view, just as patients have the right to refuse interventions, physicians should also have the right to refuse to violate their professional ethics or personal morality.

According to this reasoning, it is wrong to force health care workers to contradict their moral values or violate their conscience. Because the United States respects freedom of religion, it would be particularly repugnant to require health care workers to carry out actions that violate their religious beliefs. Practically speaking, it would be counterproductive to require physicians to act against their moral views. A grudging or antagonistic doctor–patient relationship would not be therapeutic. It would make more sense for the patient to receive care from a physician and hospital who are willing to withhold care as requested.

In this view, physicians present themselves to patients and to colleagues as following certain standards of scientific practice, professional ethics, and personal integrity. When physicians violate these standards, they lose the respect of colleagues, the trust of the public, and their own sense of integrity.

Respect the Mission of Health Care Institutions

Health care institutions may have a statement of mission that expresses their goals and values. Hospices have an explicit philosophy of palliative care. Catholic hospitals have policies that forbid abortions. Many people believe that a pluralistic society should encourage such statements of mission so that patients can seek care at institutions whose moral and spiritual views match their own (4,5).

OBJECTIONS TO INSISTENCE BY CAREGIVERS ON INTERVENTIONS

Insistence by caregivers on providing interventions over the objections of patients is ethically problematical in several ways (Table 16-1).

Undermining the Right of Refusal

If caregivers could insist on treatment, the right of competent patients to refuse medical interventions would in effect be nullified. The court in Case 16.1 ruled that the patient's refusal of treatment must be respected. "If the right of the patient to self-determination as to his own medical treatment is to have any meaning at all, it must be paramount to the interests of the patient's hospital and doctors" (2).

TABLE 16-1. *Objections to caregivers' insistence on life-sustaining interventions*

Undermining the right of refusal
Confusion between negative and positive rights
Lack of timely and clear notification of patients
Payment for unwanted services

Confusion Between Negative and Positive Rights

Philosophers make a distinction between negative and positive rights. *Negative rights* are claims to be left alone, to be free from unwanted interference or intrusions. An example is the constitutional right to be free of unreasonable searches and seizures. Negative rights may require other people to refrain from intervening, exerting control, or thwarting the person holding the rights. In refusing treatment, a patient claims the negative right to be free of unwanted medical interventions. To be exercised, this negative right requires physicians to refrain from providing the treatment. People may also claim negative rights not to be forced to act in violation of their religion and conscience. An example is refusal by physicians or nurses to perform abortions, because abortion violates their moral or religious beliefs.

Positive or affirmative rights, on the other hand, are claims to receive something or act in a certain way. Positive rights may require others to take action or provide means or resources, not simply to refrain from interfering (6). In Case 16.1, the physicians claimed the positive right to continue medical interventions, even though Mr. Bartling did not want it. This putative positive right would override the patient's negative right to refuse the intervention and thereby infringe on the patient's liberty.

Negative rights are generally considered to carry more moral weight than positive rights (7). Virtually all Western philosophers agree that people have a strong right to be free of unwanted intrusions. This right to be left alone is regarded as fundamental to the idea of an ordered society. Usually negative liberty is limited only by promises or role-specific obligations; for example, parents cannot claim a negative right to be freed from providing their children's basic needs. In contrast, positive rights are more difficult to justify and enforce, because they generally require other people to do something and interfere with the negative rights of others.

Although a distinction between negative and positive rights seems intuitively clear, they may be hard to distinguish in practice.

CASE 16.2. WITHDRAWAL OF FEEDING TUBES. *Elizabeth Bouvia, a 26-year-old quadriplegic woman with severe cerebral palsy, asked a hospital to provide pain relief and hygiene while she starved herself to death. She asserted that she was physically unable to take her own life (8,9). Many health care workers believed that Ms. Bouvia was not merely requesting to be allowed to die but also asking them to assist in her suicide. In the view of these health care workers, although Ms. Bouvia had the right to leave the hospital and starve herself to death, she had no right to compel them to be accomplices in her death. One physician declared, "The court cannot order me to be a murderer nor to conspire with my staff and employees to murder Elizabeth." In 1983, a California court rejected her request to be allowed to starve to death while hospitalized. The ruling declared that she did not have "the right to end her life with the assistance of society"(8). The court ordered the insertion of a nasogastric feeding tube, and refused to bar the hospital from discharging her.*

By 1986, Ms. Bouvia's condition worsened, and she required morphine for pain caused by contractures. An appellate court ordered physicians to remove a nasogastric tube that they had inserted over her objections, ruling that her refusal of tube feedings was not suicide (9).

The Bouvia case illustrates how the distinction between positive and negative rights may be confusing and unhelpful. The first court implicitly characterized her request as a positive right to assisted suicide. In contrast, the second court ruling implicitly framed her request as a negative right to refuse unwanted treatment, declaring that this right was virtually absolute and that the patient's motives were not a matter for review by others (9). The latter court stated, "We find nothing in the law to suggest that the right to refuse medical treatment may be exercised only if the patient's motives meet someone else's approval" (9).

Lack of Timely and Clear Notification of Patients

As in the Bartling case, physicians or institutions often do not notify patients of their insistence on certain interventions until patients indicate that they would refuse it. At that stage, however, it may be difficult to transfer care to a different physician. In the Bartling case, no other physician or hospital was willing to accept the patient in transfer. Even if transfer were possible, disruption of continuity of care might be deleterious to the patient. For these reasons, physicians who insist on providing interventions because of their religious or moral beliefs should so inform patients at the beginning of the doctor–patient relationship. Such notification would enable patients to make informed plans for their care and to seek another provider. Similarly, institutions who have policies insisting on certain interventions should notify patients on admission. The burden should be on the physician or institution to notify patients. After all, caregivers are in a much better position than patients to anticipate future scenarios and potential disagreements.

Payment for Unwanted Services

Families may refuse to pay for continued life-sustaining treatment administered against the patient's wishes. In the Elbaum case, the husband of a 63-year-old woman in a persistent vegetative state refused to pay a nursing home that insisted on providing tube feedings. He had repeatedly informed the institution that his wife had stated that she would not want her life prolonged in such a condition. The patient had "repeatedly extracted a series of promises" from her family that they would not to sustain her life if she became "a vegetable" (10). An appeals court permitted the nursing home to collect payment, because it could not have known before the case was adjudicated that the patient's previous statements were sufficient to justify withholding tube feedings (11).

The reasoning of the Elbaum court, however, seems unpersuasive. Although the physicians and nursing home subjectively believed that they were not legally obligated to remove the patient's feeding tube, the court did not analyze whether that belief was reasonable, that is, would a reasonable physician or nursing home administrator believe that the courts would regard the patient's statements as clear and convincing evidence that she would not want tube feedings in that situation? By omitting this inquiry, the court is inviting defensive medicine. Any institution could claim that they did not really know that the patient's refusal was valid and then collect payment for their services.

TRANSFERRING THE PATIENT

In the highly publicized Bartling case, transfer to another hospital was not possible. When transfer to another physician or institution who will respect the patient's refusal is feasible, the courts have taken several positions.

Transfer Is Permitted

In the Brophy case (*see* Chapter 23), the Massachusetts Supreme Court ruled that although the patient had a right to refuse tube feedings, the hospital and physicians had a right to decline to participate in such a plan. The patient's family had the burden of finding another physician willing to accept the patient. The Brophy family was able to do so.

Refusal Must Be Honored if Transfer Is Not Possible

In the Bartling case, when transfer was impossible, the court ruled that the patient's right of refusal was "paramount" to the physician's insistence on providing treatment (2).

Refusal Must Be Honored if Transfer Is Too Burdensome

Even when transfer of care can be arranged, it may place a serious burden on patients or their families. Patients may face an awful choice if they must either accept unwanted interventions or else leave caregivers with whom they have developed a long-term relationship. In the Requena case, a 57-year-old woman with amyotrophic lateral sclerosis wanted tube feedings withheld if she could no longer swallow. The hospital asserted that her decision conflicted with its pro-life values and asked her to accept transfer to another local hospital that would respect her decision. When she refused to accept the transfer, the hospital went to court to force her to leave. According to the court, because she had lived in the hospital for 17 months, transfer would be upsetting and burdensome for her. The trial court judge suggested that "by rethinking their own attitudes" the hospital staff "might find it possible to be more fully accepting and supportive of Ms. Requena's decision." The court continued, "It is fairer to ask the health care workers to bend than to ask Ms. Requena to bend" (12).

In summary, the claims of health care professionals to insist on interventions may negate the rights of competent, informed patients to refuse them. Caregivers should not expect to impose treatment on patients if they did not notify them of their insistence when care was initiated.

REFERENCES

1. Lo B. The Bartling case: protecting patients from harm while respecting their wishes. *J Am Geriatr Soc* 1986;34:44–48.
2. Bartling *v.* Superior Court. 209 Cal Rptr. 220 163 Cal. App. 3d 186 (1984).
3. Caralis PV, Hammond JS. Attitudes of medical students, housestaff, and faculty physicians toward euthanasia and termination of life-sustaining treatment. *Crit Care Med* 1992; 20:683–690.
4. Miles SH, Singer M. Conflicts between patients' wishes to forgo treatment and the policies of health care facilities. *N Engl J Med* 1989;321:48–50.
5. Engelhardt HT. *The foundations of bioethics.* New York: Oxford University Press, 1986.
6. Collopy BJ. Autonomy in long term care: some crucial distinctions. *Gerontologist* 1988;28 [Suppl]:10–17.
7. Beauchamp TL, Childress JF. *Principles of biomedical ethics,* 3rd ed. New York: Oxford University Press, 1989.
8. Steinbrook R, Lo B. The case of Elizabeth Bouvia: starvation, suicide, or problem patient? *Arch Intern Med* 1986;146:161–164.
9. Bouvia *v.* Superior Court. 225 Cal Rptr. 297, 179 Cal. App. 3d 1127 (1986).
10. Elbaum *v.* Grace Plaza of Great Neck I, 148 AD2d 244.
11. Grace Plaza of Great Neck I, v. Elbaum, 1992 N.Y. App. Div. LEXIS 10728.
12. In re Requena, 517 A. 2d 869 (N.J. 1986).

ANNOTATED BIBLIOGRAPHY

1. Miles SH, Singer PA, Siegler M. Conflicts between patients' wishes to forgo treatment and the policies of health care facilities. *N Engl J Med* 1989;321:48–50.
Emphasizes the importance of respecting the mission of health care institutions and the moral beliefs of physicians. Ideally, patients would seek care from physicians and institutions that share their values.

17

Ethics Committees
and Case Consultations

Ethical dilemmas in clinical practice often involve life-or-death decisions and may arouse wrenching emotions. Just as physicians and patients turn to medical subspecialists for consultation in difficult cases, they may also discuss perplexing ethical issues with the hospital ethics committee or an ethics consultant. Such case consultations are more timely, less adversarial, and more flexible than court proceedings as a way to resolve disputes. The Joint Commission on Accreditation of Healthcare Organizations requires institutions to have a mechanism to address ethical issues arising in the care of patients, such as an ethics committee or consultation service (1). Consultations by individuals with special training in clinical ethics have been suggested as an alternative to ethics committees.

This chapter reviews the goals of ethics committees and consultants, problems with their work, and procedures for effective case consultation. Important unresolved questions regarding ethics case consultations are also discussed.

GOALS OF ETHICS CASE CONSULTATIONS

The goal of case consultations by ethics committees or consultants is to help resolve disagreements over ethical issues. As the following case illustrates, this can occur in several ways (Table 17-1).

CASE 17.1. DECISIONS ABOUT LIFE-SUSTAINING INTERVENTIONS. *An elderly woman with severe dementia develops pneumonia and ventilatory failure. Her daughter insists that mechanical ventilation would be pointless and that her mother would not want such "heroics." However, the patient's son demands aggressive treatment, saying that they can't just let her die and have no right to call her quality of life unacceptable. The resident and outpatient doctor agree with the daughter that mechanical ventilation should be withheld. The hospital attending physician agrees with the son. The nurses feel caught between these conflicting views. The health care team asks the hospital ethics committee for a consultation.*

Clarify and Analyze the Ethical Issues

In Case 17.1, an ethics consultation can help the health care team identify and understand the ethical issues the case raises, such as the interpretation of advance directives (*see* Chapter 12), the process of surrogate decision-making (*see* Chapter 13), and the distinction between ordinary and heroic interventions (*see* Chapter 14). The ethics committee or ethics consultant can

TABLE 17-1. *Goals of ethics case consultations*

Clarify and analyze the ethical issues.
Improve communication.
Provide emotional support.
Offer specific recommendations.

identify ethical consensus where it exists. Often health care workers need to think through the ethical issues before they try to resolve disagreements with the patient or family.

Improve Communication

In Case 17.1, poor communication among members of the health care team and between the team and the family hinders decisions. To improve communication, many ethics committees will hold a meeting with the health care team and the family.

Provide Emotional Support

The attending physician, house officers, and nurses in Case 17.1 felt frustrated that they could not resolve the conflict. Unless such feelings are explicitly expressed and acknowledged, discussion of substantive issues is unlikely to be fruitful.

Offer Specific Recommendations

Some committees or consultants help the health care team analyze the ethical issues and facilitate discussions with patients or families, but stop short of giving recommendations (2). Most committees or consultants, however, offer specific recommendations for resolving ethical dilemmas. For instance, in Case 17.1, the ethics committee can recommend that clear and convincing advance directives should be respected and that more information about the patient's previous statements should be gathered. In what context did she make such statements? Did she indicate what she meant by "heroic?" Even if patient care decisions do not change after an ethics consultation, health care workers, patients, or surrogates may feel that their concerns have been addressed and better accept the rationale for the decision.

PROBLEMS WITH ETHICS CASE CONSULTATIONS

Although consultations by ethics committees or consultants may help resolve disputes, they may also be problematic (Table 17-2) (3).

CASE 17.2. LIMITED ACCESS TO THE ETHICS CONSULTANTS. *A 76-year-old widower with moderate Alzheimer's disease is cared for by his daughters and their families. For the third time*

TABLE 17-2. *Potential problems with ethics consultations*

Consultations may not be timely.
Recommendations may be unsound.
Problems may be outside the scope of the ethics consultation.
Procedures may be unfair.

in 2 months, he is hospitalized for aspiration pneumonia. His family asks that antibiotics not be administered and that he be allowed to die peacefully. The attending physician insists on treating him. "They can't let him die just because they're overwhelmed. If they didn't want him treated, why did they bring him to the hospital? It would be one thing if we were talking about intensive care, but antibiotics are basic, ordinary care." At the request of the attending physician, two members of the ethics committee review the medical record. They agree that antibiotics are basic care and should be administered. Family members are outraged. "Who are these people? They never even spoke to us." The charge nurse also objects, "How did they become experts in ethics? They want us to torture him."

In Case 17.2, family members are upset because the ethics committee has made a recommendation without talking with them. Moreover, the committee has not provided the reasoning behind its recommendation.

Consultations May Not Be Timely

In clinical medicine, ethical dilemmas often need to be resolved within hours or days. Unless ethics case consultations can be conducted promptly, they will not improve patient care decisions.

Recommendations May Be Unsound

Agreement among ethics committee members or consultants does not guarantee that their recommendations are sound. In Case 17.2, the ethics committee members adopt a view of "ordinary" care that is highly problematical (*see* Chapter 14). Furthermore, they do not consider when family members may appropriately refuse life-prolonging interventions (*see* Chapter 13). Such unsound thinking may result from lack of knowledge, unrecognized bias, or flawed committee procedures.

Problems May Be Outside the Scope of the Consultation

In some cases, the problems concern legal liability, staff conflicts, or discharge planning rather than strictly ethical issues. Nurses or house officers might want the ethics committee or consultant to resolve long-standing grievances. Consultants, however, have no power to reform individuals and institutions. It is unwise for ethics committees and consultants to take on the duties of risk managers, hospital administrators, psychiatrists, or social workers.

Procedures May Be Unfair

In Case 17.2, the family and a nurse complained that the ethics committee talked to only one side in the dispute. This lack of even-handedness is not uncommon. Some committees explicitly view themselves as providing support to the health care team, whereas others view their role as patient advocates (3). Critics charge that many ethics committees pay little attention to process and that some use procedures that undermine patient autonomy (4).

PROCEDURES FOR ETHICS CASE CONSULTATIONS

For ethics case consultations to be generally accepted, they must be regarded as accessible and fair (3).

Who Can Request Ethics Case Consultations?

Attending physicians, who are responsible for patient management, clearly should have the power to ask for ethics consultations. Beyond that, there may be controversy over whether patients, their surrogates, nurses, or house officers may request case consultations, without the agreement of the attending physician. It seems unfair if one side in a dispute may ask for an ethics consultation but the other may not. Disagreements over the need for a consultation generally indicate serious conflicts over patient care or ethical issues. Restricting access to ethics consultations is likely to exacerbate such disputes. If someone other than the attending physician requests an ethics consultation, it is prudent for the committee or the consultant to notify the attending physician.

Who Participates in Case Consultations?

Some attending physicians feel that they will lose power and control if their decisions are discussed in front of other members of the health care team. Thus some ethics committees do not permit nurses, house officers, or other health care workers who provide care to the patient to attend meetings, and some ethics consultants may not talk directly to these caregivers. On the other hand, nurses caring for the patient have close contact with the patient and family and carry out physicians' orders. In addition, nurses may view themselves as patient advocates. Their point of view may be omitted or misunderstood if they cannot talk directly with the ethics committee or consultant. As in Case 17.2, nurses may also reject the committee's recommendations if they are not allowed to express their disagreement with the attending physician. For these reasons, ethics committees and consultants should invite all health care workers directly caring for the patient to discuss the case.

Ethics committees and ethics consultants often do not talk directly to patients or their surrogates (3). Restricting discussions may help overcome resistance to the ethics committee within the medical staff and may facilitate frank discussions among health care providers. Some ethics committees consider that their primary role is to help the health care team clarify their thinking before they talk with patients or surrogates.

There are compelling reasons, however, for patients or surrogates to attend ethics committee meetings or talk with ethics consultants. As in Case 17.2, surrogates or patients may be outraged that decisions about them are being discussed behind closed doors by people they have never met (3). In addition, ethics committees or consultants are more likely to appreciate the patient's values and concerns if they hear from the patient or surrogate directly (4). For these reasons, patients or surrogates should be informed that the case will be discussed and be invited to participate in at least part of the discussions.

Does the Ethics Committee or Consultant Gather Primary Data?

Ethics committees or consultants may make mistakes if they uncritically accept second-hand data about the medical situation or the patient's preferences (3,5). First, only one view of a complicated case may be presented. Second, important information may be omitted. In Case 17.1, the committee or consultant needs to ascertain what the patient said about her preferences for future care. Third, conclusions and inferences, rather than primary data, may be presented to the committee or consultant. For instance, physicians or nurses may describe patients as "terminal" or "incompetent" without supporting evidence.

Like consultations by medical specialists, an ethics committee or consultant would optimally review medical records and talk with the patient or surrogate. Such primary data gathering, however, may be impractical given time constraints. At a minimum, however, an ethics committee or consultant should review whether the data and reasoning offered by the physician support the conclusions. In many cases, the ethics committee might decide that crucial information is lacking and recommend that the team gather it.

Does the Ethics Committee or Consultant Make a Recommendation?

Most ethics committees or consultants make specific recommendations regarding the case (6). If recommendations are based on second-hand information, this should be noted. In Case 17.1, the recommendation might be to follow the patient's oral directives, provided they are trustworthy and the daughter is acting in good faith.

Recommendations should be written in the medical record, together with their rationale. Unwritten recommendations invite misunderstandings and reduce accountability. Recommendations are more likely to be followed if they are brief and specific. Direct conversations with the team also increase acceptance of the recommendations.

As with any consultation, the attending physician retains the power to follow the recommendations or not. Although attending physicians are not obligated to follow the recommendations, ethically and legally they need to act as a reasonable physician would after receiving the recommendations.

ETHICS COMMITTEES AND ETHICS CONSULTANTS

Both ethics committees and ethics consultants have both advantages and disadvantages.

Ethics Committees

Interdisciplinary ethics committees are the most common providers of ethics case consultations. In addition to doing case consultations, ethics committees usually carry out educational activities and develop institutional policies on such ethical issues as do not resuscitate orders and withdrawal of life-sustaining interventions (6).

Composition of Ethics Committees

Interdisciplinary ethics committees typically include physicians, nurses, house officers, social workers, and clergy. Lay members can point out overlooked issues and arguments and help health care workers better understand the patient's perspective.

Personal qualities of the committee members are as important as their professional backgrounds. Committee members should be respected by colleagues for their clinical judgment and interpersonal skills. They should be willing to learn about clinical ethics, receptive to different ideas and points of view, capable of dealing with emotionally charged topics and interpersonal disagreements, and able to tolerate ambiguity.

Advantages of Ethics Committees for Case Consultations

Interdisciplinary Membership

Diverse perspectives can lead to more thorough and thoughtful discussions (7), particularly in complex, difficult cases (8). In addition, nurses and social workers often feel more comfortable raising their concerns to a committee that includes their peers than to a committee composed solely of physicians.

Demystification of Ethics

An interdisciplinary ethics committee sends an important symbolic message to the hospital (7): ethical issues are the business of everyone who cares for patients, and clinicians can learn to resolve ethical dilemmas. In addition, ethics committees can give a voice to the practical wisdom of experienced clinicians.

Disadvantages of Ethics Committees for Case Consultations

Delays

It may be difficult to mobilize an ethics committee for urgent consultations. Having a subcommittee rotate responsibility for consultations may make the committee more responsive.

Diffusion of Responsibility

Decision-making power may be so diffused through a committee that no one takes responsibility for a decision (9).

Groupthink May Impair Decision-Making

Group dynamics may pressure ethics committee members to reach consensus, avoid controversial issues, and downplay objections (3). The group may discourage members from considering fresh alternatives and seeking additional information. Such undesirable dynamics, which have been termed "groupthink" (10), may lead to grave errors in judgment.

Ethics committees are especially vulnerable to groupthink. A timely recommendation may be needed despite uncertain information and conflicting values and interests. The committee may feel pressured by attending physicians who feel their power is being usurped, nurses who believe they are being given unreasonable orders, and risk managers who wish to avoid legal liability.

Ethics Consultants as an Alternative to Ethics Committees

Instead of an ethics committee, one or two individuals with special training in clinical ethics might conduct case consultations (2,11). Such ethics consultations would be similar to consultations by medical subspecialists.

Advantages of Ethics Consultants

Greater Expertise

Ethics consultants with special training might be more skilled at case consultation than committee members who have variable training in ethics and dispute resolution.

More Timely and Detailed Consultations

Ethics consultants might provide more timely consultation than committee members. They also might have more time to obtain primary data and provide follow-up.

Disadvantages of Ethics Consultants

Undue Deference to Ethics Experts

It may be difficult for others to challenge the recommendations of ethics "experts." As a result, discussion may be stifled, and divergent viewpoints may not be considered.

Potential for Individual Bias

Practice standards and quality control are far less developed in clinical ethics than in medical subspecialties (12,13). Furthermore, ethics "experts" may disagree over recommendations in a specific case (14). An individual ethics consultant may provide idiosyncratic recommendations that would be rejected by most other recognized ethics consultants. It would be misleading to represent a private belief or opinion as the consensus of the field.

Currently no single approach to ethics consultations would be appropriate for all hospitals and situations (7,8). In some institutions, there may be several individuals who are highly skilled at ethics consultations and are willing to carry them out. In other institutions, no one person with special training or experience is available; in this situation a committee would be more sensible.

In summary, ethics committees and ethics consultants may help resolve ethical dilemmas. Because the field of medical ethics is still developing, no single format for providing case consultations is appropriate for all institutions. Each institution should carefully define its goals, needs, and resources in order to determine the best format and procedures. Persons who conduct ethics case consultations need to be aware of the potential pitfalls and the steps that can be taken to avoid them.

REFERENCES

1. McCarrick PM. Ethics committees in hospitals. *Kennedy Instit Ethics J* 1992;3:285–306.
2. Purtilo RB. Ethics consulations in the hospital. *N Engl J Med* 1984;311:983–986.
3. Lo B. Behind closed doors: promises and pitfalls of ethics committees. *N Engl J Med* 1987;317:46–50.
4. Wolf SM. Toward a theory of process. *Law Med Health Care* 1992;20:278–290.
5. Purtilo RB. A comment on the concept of consultation. In: Fletcher JC, Quist N, Jonsen AR, eds. *Ethics consultation in health care*. Ann Arbor: Health Administration Press, 1989:99–108.
6. Hoffman DE. Does legislating hospital ethics committees make a difference? A study of hospital ethics committees in Maryland, the District of Columbia, and Virginia. *Law Med Health Care* 1991;19:105–119.
7. Swenson MD, Miller RB. Ethics case review in health care institutions. *Arch Intern Med* 1991;152:694–697.
8. Cohen CB. Avoiding "Cloudcuckooland" in ethics committee case review: matching models to issues and concerns. *Law Med Health Care* 1992;20:294–299.
9. Siegler M. Ethics committees: decisions by bureaucracy. *Hastings Center Rep 1986;16:22–24.*
10. Janis IL, Mann L. *Decision-making: a psychological analysis of conflict, choice, and commitment*. New York: Free Press, 1977.
11. LaPuma J, Schiedermayer DL. Ethics consultation: skills, roles, and training. *Ann Intern Med* 1991;114:155–160.
12. Drane JF. Hiring a hospital ethicist. In: Fletcher JC, Quist N, Jonsen AR, eds. *Ethics consultation in health care*. Ann Arbor: Health Administration Press, 1989:117–134.
13. Fletcher JC, Hoffmann DE. Ethics committees: time to experiment with standards. *Ann Intern Med* 1994;120:335–338.
14. Fox E, Stocking C. Ethics consultants' recommendations for life-prolonging treatment in a persistent vegetative state. *JAMA* 1993;270:2578–2582.

ANNOTATED BIBLIOGRAPHY

1. Lo B. Behind closed doors: promises and pitfalls of ethics committees. *N Engl J Med* 1987;317:46–49.
   Discusses potential problems with ethics committees, including exclusion of patients and nurses, reliance on second-hand data, and groupthink.
2. LaPuma J, Schiedermayer DL. Ethics consultation: skills, roles, and training. *Ann Intern Med* 1991;114:155–160.
   Describes training and skills needed by ethics consultants.
3. Aulisio MP, Arnold RM, Youngner SJ. Health care ethics consultation: nature, goals and competencies. *Ann Intern Med 2000;* In press.
   Report of interdisciplinary task force to set standards for ethics consultations by ethics committees and individual consultants.
4. Cohen CB. Avoiding "Cloudcuckooland" in ethics committee case review: matching models to issues and concerns. *Law Med Health Care* 1992;20:294–299.
   Proposes how case review by an ethics committee, subcommittee, and consultant might be best suited to different types of cases.

18

Do Not Resuscitate Orders

Everyone who dies suffers a cardiac arrest. Cardiopulmonary resuscitation (CPR) may revive some patients after cardiopulmonary arrests. In severe illness, however, CPR is much more likely to prolong dying than reverse death. This chapter discusses the effectiveness of CPR, appropriate reasons for Do Not Resuscitate (DNR) orders, the interpretation of such orders, and discussions with patients or surrogates about CPR.

CPR differs from other medical interventions in several ways. When a cardiopulmonary arrest occurs, physicians or nurses who may not know the patient must decide immediately whether to initiate CPR. Otherwise the patient will certainly die. Thus CPR is attempted in every patient who suffers a cardiopulmonary arrest, unless a prior decision has been made not to do so. Unlike other medical interventions, CPR is initiated without a physician's order. Instead, a physician's order is required to withhold CPR—the DNR order, or Do Not Attempt Resuscitation (DNAR) order, or No CPR order.

THE EFFECTIVENESS OF CPR

To make informed decisions about CPR, patients (or their surrogates) need to understand the limited effectiveness of CPR in many clinical situations. When CPR is attempted on general wards of an acute care hospital, circulation and breathing are restored in about 40% of cases (1). Of those initially resuscitated, about one-third survive to discharge from the hospital. Thus about 14% of patients on whom CPR is attempted are discharged alive from the hospital (1,2). In other words, even when CPR is attempted, about 86% of patients die. CPR is more effective when patients suffer cardiopulmonary arrests in the operating room, cardiac catheterization laboratory, and intensive care units.

In certain patient groups, CPR is even less beneficial. Survival to discharge is significantly lower in patients with metastatic cancer, sepsis, and elevated serum creatinine (1). For patients with metastatic cancer, several series report zero survival after CPR (3), although two series report 9% and 14% survival rates in such patients (4,5). For patients with sepsis, survival is also highly unlikely. In one series, only 1 of 73 patients survived, whereas in another study 0 of 42 patients survived (6,7). CPR is usually ineffective in the elderly, but it is not clear whether this is due to age *per se* or comorbid diseases in the elderly (1,6,8). Outcomes for nursing home residents who receive CPR are also poor. In two series, 0% and 1.7% of nursing home residents on whom paramedics attempted CPR survived (9,10).

Complications may occur in patients who are revived by CPR. A dreaded outcome of CPR is severe neurological impairment. The brain may suffer severe anoxic damage even though circulation is restored. In one series, only 1 patient survived to discharge among 52 patients who remained unconscious 24 hours after successful initial resuscitation (11). Other medical complications may also occur during CPR. For example, fractured ribs or sternum or flail chest occur in 30% of cases (12).

JUSTIFICATIONS FOR DNR ORDERS

As with other medical interventions, there are several acceptable justifications for withholding CPR.

Patient Refuses CPR

Competent, informed patients may not want CPR. Many patients wish to die peacefully, rather than have physicians and nurses attempt to revive them. Such informed refusals should be respected. However, in a large study, when patients wanted CPR withheld, a DNR order was written in only about 50% of cases (13).

Surrogate Refuses CPR

Surrogates may decline CPR for patients who lack decision-making capacity. Surrogate decisions should be based on the patient's preferences or best interests.

CPR Is Futile in a Strict Sense

As Chapter 10 discusses, physicians may decide unilaterally to withhold interventions that are futile in a strict sense.

CPR Has No Pathophysiological Rationale

A patient may be obviously dead for a length of time incompatible with successful resuscitation. For example, a patient may have rigor mortis or dependent lividity.

Cardiac Arrest Occurs Despite Maximal Treatment

For example, a patient may have progressive hypotension despite maximal therapy.

CPR Has Already Failed in the Patient

When the standard resuscitative measures recommended in the American Heart Association (AHA) guidelines have been attempted, without success, continued CPR would be futile.

In these strictly defined situations, the decision to stop or withhold resuscitation is appropriately made by physicians, and CPR should not be offered to patients or surrogates (14–16). Instead, physicians should inform them of the DNR order or the termination of CPR and explain why. Even if a patient or surrogate were to insist on CPR in such situations, physicians and nurses have no obligation to attempt it. However, few situations are as clear as these.

Problematical Appeals to Futility

Physicians often use futility in a looser sense to justify unilateral decisions by physicians to withhold CPR.

Survival After CPR Is Highly Unlikely

Some physicians assert that CPR is "futile" when patients are highly likely to die even if CPR is attempted.

CASE 17.1. FAMILY WANTS CPR EVEN THOUGH SURVIVAL WOULD BE HIGHLY UNLIKELY. *A 54-year-old man, bedridden with squamous cell carcinoma of the lung metastatic to liver and bone, is hospitalized for pneumonia. He has never indicated his preferences regarding CPR. The family insists that he be a "full code," saying that even if he doesn't regain consciousness or survive the hospitalization, it is worth prolonging life for even a few hours or days. The physicians, however, consider CPR futile, because the medical literature reports that very few such patients are discharged alive after cardiopulmonary arrest (3). Furthermore, the doctors consider his quality of life extremely poor.*

In Case 17.1, the family regards the goal of CPR as prolonging life, even if it would be unprecedented for the patient to be discharged alive from the hospital. Most physicians, however, consider the goal of CPR to be patient survival to hospital discharge, not merely temporary restoration of circulation and breathing. They point out that society and the medical profession are not obligated to do everything that a patient requests (17,18). Prolonging the patient's life for a few hours or days is not an appropriate goal for care (15). The Guidelines for Cardiopulmonary Resuscitation and Emergency Cardiac Care of the AHA state that CPR is futile and may therefore be withheld if "no survivors after CPR have been reported under the given circumstances in well-designed studies" (16).

However, unilateral DNR orders based on low likelihood of success are problematical (*see* Chapter 9) (19). First, rigorous data outcomes exist for very few clinical conditions (20). Second, physicians are inaccurate and unreliable in predicting outcomes of CPR. One study found that physicians were no better at identifying patients who would survive resuscitation than would be expected by chance alone (1). Third, physicians often define futility far more broadly than recommended in the literature. In a study of DNR orders based on a quantitative definition of futility, in 32% of cases residents estimated the patient's probability of survival after CPR to be 5% or higher (21). This definition is far looser than the criteria for futility proposed in the literature, namely zero successes in the previous 100 cases (17,18).

The Patient's Quality of Life is Unacceptably Poor

Some physicians and ethicists claim that CPR may be withheld from patients who are in a persistent vegetative state or who cannot survive outside an intensive care unit (17,18). As discussed in Chapter 9, it is problematical for physicians to make judgments that the patient's quality of life is so poor that interventions are futile. DNR decisions based on such a qualitative notion of futility are also suspect because physicians making such judgments regarding competent patients commonly do not talk to them about their quality of life (21).

DISCUSSING DNR ORDERS WITH PATIENTS

Patients or surrogates need to discuss CPR with physicians if they are to make informed decisions about it. Physicians cannot accurately determine patients' preferences regarding CPR without asking them directly. In the large multicenter SUPPORT study, physicians misunderstood patients' preferences regarding CPR in about 50% of cases (22).

Barriers to Discussions

Some physicians believe that patients do not want to discuss DNR decisions. In fact, most ambulatory patients—between 67% and 85%—want to discuss life-sustaining treatment with physicians (23,24). Among hospitalized patients, between 42% and 81% want to discuss end-of-life decisions with their physicians (25,26).

Physicians sometimes hesitate to discuss DNR orders with patients, fearing that they will lose hope, become depressed, refuse highly beneficial treatments, or even attempt suicide. Such adverse outcomes, however, almost never occur.

Targeting Discussions

Physicians typically discuss CPR only with patients whom they believe are at high risk for cardiopulmonary arrest. The prospect of cardiopulmonary arrest becomes more salient as a patient's condition worsens. However, patients may become so sick that they are no longer capable of making medical decisions or discussing CPR with their physicians (27). Additionally, targeting sicker patients for discussions about CPR reinforces the belief that DNR discussions signify a bleak prognosis. Selective discussions may also be inequitable. Physicians discuss DNR orders more frequently with patients with the acquired immunodeficiency syndrome (AIDS) or cancer than with patients with cirrhosis, who have similarly poor prognoses (28).

For these reasons, physicians should routinely discuss CPR with all adult inpatients with serious illness. Ideally, such discussions would be initiated in the ambulatory setting. When patients lack decision-making capacity, physicians should conduct discussions about CPR with appropriate surrogates.

Patient Overestimates of Survival After CPR

Many patients misunderstand basic information about the nature of CPR. Few patients understand that mechanical ventilation is usually required after CPR and that patients on a ventilator are usually conscious but cannot talk (29). Patients substantially overestimate favorable outcomes after CPR (30). Many patients who initially accept CPR change their minds after they are informed about the nature and outcomes of CPR (30,31).

Improving Discussions About DNR Orders

Better discussions with physicians will help patients make informed decisions. Table 18-1 summarizes the following suggestions:

Place Discussions in Context

Often it is better to start with a discussion of the patient's concerns and goals for care, rather than the specific decision regarding CPR (32).

TABLE 18-1. *Improving discussions with patients or surrogates about DNR orders*

Routinely invite patients to discuss CPR.
Provide enough information for patients to make informed decisions.
Make explicit recommendations.
Place CPR discussions into a positive context of supportive care.
Repeat discussions at subsequent visits.

Routinely Invite Patients to Discuss CPR

Physicians can raise the issue of CPR in a straightforward manner. "I try to discuss with all patients what to do if they become too sick to talk with me directly. How would you feel about discussing this?" If the patient agrees, the physician can continue, "One important issue is cardiopulmonary resuscitation, or CPR. Let me explain what CPR is . . . " Some physicians try to dissuade patients from CPR by describing it in graphic detail, such as "pounding on your chest." Such biased information, however, undermines the goal of informed patient decision-making.

Provide Enough Information for Patients to Make Informed Decisions

Often doctors shroud DNR discussions in euphemisms or technical jargon (33). Physicians sometimes ask patients, "If your heart or lungs stop, would you like us to start them up again?" Such phrasing suggests that CPR is as simple and effective as jump starting an automobile battery or changing an electrical fuse. The question is whether patients want doctors to *try* to revive them, even though the likelihood of death is 86% or more. Physicians can be explicit without being blunt or offensive. To avoid bias due to framing effects, physicians should explain that if CPR is attempted, overall 14% of patients will survive the hospitalization, and 86% will die. Doctors can describe CPR (including chest compressions, electroshock, and intubation) and the possible outcomes (including survival, persistent unconsciousness, and death). Even after discussions with physicians, patients often have serious misunderstandings about CPR. For example, patients often do not realize that after resuscitation, mechanical ventilation is usually needed (29).

Make Explicit Recommendations About CPR

Physicians can offer recommendations while still allowing patients ultimate decision-making power. If CPR would be futile in a strict sense, physicians should not offer patients or surrogates a choice, but instead inform them of the DNR order and its rationale.

Reassure Patients About Ongoing Care

Some patients fear that after a DNR order, physicians will give up on them. Physicians need to emphasize plans for treating other problems, seeing the patient regularly, and providing palliative care.

Repeat Discussions

Patients or surrogates often need time to think about issues and deal with their emotions. Thus repeating discussions helps them make informed choices about CPR.

Physicians can improve their skills at DNR discussions. Currently doctors seldom observe more experienced physicians carry out such discussions, or have colleagues watch them (34). Asking the advice of colleagues about a particular situation, role playing, and reviewing videotapes of simulated discussions may be helpful.

IMPLEMENTING DNR ORDERS

Writing a DNR Order

DNR orders are common in critically and terminally ill patients. CPR is not attempted for 89% of seriously ill patients who die in acute care hospitals (35). To prevent misunderstandings, physicians should write DNR orders in the medical record. In addition, the physician should explain in a progress note the rationale for the DNR order, document the agreement of the patient or surrogate, and describe plans for further care. In an urgent situation, nurses may accept a DNR order over the telephone, with the understanding that the physician will sign the order promptly. DNR orders should be reviewed periodically, particularly if the patient's condition changes.

Oral DNR orders may lead to mistakes, misunderstandings, and confusion. They create ethical quandaries and legal jeopardy for nurses who respond to cardiac arrests. Generally the use of oral rather than written DNR orders indicates serious disagreements and a need for further discussions.

Interpretation of DNR orders

Implications of DNR Orders for Other Treatments

Strictly speaking, a DNR order means only to withhold CPR. Other treatments, such as antibiotics, transfusions, and even intensive care, may still be appropriate. However, the same reasons that make CPR inappropriate may also render other interventions unsuitable. Many hospitals now require more detailed orders than simply "no CPR." For example, the physician may have to specify on a checklist whether to provide mechanical ventilation (36,37). Such detailed orders are useful because nurses need to know whether abnormalities such as hypotension or ventricular arrhythmia should be treated or allowed to progress and lead to cardiopulmonary arrest.

"Limited" or "Partial" DNR Orders

In some cases, physicians may decide to restrict resuscitative efforts to a fixed period or withhold aspects of advanced life support, such as defibrillation or intubation (6). One rationale for physician-limited DNR orders is that patients who do not respond to basic CPR may have suffered irreversible brain damage. The fear is that resuscitation may restore breathing and circulation in a patient who will never regain consciousness. However, this rationale is problematical. During an attempted resuscitation, there are virtually no reliable signs of irreversible brain damage or brain death (16). Furthermore, stopping resuscitation after basic CPR will reduce the chances for patient recovery. Even if basic CPR is ineffective, advanced life support may restore circulation, breathing, and consciousness.

"Limited" DNR orders are appropriate, however, when the patient (or surrogate) consents to them or requests them. For instance, patients with chronic obstructive lung disease may decline mechanical ventilation but agree to other resuscitative measures.

Preventing Misunderstandings

Some physicians are reluctant to write DNR orders because they fear that other health care workers—consultants, house staff, nurses, or respiratory therapists—may cease to provide needed care to the patient. Conversely, some nurses believe that once a DNR order is made, physicians will stop rounding on patients or stop talking to them. Concerns that DNR orders may lead to suboptimal care need to be addressed openly. Everyone needs to appreciate that DNR orders do not mean "provide no care."

Slow or Show Codes

"Slow codes" or "show codes" appear to provide CPR but actually do not, or do so in a way that is known to be ineffective (38,39). For example, the code team is not paged immediately, a medical student is allowed to make repeated attempts to intubate the patient, or drugs are injected into the bed rather than into the patient. Usually such orders are given orally and not written down. Slow or show codes are commonly considered when the patient has a grim prognosis but an attending physician insists that CPR be attempted or the patient or surrogate insists that "everything" be done. Show codes are unacceptable because they deceive patients or families, compromise the ethical integrity of health care professionals, and cause confusion and cynicism among health care workers.

Special Settings

Anesthesia for Surgery and Invasive Procedures

Patients with DNR orders may undergo surgery for palliation or conditions unrelated to their primary diagnosis (40). Many physicians want to "suspend" DNR orders in the operating room, when the patient's vital functions are deliberately depressed by anesthesia and maintained using techniques similar to those of advanced cardiac life support (41–43). If resuscitation were not permitted, medications might be titrated to ensure greater hemodynamic stability but lighter anesthesia, less analgesia, and less amnesia. CPR is much more successful in the operating room than elsewhere in the hospital. In one study, 65% of patients who had a cardiopulmonary arrest in the operating room survived to discharge, and 92% of those whose arrest was caused by anesthesia survived (44). Another reason for suspending DNR orders during surgery is the physician's sense of responsibility for intraoperative deaths (*see* Chapter 39).

If patients with DNR orders undergo surgery or invasive procedures, physicians should discuss how the DNR orders will be interpreted perioperatively (40). Plans should be documented clearly in the medical record. Similar considerations apply to DNR orders in radiology departments, where medications may lead to cardiac arrest that is easily reversed (45–47).

Emergency Medical Services

When emergency medical personnel are called to the home of a patient with serious illness, CPR may not be appropriate. Paramedic policies and protocols should include provisions for DNR orders (16). DNR orders can be documented with an identification card or bracelet, a sticker on the telephone or refrigerator, a formal order sheet, or a computerized registry. A DNR order should not preclude other appropriate care, such as oxygen or transport to the hospital. Similarly, emergency departments need to establish DNR policies and procedures.

Nursing Homes

Few nursing home residents who suffer cardiopulmonary arrest are successfully resuscitated (9,10). Extended care facilities should establish institutional policies regarding the provision of cardiopulmonary resuscitation and procedures for designating residents as not to be resuscitated. Residents with DNR orders should have access to appropriate emergency services.

In conclusion, CPR is not appropriate for many patients. Physicians should elicit patients' preferences about CPR and write DNR orders in the medical record. For physicians, the question is no longer whether we should discuss DNR orders with our patients but instead how to do so with compassion and caring.

REFERENCES

1. Ebell MH, Becker LA, Barry HC, et al. Survival analysis after in-hospital cardiopulmonary resuscitation. *J Gen Intern Med* 1998;13:805–816.

2. Saklayen M, Liss H, Markert R. In-hospital cardiopulmonary resuscitation. *Medicine* 1995;74:163–175.
3. Faber-Langendorf K. Resuscitation of patients with metastatic cancer: is transient benefit still futile? *Arch Intern Med* 1991;151:235–239.
4. Vitelli CE, Cooper J, Ragatko A, et al. Cardiopulmonary resuscitation and the patient with cancer. *J Clin Oncol* 1991;9:111–115.
5. Rosenberg M, Wang C, Hoffman-Wilde S, et al. Results of cardiopulmonary resuscitation: failure to predict survival in two community hospitals. *Arch Intern Med* 1993;153:1370–1375.
6. Evans AL, Brody BA. The do-not-resuscitate order in teaching hospitals. *JAMA* 1985;253:2236–2239.
7. Bedell SE, Delbanco TL, Cook EF, et al. Survival after cardiopulmonary resuscitation in the hospital. *N Engl J Med* 1983;309:579–586.
8. Murphy DJ, Murray AM, Robinson BE, et al. Outcomes of cardiopulmonary resuscitation in the elderly. *Ann Intern Med* 1989;111:199–205.
9. Applebaum GE, King JE, Finucane TE. The outcome of CPR initiated in nursing homes. *J Am Geriatr Soc* 1990;38:197–200.
10. Awoke S, Mouton CP, Parrott M. Outcomes of skilled cardiopulmonary resuscitation in a long-term care facility: futile therapy? *J Am Geriatr Soc* 1992;40:593–595.
11. Longstreth WT, Inui TS, Cobb LA, et al. Neurologic recovery after out-of-hospital cardiac arrest. *Ann Intern Med* 1983;98:588–592.
12. Moss AH. Informing patients about cardiopulmonary resuscitation when the risks outweigh the benefits. *J Gen Intern Med* 1989;4:349–355.
13. The SUPPORT Investigators. A controlled trial to improve care for seriously ill hospitalized patients. *JAMA* 1995;274:1591–1598.
14. Blackhall LJ. Must we always use CPR? *N Engl J Med* 1988;317:1281–1285.
15. Tomlinson T, Brody H. Futility and the ethics of resuscitation. *JAMA* 1990;264:1276–1280.
16. Emergency Cardiac Care Committee and Subcommittees of the American Heart Association. Guidelines for cardiopulmonary resuscitation and emergency cardiac care, VIII: Ethical considerations in resuscitation. *JAMA* 1992;268:2282–2288.
17. Schneiderman LJ, Jecker NS, Jonsen AR. Medical futility: its meaning and ethical implications. *Ann Intern Med* 1990;112:949–954.
18. Schneiderman LJ, Jecker NS, Jonsen AR. Medical futility: response to critiques. *Ann Intern Med* 1996;125:669–674.
19. Alpers A, Lo B. When is CPR futile? *JAMA* 1995;273:156–158.
20. Rubenfeld GD, Crawford SW. Withdrawing life support from mechanically ventilated recipients of bone marrow transplants: a case for evidence-based guidelines. *Ann Intern Med* 1996;125:625–633.
21. Curtis JR, Park DR, Krone MR, et al. The use of the medical futility rationale in do not attempt resuscitation orders. *JAMA* 1995;273:124–128.
22. Teno JM, Hakim RB, Knaus WA, et al. Preferences for cardiopulmonary resuscitation: physican-patient agreement and hospital resource use. *J Gen Intern Med* 1995;10:179–186.
23. Shmerling RH, Bedell SA, Lilienfeld A, et al. Discussing cardiopulmonary resuscitation: a study of elderly outpatients. *J Gen Intern Med* 1988;3:317–321.
24. Lo B, McLeod G, Saika G. Patient attitudes towards discussing life-sustaining treatment. *Arch Intern Med* 1986;146:1613–1615.
25. Reilly BM, Magnussen CR, Ross J, et al. Can we talk? Inpatient discussions about advance directives in a community hospital. Attending physicians' attitudes, their inpatients' wishes, and reported experience. *Arch Intern Med* 1994;154:2299–2308.
26. Hoffman JC, Wenger NS, Davis RH, et al. Patient preferences for communication with physicians about end-of-life decisions. *Ann Intern Med* 1997;127:1–12.
27. Council on Ethical and Judicial Affairs, AMA. Guidelines for the appropriate use of do-not-resuscitate orders. *JAMA* 1991;265:1868–1871.
28. Wachter RM, Luce JM, Hearst N, et al. Decisions about resuscitation: inequities among patients with different diseases but similar prognoses. *Ann Intern Med* 1989;111:525–532.
29. Fischer GS, Tulsky JA, Rose MR, et al. Patient knowledge and physician predications of treatment preferences after discussions of advance directives. *J Gen Intern Med* 1998;13:447–454.
30. Murphy DJ, Burrows D, Santilli S, et al. The influence of the probability of survival on patients' preferences regarding cardiopulmonary resusctation. *N Engl J Med* 1994;330:545–549.
31. O'Brien LA, Grisso JA, Maislin G, et al. Nursing home residents' preferences for life-sustaining treatments. *JAMA* 1995;254:1175–1179.
32. Lo B, Quill T, Tulsky J. Discussing palliative care with patients. *Ann Intern Med* 1999;130:744–749.
33. Tulsky JA, Chesney MA, Lo B. How do medical residents discuss resuscitation with patients? *J Gen Intern Med* 1995;10:436–442.
34. Tulsky JA, Chesney MA, Lo B. "See one, do one, teach one?" Housestaff experience discussing do-not-resuscitate orders. *Arch Intern Med* 1996;156:1285–1289.
35. Lynn J, Teno J, Phillips RS, et al. Perceptions by family members of the dying experience of older and seriously ill patients. *Ann Intern Med* 1997;126:97–106.

36. Mittelberger JA, Lo B, Martin D, et al. Impact of a procedure-specific do not resuscitate order form on documentation of do not resuscitate orders. *Arch Intern Med* 1993;153:228–232.
37. O'Toole EE, Youngner SJ, Juknialis BW, et al. Evaluation of a treatment limitation policy with a specific treatment-limiting order page. *Arch Intern Med* 1994;154:425–432.
38. Muller JH. Shades of blue: the negotiation of limited codes by medical residents. *Soc Sci Med* 1992;34:885–898.
39. Gazelle G. The slow code—should anyone rush to its defense? *N Engl J Med* 1998;338:467–469.
40. Clemency MV, Thompson NJ. Do not resuscitate orders in the perioperative period: patient perspectives. *Anesth Analg* 1997;84:859–864.
41. Cohen CB, Cohen PJ. Do-not-resuscitate orders in the operating room. *N Engl J Med* 1991;325:1879–1882.
42. Truog RD. "Do not resuscitate" orders during anesthesia and surgery. *Anesthesiology* 1991;74:606–608.
43. Walker RM. DNR in the OR: resuscitation as an operative risk. *JAMA* 1991;266:2407–2412.
44. Olsson GL, Hall B. Cardiac arrest during anesthesia: a computer-aided study in 250,543 anaesthetics. *Acta Anaes Scand* 1988;32:653–664.
45. Jacobson JA, Gully JE, Mann H. "Do not resuscitate" orders in the radiology department: an interpretation. *Radiology* 1996;198:21–24.
46. McDermott VG. Resuscitation and the radiologist. *Ann Intern Med* 1998;129:831–833.
47. Heffner JE, Barbieri C. Compliance with do-not-resuscitate orders for hospitalized patients transported to radiology departments. *Ann Intern Med* 1998;129:801–805.

ANNOTATED BIBLIOGRAPHY

1. Tulsky JA, Chesney MA, Lo B. How do medical residents discuss resuscitation with patients? *J Gen Intern Med* 1995;10:436–442.
   In discussions with patients regarding CPR, residents failed to provide key information about CPR and missed opportunities to discuss the patient's values and goals.
2. Murphy DJ, Burrows D, Santilli S, et al. The influence of the probability of survival on patients' preferences regarding cardiopulmonary resusctation. *N Engl J Med* 1994;330:545–549.
   Patients overestimate survival after CPR; when such misunderstandings are corrected, patients are less likely to accept CPR.
3. Tomlinson T, Brody H. Futility and the ethics of resuscitation. *JAMA* 1990;264:1276–1280.
   Argues that in certain situations, CPR may be futile and DNR orders may be written by physicians over the objections of patients or surrogates.
4. Curtis JR, Park DR, Krone MR, et al. The use of the medical futility rationale in do not attempt resuscitation orders. *JAMA* 1995;273:124–128.
   Empirical study documenting problems and mistakes that occur when physicians claim that CPR would be futile.

19

Physician-Assisted Suicide
and Active Euthanasia

Although traditional medical ethics prohibits assisted suicide and active euthanasia, public opinion and policies in the United States are sharply divided. In 1994, Oregon legalized physician-assisted suicide. However, several states recently passed laws criminalizing physician-assisted suicide. In 1996, the Supreme Court ruled that there is no constitutional right to physician-assisted suicide and that states may prohibit it (1). Studies document that physician-assisted suicide and active euthanasia are carried out despite legal prohibitions (2). Several juries have refused to convict Jack Kevorkian, a nonpracticing pathologist who has publicized numerous cases in which he provided physician-assisted suicide or active euthanasia.

DEFINING TERMS CLEARLY

The debate over assisted suicide and euthanasia is marred by imprecise terminology and rhetorical slogans. Several actions should be distinguished.

Active Voluntary Euthanasia

In active euthanasia, the physician administers a lethal dose of medication, such as potassium chloride. The physician both supplies the means of death and is the final human agent in the events leading to the patient's death. Active euthanasia is sometimes called mercy killing. Euthanasia is called *voluntary* when the patient requests it, *involuntary* when he opposes it, and *nonvoluntary*, when the patient lacks decision-making capacity and cannot express a preference. There is general agreement that involuntary euthanasia is wrong because it violates a patient's right not to be killed. Nonvoluntary euthanasia is also generally considered unacceptable because it may be selectively applied to the disadvantaged and vulnerable.

Assisted Suicide

In assisted suicide, the patient swallows a lethal dose of drugs or activates a device to administer the drugs. Physicians might assist in a variety of ways. They might provide the means for suicide, provide information on it, or refer the patient to the Hemlock Society for information.

Many people consider assisted suicide less ethically problematical than active euthanasia. Although the physician provides the means of death, the patient must carry out an independent act. Indeed, many patients may want a lethal dose of medication so they have control over their death, not because they want to end their lives soon. This fact may have several important eth-

156

ical implications. First, the moral responsibility of the physician may be lessened by the subsequent intervening action by the patient. In this view, patients, who have free will, are morally responsible for their acts. Although other people may influence the patient, they are not regarded as causing his actions, unless there is coercion. Second, the justification may be stronger because taking an action to commit suicide is a more direct expression of the patient's autonomy than a request for active euthanasia. Third, there may be less danger of abuse. If the patient changes his mind about suicide, he simply does not take the pills. In contrast, a patient may feel pressure to go through with arrangements for active euthanasia.

Physicians, however, must not underestimate their moral responsibility if they assist a patient to commit suicide. The motive, intent, justification, and outcome are the same as in active euthanasia. In other situations, people may be held morally responsible for assisting or encouraging another person to commit an immoral act.

Some physicians who prescribe a lethal dose of medications may claim that they did not know that the patient planned to kill himself. For example, some doctors may prescribe secobarbital upon a patient's request without discussing the topic of suicide. It would be disingenuous to abjure responsibility in this situation, however. Doctors almost never prescribe secobarbital, except as a means for suicide. Most important, by not broaching the topic of suicide, physicians forego an opportunity to provide better palliative care, which often leads patients to change their minds about suicide.

Withholding or Withdrawing Medical Interventions

Active euthanasia and assisted suicide are usually distinguished from withholding or withdrawing interventions, which are also termed "allowing to die" or "passive euthanasia." Ethically and legally, medical interventions may be withheld or withdrawn if a competent patient or an appropriate surrogate refuses them (*see* Chapter 14). A patient's refusal of life-sustaining treatment is honored because patients have a right to be free of unwanted bodily invasions. Under such circumstances, the underlying *illness*, not the action or inaction of the *physician*, is considered the cause of death. Therefore concern that assisted suicide or active euthanasia is improper should not lead physicians to impose interventions that are not wanted by the patient or surrogate.

This clear line between killing and allowing to die provides practical guidance, but it is problematical for several reasons (3,4). First, some patients who refuse life-prolonging interventions want to hasten their death, not just to be free of unwanted medical interventions (5). Second, many philosophers have rejected the distinction between acting and refraining from action, pointing out that withholding effective treatment would be condemned if done against the wishes of the patient or for malicious motives. However, even though *some* cases of foregoing life-sustaining interventions are hard to distinguish from physician-assisted suicide, it does not follow that *all* cases of foregoing life-sustaining interventions are equivalent to physician-assisted suicide.

Administering Appropriate Doses of Narcotics or Sedatives

Active euthanasia and assisted suicide can be distinguished from providing high doses of narcotics or sedatives to relieve severe pain in patients with terminal illness or to relieve dyspnea when patients forego mechanical ventilation (1). As Chapter 14 discusses, the appropriate goal of care in these situations is to relieve suffering. In rare cases, the dose required to relieve distress may hasten death. Concerns about active euthanasia and assisted suicide should not deter physicians from providing aggressive palliative care (6). Indeed, fears that terminal distress will not be adequately relieved impels some patients to seek active euthanasia and assisted suicide (7,8).

REASONS IN FAVOR OF ASSISTED SUICIDE AND ACTIVE EUTHANASIA

Proponents of these acts offer several justifications for their position (9,10).

Respect for Patient Autonomy

Many persons are horrified at the prospect of a long, debilitating illness that would destroy their sense of identity and dignity. People may fear loss of privacy and increased dependence on others for such basic needs as feeding, bathing, and toilet. They also may not want their family and friends to remember them as progressively debilitated. Proponents contend that competent patients with terminal illness should have control over the time and manner of their death. In this view, it is inconsistent to permit patients to end their life by refusing medical interventions after a complication occurs, but not to end it more directly beforehand.

Compassion for Patients Who Are Suffering

Some argue that assisted suicide and active euthanasia show compassion for patients in the final stages of a terminal illness. Many people regard it as inhumane to require such patients to suffer a progressively downhill course, while waiting to die from complications. As one author put it, "People who want an early peaceful death for themselves or their relatives are not rejecting or denigrating the sanctity of life; on the contrary, they believe that a quicker death shows more respect for life than a protracted one" (11). Some terminally ill patients have refractory symptoms despite optimal palliative care. For example, some patients with cancer of the esophagus or head and neck cannot swallow their secretions, some patients with the acquired immunodeficiency syndrome suffer refractory diarrhea, and some cancer patients experience intractable bleeding. Such patients can be sedated so that they are no longer conscious of their symptoms, but they will not have dignified or peaceful deaths.

Proponents of assisted suicide also argue that physicians cannot prevent people from killing themselves; they can only alter the means by which patients end their lives. If lethal drugs are not available, patients may resort to hanging or guns. Such means of death are gruesome and distress family members and friends. Advocates contend that terminally ill patients should have a more humane means of ending their lives.

REASONS AGAINST ASSISTED SUICIDE AND ACTIVE EUTHANASIA

Traditional codes of medical ethics prohibit physician participation in assisted suicide or active euthanasia (12–14). Active euthanasia is illegal in all states, and most states explicitly prohibit assisted suicide.

The Sanctity of Life

Many people assert that assisted suicide and active euthanasia demean the sacredness of human life and violate fundamental moral prohibitions against killing human beings.

Suffering Can Almost Always Be Relieved

Palliative care is often inadequate in terminally ill patients. Opponents fear that assisted suicide and active euthanasia will allow physicians to avoid the difficult task of providing physical and spiritual comfort to dying patients. Some people suggest that suffering can be redemptive and that patients have a duty to endure it or cope courageously (13).

Requests for Assisted Suicide Are Not Autonomous

Most terminally ill patients change their minds about suicide after receiving better palliative care or treatment for depression. Thus, their requests are not truly autonomous. Physicians have an ethical obligation to prevent suicide because the vast majority of patients who attempt suicide have a psychiatric illness, such as major depression, that can be treated (*see* Chapter 42). After treatment for depression, few patients still wish to kill themselves. Even among patients with cancer, most suicidal individuals are clinically depressed, and major depression can be treated (15,16).

Fears of Abuse

A slippery slope might occur: if physician-assisted suicide is permitted for competent terminally ill patients, there are no logical reasons to prohibit it for patients who are not competent or not terminally ill or to prohibit active euthanasia. For example, if competent patients have a right to physician-assisted suicide, it would be inconsistent to deny it to patients who have previously requested it but have lost decision-making capacity. A patient with mild Alzheimer's disease may not want to live if she could no longer recognize her family. At that stage, however, she would no longer be capable of making an informed request. Thus, if she is not permitted to request physician-assisted suicide or active euthanasia through an advance directive, she would face a cruel dilemma: to end her life when it is still meaningful to her or to live in an unacceptably dehumanized condition. Furthermore, some patients with severe amyotrophic lateral sclerosis may want to hasten their death in order to avoid further dependency and to relieve their suffering. However, such patients are not terminally ill and may lack the physical ability to ingest medication without assistance. Thus respecting their wishes to hasten death may require active euthanasia.

A second type of slippery slope might also occur. At the onset, physicians who participate in assisted suicide might carefully ensure that every case is appropriate, but over time, they might become less diligent in providing palliative care or checking that the patient's request is voluntary. Eventually, assisted suicide might occur when palliative care was grossly inadequate or major depression unaddressed.

Active euthanasia raises particular fears regarding abuse. Euthanasia for competent patients logically leads to euthanasia of patients who lack decision-making capacity, as discussed previously. In other cases, relief of unbearable suffering might be used to justify active euthanasia in mentally incapacitated patients who had never requested it. Another fear is that pressures to control health care costs will result in nonvoluntary euthanasia of persons whose care is regarded as too burdensome or too expensive (17). Patients with chronic illness or disability may feel pressured by family members or physicians into terminating their lives.

The Role of the Physician

Opponents argue that active euthanasia and assisted suicide are incompatible with the physician's role as healer. In this view, patients would lose trust in physicians if these practices were permitted. People might be reluctant to seek medical care because they fear that physicians might be more interested in helping them to die than in helping them to recover.

LEGALIZATION OF PHYSICIAN-ASSISTED SUICIDE IN OREGON

In Oregon, terminally ill, competent adults may request medication to end their life (18,19). The patient must make a written request that is witnessed by two individuals who attest that the patient is competent, acting voluntarily, and not coerced. Fifteen days after this written request, the patient must repeat the request orally. An additional 48 hours must elapse before the prescription can be filled. The patient may rescind the request at any time.

Physicians must ensure that patients are informed about their diagnosis, prognosis, and therapeutic alternatives, including palliative care. A consultant must confirm that the patient has a terminal disease, is capable of making health care decisions, is informed, and is acting voluntarily. Patients with a psychiatric disorder that impairs judgment must be referred for counseling.

Physicians who comply with the provisions of the law are granted legal immunity from criminal, civil, and professional disciplinary actions. Physicians and other health care workers may refuse to participate. If a patient ingests a lethal dose of medication under this law, life insurance policies are not voided.

Several groups of patients fall outside the coverage of this law. The law specifically prohibits active euthanasia, mercy killing, and lethal injection. Physicians are not allowed to provide assistance to patients who are too incapacitated to take lethal medication themselves. Patients are excluded if they suffer from nonterminal illnesses, lack decision-making capacity, or are too sick to survive the waiting periods. Patients may not request suicide assistance through advance directives or surrogate decision-makers.

In Oregon, 23 terminally ill persons in 1998 were reported to the state as receiving prescriptions for lethal medications (20). Compared with other terminal patients, these patients were more concerned about loss of autonomy and loss of control over bodily functions as a result of their illness (20). These patients were not disproportionately uneducated, poor, uninsured, or fearful of the financial impact of their illness (20). Forty percent of these patients did not receive the requested prescription from the first doctor they asked (20). Some physicians who participated in physician-assisted suicide reported a large emotional toll (20).

THE PRACTICE OF PHYSICIAN-ASSISTED SUICIDE AND ACTIVE EUTHANASIA IN THE UNITED STATES

Several well-designed empirical studies demonstrate that despite legal prohibitions, physician-assisted suicide and active euthanasia are practiced in the United States.

Requests for Physician-Assisted Suicide and Active Euthanasia Are Common

In a national sample, 18% of physicians report that in their careers they had received a request for physician-assisted suicide and 11% a request for active euthanasia. In another study, over 50% of oncologists had received a request for physician-assisted suicide and 38% a request for active euthanasia (21). Twelve percent of cancer patients report serious discussions about active euthanasia or physician-assisted suicide with their family or physician, and 3.4% hoarded drugs (21).

Requests Are More Common in Depressed Patients

Nineteen percent of patients who received physician-assisted suicide and 39% of patients who received active euthansia were depressed (2). In another study, cancer patients who were depressed were 4.6 times more likely to have discussed euthanasia (21).

Physicians Provide Requested Assistance Even When it Is Illegal

Among physicians, 3.3% had written a prescription to be used to hasten death, and 4.7% had administered a lethal injection (2). Among oncologists, 13% had performed physician-assisted suicide and 1.8% active euthanasia. When oncologists prescribed a lethal dose of medications, the patient did not commit suicide in 20% of cases, and in another 15% of such cases the suicide attempt failed (22).

Physicians Are Confused About What Constitutes Physician-Assisted Suicide and Active Euthanasia

When physicians characterized a case as physician-assisted suicide or active euthanasia, they actually provided high doses of narcotics for pain relief in 13% of cases, and in another 9% of cases patients overdosed without asking the physician for a prescription for a lethal dose (22). Furthermore, 12% of physicians who report that they had performed physician-assisted suicide actually ordered a nurse to inject medications to end the patient's life; this action is more accurately characterized as active euthanasia (22).

Proposed Safeguards Are Often Violated

When physicians prescribe a prescription for physician-assisted suicide, suggested safeguards, such as persistent requests and second opinions, are often not followed. In the two studies, patients repeat their request in only 51% and 60% of cases (2,22). Doctors obtained a second opinion in only 1% and 40% of cases (2,22).

In cases of active euthanasia, a family member or partner made the request rather than patient in 54% of cases (2). A second opinion was obtained in only 32% of cases. In 94% of cases, immediate assistance was requested.

Patients Frequently Do Not Use Prescriptions for Lethal Doses of Medication

Approximately 40% of patients who receive prescriptions for lethal doses of medication do not use it (2,23). Presumably the prescription provided reassurance that the patient was in control over their final days.

Physician-Assisted Suicide May Adversely Affect the Doctor–Patient Relationship

Nineteen percent of oncology patients say they would change physicians if their physician told them they had provided active euthanasia or physician-assisted suicide for other patients (22).

Physician-Assisted Suicide Has an Emotional Impact on the Physician

In one study, 18% of physicians who had provided physician-assisted suicide were uncomfortable with that role (2). In the other study, although 53% of respondents received comfort from providing physician-assisted suicide or active euthanasia, 24% regretted performing it (22).

DE FACTO LEGALIZATION OF ASSISTED SUICIDE AND ACTIVE EUTHANASIA IN THE NETHERLANDS

In the Netherlands, active euthanasia and assisted suicide, although prohibited, are not prosecuted in certain situations (24). A competent patient with a terminal illness must make a voluntary and persistent request for active euthanasia or assisted suicide, and two physicians must certify that the patient is terminally ill. In the Netherlands, active euthanasia occurs in between 2.3% and 2.4% of deaths and assisted suicide in 0.2% to 0.4% (25).

Most Patients Withdraw Their Requests for Euthanasia or Assisted Suicide

Patients' requests for active euthanasia or assisted suicide usually do not persist over time. When patients ask physicians to help them to die, only one-third of requests are serious and persistent. Of these, only one-third actually receive active euthanasia or assisted suicide; most change their minds after obtaining better palliative care. Thus only 11% of patients who initially request active euthanasia or assisted suicide receive it (26).

Procedural Safeguards Are Violated

In 0.7% of deaths, physicians ended the patient's life without the explicit, concurrent request of the patient (25). In about one-half of these cases, the patient had previously discussed these decisions with the physician. In a few cases, however, the physician did not discuss these actions with anyone, including relatives or colleagues.

POLICY OPTIONS

Several public policies are possible regarding physician-assisted suicide and active euthanasia. One is to continue traditional prohibitions. However, these practices occur even though they are illegal. Abuses may be more likely to occur if decisions remain secret than if they are discussed openly. Furthermore, prosecutors are reluctant to bring charges against physicians who convincingly assert that they were relieving the patient's suffering, and juries are reluctant to convict such doctors. This discrepancy between the law on the books and in practice is problematical because enforcement may be inconsistent or biased (6). A second option is to legalize these practices under certain conditions, such as in Oregon. The challenge is whether effective safeguards against abuses can be developed. A third option is to keep active euthanasia and assisted suicide illegal, but to acknowledge that in exceptional cases, such practices may be ethically justified and legally condoned (27). The risk of legal sanctions would help deter these actions in questionable or inappropriate cases.

HOW SHOULD PHYSICIANS RESPOND TO REQUESTS FOR ASSISTED SUICIDE OR ACTIVE EUTHANASIA?

Physicians must be prepared for questions from patients about assisted suicide or active euthanasia. Like the general public, doctors will disagree over the morality of these controversial actions (2). Regardless of their personal views, physicians can respond in certain ways (Table 19-1) (28–30).

Find Out the Reasons for the Request

Why is the patient asking a question or making a request at this time? A request or question may represent a response to unrelieved suffering, a demand for more control, emerging psy-

TABLE 19-1. *Responding to requests for assisted suicide or active euthanasia*

Find out the reasons for the request.
Provide more intensive palliative care.
Reaffirm patient control over treatment decisions.
Do not impose your values on patients.
Consult a trusted and wise colleague.

chosocial problems, a spiritual crisis, or fear of abandonment (29,31). Requests may be triggered by loss of dignity, pain, and dependence on others (26). Only rarely is pain the sole reason for a patient's request. Physicians also need to screen patients for major depression, which can be treated even in terminally ill patients (16).

Some physicians fear that talking about assisted suicide or active euthanasia will encourage patients to carry out these acts. Such fears are unfounded. Most terminally ill patients have already thought about these issues and feel relieved that physicians are willing to discuss them. Suicidal patients with terminal illness deserve the same careful evaluation and mobilization of resources as patients who are not terminally ill (32).

Provide More Intensive Palliative Care

If their suffering or concerns are addressed, most patients find life worth living. Pain relief can be improved through using higher and more frequent doses of narcotics, administering them on a regular schedule rather than as needed, and giving patients more control over dosage. In addition to alleviating physical suffering, physicians can help patients come to terms with their mortality and to find meaning in the final stage of their life. Instead of trying prematurely to resolve problems or reassure patients, doctors can explore the patient's suffering using open-ended questions and empathic comments: "That sounds very distressing. Can you tell me more?" (33). Attentive listening validates the patient's emotions and shows the patient that he or she has been understood. The physician should consult with palliative care specialists, psychiatrists or psychologists, social workers, chaplains, and hospice workers as needed. Physicians also can arrange hospice-type home care, mobilize family members and friends, and be available during patients' final weeks and days.

Reaffirm Patient Control Over Treatment Decisions

Some patients may seek to hasten death because they fear they will be subjected to unwanted life-prolonging interventions. Physicians need to reassure patients that their decisions to forego life-sustaining interventions will be respected.

Do not Impose Your Own Values on Patients

Proponents of assisted suicide should not write a lethal prescription on request, without evaluating the patient for depression and inadequate palliative care. Conversely, opponents of these actions should not denigrate the patient's request, but rather communicate empathy and compassion for the patient's plight.

Consult a Trusted and Wise Colleague

Most physicians find patient requests for assisted suicide or active euthanasia to be highly stressful. As with any other difficult case, a second opinion or discussion with a colleague is generally helpful. Often a colleague can suggest how to improve palliative care or how to talk with the patient.

Declining to Give Assistance

Physicians should not participate in assisted suicide or active euthanasia against their conscience or religious beliefs. When communicating their refusal, physicians need to elicit and address the patient's concerns and show empathy for the patient's plight. The physician might say, "I hear that you are deeply distressed by your illness. I'll try my best to relieve your suffering. But I can't help you kill yourself. My conscience won't allow me to do that." Such physicians need to emphasize their commitment to provide ongoing palliative care.

Situations in Which Assisted Suicide Might Be Justified

Many physicians can conceive of a case in which they would consider assisted suicide morally permissible (34). The following circumstances would constitute the strongest case for agreeing to a patient's request (9,10).

- *The patient has a terminal illness* or a progressive, incurable condition causing unrelenting suffering, such as advanced multiple sclerosis.
- *The patient is experiencing intractable symptoms* despite optimal palliative care. Actual distress is more compelling than anticipated future symptoms. Many physicians are more sympathetic to patients with physical distress than to patients with mental distress. The distinction between physical and mental suffering may be philosophically untenable. However, it may be helpful for pragmatic reasons because mistakes and abuse are less likely with physical distress.
- *The patient's request is voluntary, informed, and repeated.* Ideally, the patient raises the issue and is willing to discuss it with family members, friends, or religious advisors.
- *The physician has a long-term relationship with the patient* that started before the patient requested assistance with suicide.
- *The physician has obtained second opinions* regarding the adequacy of palliative care and the absence of depression.

In the rare cases in which these conditions are present, I believe that it is not unethical for physicians to assist in suicide. Active euthanasia is more problematical because it presents greater potential for abuse.

Patients who have lost decision-making capacity present dilemmas. Although requests by surrogates for active euthanasia are usually motivated by compassion, surrogates may confound their own values and desires with those of the patient. They may interpret a gesture or a look as an unspoken request to hasten death, saying, for example, "I looked into his eyes and I just knew what he was asking me to do." The risk of projection, misinterpretation, and abuse are great in this situation. Prohibiting active euthanasia for patients who lack decision-making capacity is sound public policy.

In conclusion, it should never be easy for a physician to respond to the request of a patient who is dying in great suffering despite excellent palliative medicine. Even in the most compelling case, decisions will be difficult, and conscientious and reasonable persons will disagree. Ultimately, physicians will find answers in their own conscience, personal morality, and religious beliefs. Regardless of the physician's decision, however, patients deserve an honest answer to their questions or request. More importantly, physicians must demonstrate their dedication to relieving suffering and their willingness to be with patients during the process of dying.

REFERENCES

1. Alpers A, Lo B. The Supreme Court addresses physician-assisted suicide: can its decisions improve palliative care? *Arch Fam Pract* 1999;8:200–205.
2. Meier DE, Emmons CA, Wallenstein S, et al. Physician-assisted death in the United States: a national prevalence survey. *N Engl J Med* 1998;338:1193–1201.

3. Brock D. Forgoing life-sustaining food and water: is it killing? In: Lynn J, ed. *By no extraordinary means* (expanded edition). Bloomington: Indiana University Press, 1989:117–131.

4. Alpers A, Lo B. Does it make clinical sense to equate terminally ill patients who require life-sustaining interventions with those who do not? *JAMA* 1997;277:1705–1708.

5. Kadish SH. Letting patients die: legal and moral reflections. *Cal Law Rev* 1992;80:857–888.

6. Alpers A. Criminal act or palliative care: prosecutions involving the care of the dying. *J Law Med Ethics* 1998;26:308–331.

7. Angell M. Euthanasia. *N Engl J Med* 1988;319:1348–1350.

8. Foley KM. The relationship of pain and symptom management to patient requests for physician-assisted suicide. *J Pain Symptom Manage* 1991;6:289–297.

9. Quill TE, Cassel CK, Meier DE. Care of the terminally ill: proposed clinical criteria for physician-assisted suicide. *N Engl J Med* 1992;327:1380–1384.

10. Miller FG, Quill TE, Brody H, et al. Regulating physician-assisted death. *N Engl J Med* 1994;331:119–123.

11. Dworkin R. *Life's dominion.* New York: Alfred A. Knopf, 1993:328.

12. Singer PA, Siegler, M. Euthanasia—a critique. *N Engl J Med* 1990;322:1881–1883.

13. Pellegrino ED. Doctors must not kill. *J Clin Ethics* 1992;3:95–102.

14. Foley K. Competent care for the dying instead of physician-assisted suicide. *N Engl J Med* 1997;336:54–58.

15. Conwell Y, Caine ED. Rational suicide and the right to die: reality and myth. *N Engl J Med* 1991;325:1100–1102.

16. Block SD. Assessing and managing depression in the terminally ill patient. *Ann Intern Med* 2000 (*in press*).

17. Sulmasy DP. Managed care and managed death. *Arch Intern Med* 1995;155:133–136.

18. Oregon Death with Dignity Act, Ballot Measure 16 (November 8, 1994 general election).

19. Alpers A, Lo B. Physician-assisted suicide in Oregon: a bold experiment. *JAMA* 1995;274:483–487.

20. Chin AE, Hedberg K, Higginson GK, et al. Legalized physician-assisted suicide in Oregon—the first year's experience. *N Engl J Med* 1999;340:577–583.

21. Emanuel EJ, Fairclough DL, Daniels ER, et al. Euthanasia and physician-assisted suicide: attitudes and experiences among oncology patients, oncologists, and the general public. *Lancet* 1996;347:1805–1810.

22. Emanuel EJ, Daniels ER, Fairclough DL, et al. The practice of euthanasia and physician-assisted suicide in the United States: adherence to proposed safeguards and effects on physicians. *JAMA* 1998;280:507–513.

23. Back AL, Wallace JI, Starks HE, et al. Physician-assisted suicide and euthanasia in Washington state: patient requests and physician responses. *JAMA* 1996;275:919–925.

24. Griffiths J, Bood A, Weyers H. *Euthansia and the law in the Netherlands.* Amsterdam: Amsterdam University Press, 1998.

25. van der Maas PJ, can der Wal G, Haverkate I, et al. Euthanasia, physician-assisted suicide, and other medical practices involving the end of life in the Netherlands, 1990–1995. *N Engl J Med* 1996;335:1699–1705.

26. van der Maas PJ, van Delden JJM, Pijnenborg L, et al. Euthanasia and other medical decisions concerning the end of life. *Lancet* 1991;338:669–674.

27. Tulsky JA, Alpers A, Lo B. A middle ground on physician-assisted suicide. *Cambridge Q Healthcare Ethics* 1996;5:33–43.

28. Emanuel LL. Facing requests for physician-assisted suicide: toward a practical and principled clinical skill set. *JAMA* 1998;280:643–647.

29. Quill TE. Doctor, I want to die. Will you help me? *JAMA* 1993;270:870–873.

30. Block SD, Billings JA. Patient requests to hasten death: evaluation and management in terminal care. *Arch Intern Med* 1994;154:2039–2047.

31. Muskin PR. The request to die: role for a psychodynamic perspective on physician-assisted suicide. *JAMA* 1998;279:323–328.

32. Hirschfeld RMA, Russell JM. Assessment and treatment of suicidal patients. *N Engl J Med* 1997;337:910–915.

33. Lo B, Quill T, Tulsky J. Discussing palliative care with patients. *Ann Intern Med* 1999;130:744–749.

34. Bachman JG, Alcser KH, Doukas DJ, et al. Attitudes of Michigan physicians and the public toward legalizing physician-assisted suicide and voluntary euthanasia. *N Engl J Med* 1996;334:303–309.

ANNOTATED BIBLIOGRAPHY

1. Quill TE, Cassel CK, Meier DE. Care of the terminally ill: proposed clinical criteria for physician-assisted suicide. *N Engl J Med* 1992;327:1380–1384.
   Proposes circumstances in which assisted suicide would be ethically permissible.

2. Pellegrino ED. Doctors must not kill. *J Clin Ethics* 1992;3:95–102.
   Eloquent summary of reasons for opposing assisted suicide and active euthanasia.

3. Alpers A, Lo B. Physician-assisted suicide in Oregon: a bold experiment. *JAMA* 1995;274:483–487.
   Describes the Oregon law legalizing physician-assisted suicide and analyzes the ethical and practical problems in implementing the law.

4. Quill TE. Doctor, I want to die. Will you help me? *JAMA* 1993;270:870–873.
   Emanuel LL. Facing requests for physician-assisted suicide: toward a practical and principled clinical skill set. *JAMA* 1998;280:643–647.

Suggestions for how doctors can respond when terminally ill patients request physicians to hasten their death. These papers are by a proponent and opponent of physician-assisted suicide, respectively.

5. Meier DE, Emmons CA, Wallenstein S, et al. Physician-assisted death in the United States: a national prevalence survey. *N Engl J Med* 1998;338:1193–1201.

6. Emanuel EJ, Daniels ER, Fairclough DL, et al. The practice of euthanasia and physician-assisted suicide in the United States: adherence to proposed safeguards and effects on physicians. *JAMA* 1998;280:507–513.

Well-designed empirical studies elucidating the practice of physician-assisted suicide and active euthanasia in the United States, despite legal prohibitions.

20

Tube and Intravenous Feedings

Tube and intravenous feedings can prolong life in patients who cannot take adequate nutrition by mouth. However, in severe, progressive illness such as advanced dementia or metastatic cancer, tube and intravenous feedings may merely prolong the process of dying and subject patients to indignity.

CASE 20.1. TUBE FEEDINGS IN A PATIENT WITH SEVERE DEMENTIA (1). *The phone message from the patient's daughter is ominous. "Mrs. F. has eaten nothing all weekend. What should we do?" A 70-year-old woman with severe dementia, Mrs. F. rarely speaks, is confined to a wheelchair, and requires diapers for incontinence. She has been kept out of a nursing home by the efforts of a devoted family and daily attendance at a geriatric day care center. During the past year, her social actions have decreased, and her food intake has become increasingly erratic. First, she stopped feeding herself. Now, although her family feeds her by hand, her intake continues to decline. Once she required overnight hospitalization for dehydration. During the past week, she has been clamping her mouth shut, pushing the spoon away with her hand, and spitting out food. Over the weekend, even coaxing with her favorite foods was unsuccessful. Those who care for her must now face a dreaded question: If hand feedings continue to fail, should she be fed through a feeding tube? The situation evokes strong and conflicting reactions. The patient's sister says, "We can't let her starve to death!" The daughter, however, says, "She's telling us to stop. We're just torturing her."*

This chapter discusses the reasons for providing or withholding tube and intravenous feedings in severe, progressive illness. Tube and intravenous feedings should be considered medical interventions whose benefits and burdens need to be assessed for each individual patient.

DEFINING THE GOALS OF CARE

Tube and intravenous feedings can accomplish different goals of care. They may permit reversible problems to be treated, prolong life, or provide comfort.

Allowing Physicians to Identify and Treat Causes of Feeding Problems

Decreased oral intake may result from medical problems, such as intercurrent illness, mouth lesions, or side effects of medications. Feeding problems may also be caused by psychosocial problems, such as a desire for more control, depression, or a change of caregivers. Sometimes refusals to eat can be addressed by making hand feedings more acceptable to the patient. The caregiver can slow the pace of feeding, offer smaller bites, alter the taste or consistency, remind the demented patient to swallow, or gently touch the patient (1,2). Temporary use of tube or intravenous feedings may resolve the crisis and allow the underlying problem to be identified and treated.

Prolonging Life

Many patients with irreversible feeding problems, such as patients with head and neck cancer or short bowel syndrome, may want their lives prolonged with long-term artificial nutrition.

Providing Comfort and Alleviating Symptoms

For patients who are fully conscious but unable to take food by mouth, such as some patients with head and neck cancer, tube feedings may relieve symptoms of hunger and thirst.

REASONS TO PROVIDE TUBE AND INTRAVENOUS FEEDINGS

Withholding Tube and Intravenous Feeding Would Starve People to Death

Many people are horrified at not feeding patients with severe dementia or metastatic cancer who are unable to maintain oral intake. If tube and intravenous feedings are withheld, they fear such patients may suffer from thirst or hunger. Everyone has temporarily experienced these distressing sensations and can imagine how agonizing it must be to starve to death. Similarly, everyone appreciates how upset infants become when they are not fed. By analogy, advocates of tube feedings conclude that adult patients with terminal illness suffer when feeding tubes are withheld.

Tube and Intravenous Feedings Are Ordinary Care

Some people assert that feeding is ordinary, basic nursing care, not medical treatment. To them, feeding is an essential part of caring for the helpless, just like providing a warm, clean bed. Withholding tube feedings seems as cruel as not changing dirty linens.

Tube and Intravenous Feedings May Be Withheld but Not Withdrawn

Although some physicians and families do not believe that tube feedings must be given in every case, they feel obligated to continue artificial feedings once they have started. They may believe that they have made an implicit promise to the patient or created an expectation that nutritional support will continue. Other physicians would not directly stop artificial fluids or nutrition but are willing to forego restarting an intravenous line if it becomes infiltrated, or to forego reinserting a feeding tube if it is pulled out (3). Finally, some physicians believe that discontinuing tube or intravenous feedings makes them the direct cause of the patient's death.

Tube and Intravenous Feedings Symbolize Caring

In one survey, 16% of physicans agreed that tube feedings are basic humane care (4). One ethicist has declared that feeding the hungry is "the perfect symbol of the fact that human life is inescapably social and communal" (5). Feeding symbolizes concern for helpless people, a sense of community, and interdependence. Tube feedings, then, are a means of expressing compassion, caring, and love.

Withholding Tube and Intravenous Feedings Would Lead to Abuses

Fears of abuses and slippery slopes cause some people to insist on providing artificial feedings. Suppose artificial feedings are withheld in a case in which the reasons seem compelling. Some fear this precedent makes it easier to withhold artificial feedings in another case, even if the reasons are not as convincing. The next patient's family might not be so loving, or the next physician might not be so careful to search for treatable feeding problems. Eventually, artificial feedings might be withheld in cases in which it would previously have been regarded as inappropriate. Similarly, persons with end-stage illness who are "biologically tenacious" and do not die as promptly as expected may be vulnerable to having artificial feedings withheld (5). According to this line of argument, the only way to prevent the loosening of standards is to prohibit the action under all circumstances.

REASONS TO WITHHOLD TUBE AND INTRAVENOUS FEEDINGS

Those who would allow artificial feedings to be withheld from patients with severe, progressive illness object to the images and terms used by proponents. They agree that it is morally obligatory to give bottles to infants, provide groceries to homebound persons, and place spoonfuls of food in the mouth of a person with dementia. Indeed, it is obligatory to continue to offer food and fluids to patients like Mrs. F. in Case 20.1, even though they refuse to eat or they spit out food. However, opponents offer the following reasons for withholding tube feedings from patients like Mrs. F.

Tube and Intravenous Feedings Merely Prolong Dying

Many people believe that tube and intravenous feedings only prolong the process of dying for terminally ill patients. They consider it inhumane to force-feed people with severe dementia or metastatic cancer, only to have them succumb to pneumonia or some other complication. Furthermore, it is problematical to say that withholding artificial feedings causes death in such patients. Determining *a single* cause of death when there are many factors contributing to the patient's death is a controversial philosophical topic (6). Nonetheless, death is usually attributed to the underlying dementia or cancer in such cases, not to forgoing medical interventions, provided that the reasons for withholding treatment are ethically acceptable. Chapter 14 discusses these distinctions in more detail.

Such Patients Do Not Suffer if Tube and Intravenous Feedings Are Withheld

Patients with severe dementia or metastatic cancer do not suffer thirst or hunger if they continue to refuse oral intake (7). In a comfort care unit, almost all such patients reduced intake of food and fluids, less than their nutritional needs. About two-thirds never experienced hunger, while about one-third experienced hunger only initially. Symptoms of thirst or dry mouth were more common, with 36% experiencing them until death. In all patients, symptoms of hunger and dry mouth were relieved with small intake of food and fluids, ice chips, and meticulous mouth care (8). With reduced oral intake, symptoms such as nausea, vomiting, edema, cough, and incontinence are reduced (2). Furthermore, pain medications should be given if needed, just as they are provided to patients with respiratory failure who decline mechanical ventilation.

Tube and Intravenous Feedings Cannot Be Considered Ordinary Care

Labeling artificial feedings as "ordinary" care is questionable. To begin with, it is historically inaccurate. Cessation of the desire for food and drink is part of the natural history of severe illnesses such as severe dementia or metastatic cancer. In other Western societies, such as the United Kingdom and Sweden, tube feedings are rarely administered to patients with severe dementia (9). In addition, long-term intravenous or nasogastric tube feedings have become technically possible only in the past 20 years. The Food and Drug Administration regulates artificial feedings as drugs and medical devices, not as foods. Furthermore, feeding gastrostomy or jejunostomy tubes require a surgical or endoscopic procedure for insertion.

More fundamentally, most writers on medical ethics and virtually all court decisions reject the distinction between "extraordinary" and "ordinary" care (10–12). The issue is not whether an intervention can be considered "extraordinary" or "ordinary," but whether its benefits outweigh its burdens for the individual patient (11). As with other interventions, tube and intravenous feedings should not be provided simply because they are technically feasible or may prolong life. Chapter 14 analyzes these issues in further detail.

Tube and Intravenous Feedings Have Burdens and Benefits

Tube and intravenous feedings have burdens as well as benefits, just like any other intervention. For patients with severe dementia or metastatic cancer, the benefits may be limited. Few such patients are able to discontinue tube feedings because treatable conditions have been found and corrected (13). In addition, the burdens of tube feedings may be substantial. In one study of tube feedings in a nursing home, the stated goal of care was patient comfort in 38% of cases (13). However, feeding tubes may cause distress rather than comfort. Restraints were applied in over 50% of patients to prevent them from pulling out their feeding tubes. Patients who pull out feeding tubes may be communicating refusal, expressing discomfort or anger, seeking attention or control, or acting in a purely reflexive manner.

Restraining demented patients to prevent them from pulling out tubes compromises their independence and dignity, particularly because they cannot appreciate how the feeding tube will help them (1). Restraints also increase patient agitation. Sedation or "chemical restraint," which might appear to be more acceptable, also compromises patient dignity. Patients may not want to be restrained. In a study of nursing home residents, 33% said they wanted tube feedings if they were unable to eat because of permanent brain damage that also left them unable to recognize people. However, after learning that physical restraints are sometimes applied to patients receiving tube feedings, 25% of residents who initially wanted tube feedings or were not sure changed their minds and preferred not to have them (14).

Tube feedings may not reduce the risk of aspiration pneumonia, which has been reported to occur in 47% in patients with feeding tubes (15). Aspiration pneumonia appears to be as common with gastrostomy tubes as with nasogastric tubes (16).

Withdrawing Interventions May Be Appropriate

If interventions are not wanted by patients or not in their best interests, it is as appropriate to discontinue them as not to start them in the first place, as discussed in Chapter 14.

Care Should Be Provided Directly, not Through Symbols

If the goal of care is to provide comfort and compassion, caregivers should do so directly (1). Ironically, artificial feedings may be impersonal. With tube feedings, the caregiver may focus more attention on technical issues, such as positioning the feeding tube and checking the residual volume, than on the patient. If tube feedings proceed without complication, social interaction between the caregiver and patient can be minimal. Moreover, the patient has no control over tube feedings except to pull out the tube. In contrast, with hand feedings, patients determine the timing, pace, and even the content of feedings. Patients are in control if they turn away or clamp their mouths shut. Thus hand feedings that provide inadequate nutrition may meet more of the patient's human needs than tube feedings that deliver adequate calories impersonally.

Sometimes tube and intravenous feedings are used in a purely symbolic fashion. For instance, physicians may order intravenous fluids at a "keep open" rate, which do not provide sufficient fluids to prevent dehydration (3). Such measures serve only to comfort the caregivers, not the patient.

If tube feedings are intended to symbolize compassion and caring, then it might be better to provide comfort measures directly. Simply being with the patient, offering food and water by hand, moistening her mouth, holding her hand, or giving a backrub might be more effective than forcing calories.

Slippery Slope Arguments Are Unpersuasive

Slippery slope arguments shift attention away from the individual patient to future patients or to society as a whole. The patient's family and physicians may assert that the proper focus should be on what is best for the individual patient, not on what precedent is set. The duty of beneficence has traditionally obliged physicians to act for the benefit of the individual patient, not for the benefit of third parties, such as future patients. It seems cruel to impose interventions that are not in the patient's best interests to protect other people from harm. A better approach would be to develop adequate safeguards to protect other patients.

Another rebuttal to slippery slope arguments is empirical: there is little evidence that feeding tubes are withheld in acute care hospitals for inappropriate reasons. Furthermore, in other countries, such as the United Kingdom and Sweden, withholding tube feedings from severely demented patients has not led to inappropriate withholding of care in other situations.

A final problem with slippery slope objections is that they also apply to withholding any form of life-sustaining intervention. Singling out artificial feedings as leading to a slippery slope implicitly assumes that they differ in significant ways from other interventions. As discussed above, this distinction is untenable.

LEGAL ISSUES

According to court decisions, artificial feedings are similar to other medical interventions, which have benefits and burdens for the patient (12,17). The predominant judicial opinion is that artificial feedings are medical interventions that may be withheld under appropriate circumstances, not comfort measures that must always be given.

Several states have living will statutes that preclude patients from refusing artificial nutrition through a living will. However, artificial nutrition may still be withheld if a patient who lacks decision-making capacity has provided clear and convincing evidence that she would not want tube feedings.

CLINICAL RECOMMENDATIONS

When patients with conditions such as severe dementia stop eating and cannot be fed by hand, physicians and surrogates need to discuss the goals of care as well as the benefits and burdens of tube feedings. Decisions are difficult when patients have not provided advance directives. If there are reversible problems that impair oral intake, temporary intravenous or tube feedings are appropriate. Long-term tube feedings are appropriate if the patient has no irreversible life-threatening problems and would consider her quality of life acceptable. However, tube feedings are not indicated if the patient has irreversible life-threatening medical problems and a poor quality of life, and a caring surrogate agrees that the goal should be to provide comfort rather than prolong life.

Many cases will fall into a gray zone. A trial of tube feedings may be helpful. If they are well tolerated, the benefits probably outweigh the burdens. If the patient repeatedly pulls out a nasogastric tube, the goals need to be reconsidered. If prolonging life is still deemed the goal, a feeding gastrostomy or jejunostomy would be appropriate. Such tubes are less obtrusive than nasogastric tubes and more difficult to remove. Tying the patient down or sedating her to keep the tube in place is difficult to reconcile with the goal of providing humane care (1). Instead, it might be appropriate to withhold tube feedings. Although food and water should still be offered by hand, compassion and comfort are probably better expressed through direct attention and affection than by forced feedings.

REFERENCES

1. Lo B, Dornbrand L. Guiding the hand that feeds: caring for the demented elderly. *N Engl J Med* 1984;311: 402–404.
2. Billings JA. Comfort measures for the terminally ill: is dehydration painful? *J Am Geriatr Soc* 1985;33:808–810.
3. Micetich KE, Steinecker PH, Thomasma DC. Are intravenous fluids morally required for a dying patient? *Arch Intern Med* 1983;243:975–980.
4. Hodges MO, Tolle SW, Stocking C, et al. Tube feedings: internists' attitudes regarding ethical obligations. *Arch Intern Med* 1994;154:1013–1020.
5. Callahan D. On feeding the dying. *Hastings Center Rep* 1983;13:22.
6. Brock D. Forgoing life-sustaining food and water: is it killing? In: Lynn J, ed. *By no extraordinary means* (expanded edition). Bloomington: Indiana University Press, 1989:117–131.
7. Sullivan RJ. Accepting death without artificial nutrition and hydration. *J Gen Intern Med* 1993;8:220–224.
8. McCann RM, Hall WJ, Groth-Juncker A. Comfort care for terminally ill patients: the appropriate use of nutrition and hydration. *JAMA* 1994;272:1263–1266.
9. Norberg A, Norberg B, Gippert H, et al. Ethical conflicts in long-term care of the aged: nutritional problems and the patient-care worker relationship. *BMJ* 1980;1:377–378.
10. Steinbrook R, Lo B. Artifical feedings: solid ground, not slippery slope. *N Engl J Med* 1988;318:286–290.
11. President's Commission for the Study of Ethical Problems in Medicine and Biomedical and Behavioral Research. *Deciding to forego life-sustaining treatment.* Washington: US Government Printing Office, 1983:82–89.
12. Meisel A. A retrospective on Cruzan. *Law Med Health Care* 1992;20:340–353.
13. Quill TE. Utilization of nasogastric feeding tubes in a group of chronically ill, elderly patients in a community hospital. *Arch Intern Med* 1989;149:1937–1941.
14. O'Brien LA, Siegert EA, Grisso JA, et al. Tube feeding preferences among nursing home residents. *J Gen Intern Med* 1997;12:364–371.
15. Ciocon JO, Sliverstone FA, Graver LM, et al. Tube feedings in elderly patients. *Arch Intern Med* 1988;148:429–443.
16. Finucane TE, Christmas C, Travis K. Tube feeding in paients with advanced dementia. *JAMA* 1999;282:1365–1370.
17. Meisel A. *The right to die*, 2nd ed. New York: John Wiley & Sons, 1995:592–608.

ANNOTATED BIBLIOGRAPHY

1. Lo B, Dornbrand L. Guiding the hand that feeds: caring for the demented elderly. *N Engl J Med* 1984;311:402–404.
   Argues that tube feedings may not be appropriate for severely demented patients who refuse feedings by hand, particularly if patients are tied down to prevent them from pulling out the tubes.
2. Gillick MM. Rethinking the role of tube feeding in patients with advanced dementia. *N Engl J Med* 2000; 342:206–210.
   Finucane TE, Christmas C, Travis K. Tube feeding in paients with advanced dementia. *JAMA* 1999;282:1365–1370.
   These two articles argue that tube feedings should be discouraged in patients with advanced dementia.

21

The Persistent Vegetative State

Patients in the persistent vegetative state (PVS) are alive because their hearts are beating and they are breathing. However, they are not alive in the broader senses of the term: they are not aware of their environment and cannot respond to other people or communicate with them. Although PVS is uncommon, the cases of Karen Ann Quinlan and Nancy Cruzan, patients in PVS, dramatized fundamental questions about the goals of medicine and the definition of human life.

This chapter describes the clinical features of PVS, discusses some of the philosophical quandaries it presents, and analyzes appropriate justifications for limiting life-prolonging interventions for patients in this condition.

CLINICAL FEATURES

Definition of Vegetative State

Patients in a vegetative state have no cortical function but preserved brainstem function. As far as can be determined, they are unconscious, with no awareness of their environment (1). They show no purposeful activity and cannot obey verbal commands. Because their cortical structures have been destroyed, they cannot experience pain. However, it is important for physicians and family members to appreciate that some neurological functions are maintained. "Vegetative" functions, such as breathing and circulation, remain intact. Thus patients in a vegetative state usually do not require mechanical ventilation. In addition, these patients are not comatose because they have cycles of sleeping and waking. While awake, their eyes may be open. Roving eye movements are present, and tracking may occasionally occur. Reflexes such as sucking, chewing, and swallowing may also be present. Pupillary, oculocephalic, and deep tendon reflexes are sometimes preserved. Patients may withdraw or posture in response to noxious stimuli and startle and turn in the direction of sudden loud noises. Such patients may grunt, grimace, smile, and have tears. Because of these preserved neurological functions, some observers believe that patients in a vegetative state are aware of the surroundings or have responded to them. Some observers may claim that the patient watched them cross the room or cried when they talked to them. These "responses," however, cannot be replicated in any consistent manner at other times or by other observers.

The diagnosis of a vegetative state requires repeated examinations by an experienced neurologist. The diagnosis is clinical, and diagnostic tests are not essential. Positron emission tomography scans in patients in a PVS show low brain metabolism, similar to what is seen in patients under general anesthesia.

Definition of Persistent Vegetative State

A PVS is defined as a vegetative state that has lasted for 1 month (1). In the United States, about 10,000 to 25,000 adults and 4,000 to 10,000 children are in a PVS (1). A crucial issue is determining when a PVS has become permanent.

Prognosis for recovery of consciousness can be accurately established only after the patient has been in a vegetative state for some time (1). The required time of observation will depend on the etiology. After nontraumatic injury, such as anoxic brain damage during a cardiac arrest, very few patients awaken after 3 months. After trauma, patients rarely awaken after 12 months in a vegetative state.

No intervention has been shown to be effective in restoring consciousness. Cases of late recovery of consciousness by patients in a PVS have been reported (2). In a few well-documented cases, however, patients in true PVS have recovered consciousness more than 3 months after anoxic injury or more than 12 months after traumatic injury (1). Patients who recover consciousness have moderate or severe residual neurological impairments.

The mean survival of patients in a PVS is 2 to 5 years. A few patients have been reported to survive longer than 15 years. Patients in a PVS require tube feedings because they are unable to swallow and protect their airway. They are incontinent and require total nursing care. Common complications include decubitus ulcers, aspiration pneumonia, and urosepsis.

PVS needs to be distinguished from other catastrophic neurological conditions. In *brain death*, there is neither cortical nor brainstem function (*see* Chapter 22). Thus the electroencephalogram (EEG) shows no activity. In the *locked-in syndrome*, patients are conscious but have no motor function. Such patients may be able to communicate by blinking their eyes. Patients with *severe dementia* may be virtually unresponsive. However, they are conscious and may have some motor function.

WHAT TREATMENT IS APPROPRIATE?

To many persons, the prospect of being kept alive when there is no likelihood of regaining consciousness is abhorrent. To them, life as a "vegetable" is not really living and may seem a fate worse than death. Many health care workers and family members of patients in a PVS question whether it is appropriate to keep such persons alive by tube feedings and other medical interventions.

On other hand, some people believe that persons in a PVS should receive life-prolonging interventions. Some family members reject the diagnosis that the patient is unconscious, claiming that the patient responds to them. Others reject the prognosis, believing that the patient will recover despite unfavorable odds. Still others believe a life without consciousness is still sacred and that quality of life judgments invite discrimination.

Within these disputes, however, there are certain areas of general agreement.

Medical Interventions May Be Withheld or Withdrawn

Ethical guidelines regarding patients who lack decision-making capacity should be followed. Interventions ranging from cardiopulmonary resuscitation to antibiotics for infection may be withheld, based on advance directives or decisions by appropriate surrogates (1). It is worth noting how a consensus has developed since the Karen Ann Quinlan case (*see* Chapter 23). In that case, the issue was whether to discontinue a ventilator. (At the time, doctors did not know that patients in a PVS do not require ventilatory assistance.) In recent cases, decisions to withhold CPR or antibiotics from patients in a PVS were not challenged. More recent discussions have focused on whether feeding tubes should be regarded differently from other medical interventions.

Tube Feedings Are a Medical Intervention, Which May Be Withheld or Withdrawn

As Chapter 14 discusses, it is permissible to withhold or withdraw tube feedings from persons in a PVS, provided that such decisions are consistent with the patient's prior directives or best interests (1,3,4). Feeding tubes have benefits and burdens that must be assessed for the individual patient. They should not be considered "ordinary" nursing care that must always be provided. In practice, many people are ambivalent about tube feedings in PVS. In a survey of neurologists, 88% believed that it is ethical to forego artificial nutrition in PVS; however, 47% also believed that generally artificial nutrition should be provided. Despite extensive clinical evidence that patients in a PVS lack the cortical capacity to be conscious of pain (1), 25% of neurologists believed that patients in a vegetative state experience feelings of pain, and 22% believed that such patients are more comfortable with tube feedings (5).

A more radical and controversial position is that all medical interventions should be withheld or withdrawn from patients in a PVS. In this view, it is not merely *permissible* to withdraw tube feedings from patients in a PVS, but *mandatory* to do so. Several arguments are offered to support this position (6,7). First, patients with a PVS cannot receive any benefit from feeding tubes or any other medical intervention, because consciousness is a prerequisite for having interests, or receiving benefit from medical interventions. Second, patients in a PVS have lost the essential characteristics of being human, including social interactions with other people and the ability to respond or reason. In this view, it is pointless to prolong mere biological existence when there is no hope of regaining these primary human qualities. Many people, however, particularly those holding "right to life" views, reject these arguments. In addition, many philosophers contend that people can receive benefit or be harmed even if they are not aware of it (8).

Controversies over interventions in a PVS are not technical issues to be decided solely by physicians. Value judgments about the definition of a human being are unavoidable. Ultimately these issues are not susceptible to logical proof or refutation. They can be resolved only by appealing to deeply personal or religious beliefs. One of the most divisive aspects of debates over appropriate care of patients in a PVS is that these beliefs may lead people to strikingly different conclusions.

In summary, physicians need to understand the clinical features of PVS and the criteria for diagnosing it. Many ethical dilemmas regarding PVS can be resolved by applying guidelines for decisions in patients who lack decision-making capacity. It is permissible to withdraw feeding tubes and other interventions in accordance with advance directives or decisions by appropriate surrogates.

REFERENCES

1. The Multi-Society Task Force on PVS. Medical aspects of the persistent vegetative state. *N Engl J Med* 1994;330:1499–1508, 1572–1579.
2. Childs NL, Mercer WN. Late improvement in consciousness after post-traumatic vegetative state. *N Engl J Med* 1996;334:24–25.
3. President's Commission for the Study of Ethical Problems in Medicine and Biomedical and Behavioral Research. *Deciding to forego life-sustaining treatment.* Washington: US Government Printing Office, 1983.
4. Council on Scientific Affairs and Council on Ethical and Judicial Affairs. Persistent vegetative state and the decision to withdraw or withhold life support. *JAMA* 1990;263:426–430.
5. Payne K, Taylor RM, Stocking C, et al. Physicians' attitudes about the care of patients in the persistent vegetative state: a national survey. *Ann Intern Med* 1996;125:104–110.

6. Schneiderman LJ, Jecker NS, Jonsen AR. Medical futility: its meaning and ethical implications. *Ann Intern Med* 1990;112:949–954.
7. Schneiderman LJ, Jecker NS, Jonsen AR. Medical futility: response to critiques. *Ann Intern Med* 1996;125:669–674.
8. Feinberg J. *Harm to others.* New York: Oxford University Press, 1984:79–95.

ANNOTATED BIBLIOGRAPHY

1. The Multi-Society Task Force on PVS. Medical aspects of the persistent vegetative state. *N Engl J Med* 1994;330:1572–1579.
Comprehensive review of clinical features and prognosis.
2. American Neurological Association Committee on Ethical Affairs. Persistent vegetative state: report of the American Neurological Association Committee on Ethical Affairs. *Ann Neurol* 1993;33:386–390.
Excellent recent review of clinical and ethical issues.
3. Payne K, Taylor RM, Stocking C, et al. Physicians' attitudes about the care of patients in the persistent vegetative state: a national survey. *Ann Intern Med* 1996;125:104–110.
Documents widespread misconceptions about PVS among physicians.

22

Determination of Death

Before the development of intensive care, patients were declared dead when breathing and circulation stopped. However, such traditional concepts of death are now problematical because a patient's breathing and circulation can be sustained on life support after all cerebral functions have been permanently lost. Thus criteria for brain death have been developed and are widely accepted. Accurate and consistent determinations of death are essential because declaring a patient dead has profound emotional and practical consequences (1–3). Mourning commences, and funeral services are held. Dead persons are buried or cremated. Their organs may be removed for transplantation. Their spouses may remarry, pensions and health insurance coverage are terminated, their property passes on to heirs, and their life insurance policies are paid. Defining death is controversial because it involves cultural, social, and religious values, as well as scientific judgment. Furthermore, discussions are complicated by frequent misunderstandings about brain death.

This chapter discusses ethical issues regarding traditional, whole-brain, and higher brain criteria for death.

PROBLEMS WITH CARDIOPULMONARY CRITERIA FOR DEATH

Brain function ceases minutes after cessation of heartbeat and breathing in the absence of artificial life support. With the development of intensive care units, however, circulation and breathing can be sustained for months even though the brain has irreversibly ceased to function and the patient will never recover. Most people believe it would be pointless to sustain vital functions in such a situation.

Organ transplantation has also raised ethical issues regarding the declaration of death. Transplantation of vital organs, which is potentially life-saving to recipients, cannot be performed without clear agreement that the organ donor has died. Transplant teams want to retrieve organs as soon as possible. On the other hand, relatives and the public want assurance that organs are not harvested prematurely from persons who are not truly dead.

Disputes about the determination of death may also arise with victims of criminal acts. Some defendants in murder trials have contended that the victim's death was caused by discontinuation of life-sustaining treatment, not by their actions (4).

Because of these problems with traditional cardiopulmonary criteria for death, the concept of brain death was developed.

THE CONCEPT OF BRAIN DEATH

Patients who have permanently lost all brain function are considered dead, even though their circulation and breathing were supported by medical technology. Brain death is defined as irreversible loss of functioning in the entire brain, both cortex and brainstem. This is also called whole-brain death. Brain death is tantamount to "permanent cessation of the functioning of the organism as a whole" (5). Because the brain is the coordinating and integrating center of the body, death of the brain ensures that the organism as a whole can no longer function. Destruction of the brain generally leads to cessation of spontaneous cardiac function within a week (6).

Currently, the clinical tests for brain death include coma, absence of brainstem function, and apnea (7). Potentially reversible, confounding causes of coma, such as drug overdose or hypothermia, must be ruled out. Circulation and spinal cord reflexes may be intact in brain death. Confirmatory testing with an electroencephalogram (EEG) or angiography may be helpful but is not required. In children, the determination of brain death is more complicated because prognosis is more difficult to establish (8,9).

In recent years, these criteria for brain death have been called into question. In some brain-dead patients, there may be persistence of some cerebral blood flow, oxygen and glucose metabolism, EEG activity, brainstem evoked potentials, and secretion of antidiuretic hormone (10). In exceptional cases, there may be substantial discrepancy between determinations of death using brain death criteria and traditional cardiopulmonary criteria. Several pregnant women meeting brain death criteria had their vital functions sustained for months until the fetus could be delivered (11).

CONTROVERSIES REGARDING BRAIN DEATH

A recent survey showed widespread confusion over brain death (12). Only 35% of physicians who were responsible for declaring death were able to identify irreversible loss of all brain function as the criterion for determining death and apply it to simple case vignettes. Among other health care workers involved in the care of persons declared brain dead, over 70% were unable to identify the legal and medical criteria for brain death. When asked to explain their personal opinions about two case vignettes, 58% of all respondents did not use a coherent concept of death consistently. Fully 36% believed that it was appropriate to retrieve organs from a patient in a vegetative state who does not meet criteria for whole-brain death.

Whole-brain death criteria have been criticized for being both too narrow and too inclusive. These controversies illustrate the impact of cultural, social, and religious values on the definition of death.

Higher Brain Death

Some writers criticize the whole-brain definition of death because it regards as alive individuals in a persistent vegetative state (PVS), who have no cortical function and therefore no consciousness or cognition. Such patients are considered alive according to whole-brain criteria because they have intact brainstem function. These critics argue that qualities such as a "will of its own, awareness of actions, or reactive feelings" characterize living human beings (13). Under a "higher brain" or neocortical definition of death, individuals with irreversible loss of function in the cerebral cortex would be considered dead.

Higher brain criteria for death, however, are rejected by most writers (14). Reliable clinical tests for higher brain death are not available. Slippery slopes are also a concern: would severely demented patients be considered dead by a higher brain standard? The concept of higher brain death seems to confuse what it means to be a person with what it means to be alive. It may be appropriate to say that individuals without cortical function are no longer persons in the philosophical sense of having rights and interests. However, it does not follow logically that they should be considered dead. Finally, higher brain criteria contradict deeply held beliefs about death. Burying or cremating an individual who is still breathing and has a pulse seems intuitively wrong.

Rejection of the Concept of Brain Death

Some persons reject the concept of brain death for religious or philosophical reasons (15,16). For example, some orthodox Jews, Native Americans, and Japanese believe that a person is alive until he or she literally stops breathing (17). No distinction is made between mechanical ventilation and spontaneous breathing. In this view, a person on a ventilator who meets the standards for brain death is not dead.

Legal Status of Brain Death

Most states have adopted the Uniform Determination of Death Act. It declares, "Any individual who has sustained either (1) irreversible cessation of circulatory and respiratory functions, or (2) irreversible cessation of all functions of the entire brain, including the brain stem, is dead. A determination of death must be made in accordance with accepted medical standards" (4). Thus a person may be declared dead if he or she meets either cardiopulmonary criteria (absence of breathing and pulse) or brain death criteria. For the vast majority of patients who are not on life support, these two criteria are equivalent.

New Jersey authorizes the declaration of brain death, except in cases in which the physician has "reason to believe" that "such a declaration would violate the personal religious beliefs of the individual" (18). For such individuals, death must be declared according to traditional cardiorespiratory criteria. Similarly, New York requires "reasonable accommodation of the individual's religious or moral objection" to brain death criteria (19).

PRACTICAL SUGGESTIONS REGARDING BRAIN DEATH

Consultation from an experienced neurologist should be obtained before a patient is declared brain dead. Once the determination of brain death has been made, relatives need to be told. Such discussions require sensitivity and patience. Some family members may believe the patient will regain consciousness, particularly if the death was sudden or unexpected. In almost all cases, compassionate explanations and emotional support from health care workers help the family accept the situation.

If organ transplantation is feasible, death should be declared by a physician not associated with the transplantation team, to avoid even the appearance of conflict of interest (20,21). Discussion of the possibility of organ donation with the survivors wait until after the declaration of death, unless the family first raises the issue.

After a patient has been declared dead by brain death criteria, all life-sustaining interventions should be discontinued, with certain exceptions. Maintaining life support may be appropriate until family members can come to the hospital, until organs for transplantation can be harvested or, under exceptional circumstances, until a fetus can be delivered.

In summary, the development of intensive care and organ transplantation has made traditional definitions of death untenable in some cases. Physicians need to understand the clinical criteria for brain death and controversies regarding the concept. Ultimately the definition of life and death depends on cultural, social, and religious beliefs as well as medical expertise.

REFERENCES

1. Charo RA. Dusk, dawn, and defining death: legal classifications and biological categories. In: Youngner SJ, Arnold RM, Schapiro R, eds. *The definition of death*. Baltimore: Johns Hopkins University Press, 1999:277–292.
2. Veatch RM. An ethical framework for terminal care decisions. *J Am Geriatr Soc* 1984;32:665–669.
3. Burt RA. Where do we go from here? In: Youngner SJ, Arnold RM, Schapiro R, eds. *The definition of death*. Baltimore: Johns Hopkins University Press, 1999:332–339.
4. Defining death. In: Furrow BR, Johnson SH, Jost TS, Schwartz RL, eds. *Health law: cases, materials, problems*. St. Paul, MN: West Publishing, 1991:1034–1055.
5. Bernat JL. How much of the brain must die in brain death? *J Clin Ethics* 1992;3:21–26.
6. Plum F, Posner JB. *The diagnosis of stupor and coma*, 3rd ed. Philadelphia: FA Davis, 1980.
7. Wijdicks EFM. Determining brain death in adults. *Neurology* 1995;45:1003–1011.
8. Task Force for the Determination of Brain Death in Children. Guidelines for the determination of brain death in children. *Pediatrics* 1987;80:298–300.
9. Mejia RE, Pollack MM. Variability in brain death determination practices in children. *JAMA* 1995;274:550–553.
10. Halevy A, Brody B. Brain death: reconciling definitions, criteria, and tests. *Ann Intern Med* 1993;119:519–525.
11. Field DR, Gates EA, Creasy RK, et al. Maternal brain death during pregnancy: medical and ethical issues. *JAMA* 1988;260:816–822.
12. Youngner SJ, Landefeld CS, Coulton CJ, et al. "Brain death" and organ retrieval: a cross-sectional survey of knowledge and concepts among health professionals. *JAMA* 1989;261:2205–2210.
13. Youngner SJ, Bartlett ET. Human death and high technology: the failure of whole-brain formulations. *Ann Intern Med* 1983;99:252–258.
14. Lynn J. The determination of death. *Ann Intern Med* 1983;99:264–266.
15. Olick RS. Brain death, religious freedom, and public policy: New Jersey's landmark legislative initiative. *Kennedy Inst Ethics J* 1991;1:275–288.
16. Kimura R. Japan's dilemma with the definition of death. *Kennedy Inst Ethics J* 1991;1:123–131.
17. Youngner SJ, Arnold RM, Schapiro R, eds. *The definition of death*. Baltimore: Johns Hopkins University Press, 1999.
18. The New Jersey Declaration of Death Act, revised statutes 1991 Title 26, Chapter 6A.
19. New York Codes 1987, §400.16(e)(3).
20. Youngner SJ, Allen M, Bartlett ET, et al. Psychosocial and ethical implications of organ retrieval. *N Engl J Med* 1985;313:321–324.
21. Tolle SW, Bennett WM, Hickam DH, et al. Responsibilities of primary physicians in organ donation. *Ann Intern Med* 1987;106:740–744.

ANNOTATED BIBLIOGRAPHY

1. Youngner SJ, Arnold RM, Schapiro R. *The definition of death*. Baltimore: Johns Hopkins University Press, 1999. Collection of essays on current controversies on defining death.
2. Halevy A, Brody B. Brain death: reconciling definitions, criteria, and tests. *Ann Intern Med* 1993;119:519–525. Discusses whole-brain and higher brain formulations of death, emphasizing that patients who satisfy clinical tests for brain death may still have some brain function.
3. Youngner SJ, Landefeld CS, Coulton CJ, et al. "Brain death" and organ retrieval: a cross-sectional survey of knowledge and concepts among health professionals. *JAMA* 1989;261:2205–2210. Survey showing that many health care workers are confused about brain death.

23

Legal Rulings on Life-Sustaining Interventions

Dramatic legal cases regarding life-sustaining interventions have received prominent coverage in the news media. Such landmark court rulings have shaped clinical practice and stimulated people to discuss their preferences for such interventions.

THE QUINLAN CASE

In 1976, the Karen Ann Quinlan case dramatized the dilemma of whether it might be more humane to withdraw life support, rather than prolong life when there was no hope of regaining consciousness (1).

The Case

Karen Ann Quinlan was a 22-year-old woman in a persistent vegetative state (PVS) due to an unknown illness. Her physicians agreed that she would never regain consciousness. She was on mechanical ventilation, and her physicians believed that she would die if the ventilator was withdrawn. Her father, after consulting with his priest and the hospital chaplain, asked that the ventilator be withdrawn. When the physicians refused, he asked the courts to appoint him Karen's legal guardian, with the authority to terminate the ventilator. The Catholic bishops of New Jersey supported his request. However, physicians testified that discontinuing the ventilator "would not conform to medical practices, standards, and traditions" (1).

The Court Ruling

The New Jersey Supreme Court ruled that Karen Ann Quinlan's right to privacy included a right to decline medical treatment and that her father as guardian could exercise this right on her behalf. Her guardian and family should be permitted "to render their best judgment" as to whether she would have chosen herself to decline treatment. The countervailing state interest in protecting life and maintaining the right of physicians to exercise their best judgment "weakens and the individual's right to privacy grows as the degree of bodily invasion increases and the prognosis dims" (1). The court rejected the argument of the physicians that withdrawal of the ventilator was contrary to medical ethics. The ruling noted that the physicians had conceded that in other cases they had "refused to inflict an undesired prolongation of the process of dying on a patient in irreversible condition. . . " (1).

The court held unanimously that if Karen's guardian and family, her attending physician, and a hospital "ethics committee" agreed that "there is no reasonable possibility" of recovering a "cognitive and sapient state," the ventilator may be withdrawn. In advocating hospital ethics committees, the court wrote, "In the real world and in relationship to the momentous decision contemplated, the value of additional views and diverse knowledge is apparent" (1). No party would face any civil or criminal liability for discontinuing the ventilator. The court also declared that generally such decisions need not be brought to court "not only because that would be a gratuitous encroachment upon the medical profession's field of competence, but because it would be impossibly cumbersome."

Implications of the Case

As the first "right to die" case to gain widespread publicity, the Quinlan case had a profound impact on medical ethics.

Public Awareness of Ethical Dilemmas in Medicine

The Quinlan case stimulated discussion about ethical dilemmas regarding life-sustaining interventions. The ruling legitimized the idea that life-sustaining interventions might be inappropriate in some situations.

Decision-Making by Patients, Families, and Physicians

The Quinlan court gave judicial support to decision-making by patients, families, and physicians. Having set general guidelines for making decisions regarding life-sustaining treatment, the ruling rejected routine involvement of the courts in cases about life-sustaining treatment.

Ethics Committees

The Quinlan decision helped stimulate the development of hospital ethics committees. Strictly speaking, the court intended such committees to review prognosis, to ensure that patients like Ms. Quinlan are truly in a PVS. However, the ruling also encouraged physicians and families to use committees to facilitate discussion of the ethical issues raised by such cases.

The Fallibility of Medicine

In hindsight, the Quinlan case makes clear that medical judgments about prognosis are fallible. Her physicians expected her to die after the ventilator was discontinued. In fact, she survived for 10 years in a PVS without ventilatory support. Physicians now understand that most patients in a PVS, having intact brainstem function, breathe without assistance.

THE HERBERT CASE

In 1982, two California physicians were charged with murder for discontinuing mechanical ventilation and intravenous fluids in a patient who remained comatose after a cardiopulmonary arrest (2,3). This case dramatized physicians' worst fears about legal liability for discontinuing life-sustaining interventions.

The Case

Clarence Herbert was a 55-year-old security guard who had an intestinal obstruction requiring an ileostomy. Following surgery to close the ileostomy, he suffered a cardiopulmonary arrest in the recovery room and was resuscitated, but never regained consciousness. Three days after the arrest, the physicians judged his condition "hopeless." His wife and eight children wanted "all machines taken off that are sustaining life." The wishes of the family were consistent with Mr. Herbert's previous statements that he did not want to be kept alive by machines. The physicians and family decided to discontinue the ventilator. After withdrawal, he continued to breathe but remained comatose. Five days after the arrest, the family asked that intravenous fluids be discontinued. Mr. Herbert died 6 days later.

After a heated confrontation with one of the physicians, a nurse brought the case to the attention of the district attorney. The district attorney alleged that the physicians murdered the patient to cover up malpractice and to save money for a health maintenance organization.

The Court Ruling

The ruling dismissed all criminal charges against the physicians. The court decided that discontinuing intravenous fluids was not murder, even though the physicians knew that the patient would die. The ruling rejected the prosecutor's argument that although the ventilator was extraordinary care, intravenous fluids were ordinary care that must be continued. It declared that the benefits of artificial nutrition and hydration for the particular patient should be weighed against the burdens, just as with any other medical intervention. "A treatment course which is only minimally painful or intrusive may nonetheless be considered disproportionate to the potential benefits if the prognosis is virtually hopeless of any significant improvement in condition" (2,3). The court also ruled that stopping a life-sustaining intervention is not equivalent to active euthanasia and that a physician is not obligated to continue an intervention once it has proved ineffective.

The ruling affirmed that competent patients may refuse life-sustaining interventions and that families of incompetent patients may act as surrogate decision-makers. Surrogates should try to follow the patient's wishes. The court ruled that a conversation between the patient and his wife was sufficient to establish those wishes, even though he had not written a "living will." If a patient's wishes are unclear or unknown, his surrogates should be guided by his best interests. In irreversible illness, the surrogate may consider the quality as well as the duration of the patient's life and, in particular, the likelihood of return to "cognitive and sapient" function. The ruling also circumscribed the role of the courts in such cases, saying that guardianship procedures to appoint the family as surrogates and prior judicial approval of decisions to withdraw interventions are not routinely required.

Implications of the Case

Guidelines for Making Decisions

The Herbert ruling affirmed that competent patients or surrogates for incompetent patients may refuse life-prolonging interventions. Families may base their decisions to withhold interventions on an incompetent patient's previously stated wishes or best interests. Physicians and families may make such decisions without involving the courts.

Legal Reassurance about Discontinuing Life-Sustaining Interventions

The ruling rejected criminal liability for decisions to withdraw life-sustaining interventions made in accordance with these guidelines.

Clarification of Terms

The ruling rejected commonly drawn distinctions between ordinary and extraordinary care and between artificial nutrition and hydration and other medical interventions.

The Role of Nurses

The Herbert case illustrates why physicians should seek the agreement of the nursing staff in decisions to withdraw life-sustaining interventions. Doctors should seriously consider nurses' concerns and objections, not merely to avoid legal problems but also to improve the decision-making process.

THE CRUZAN CASE

In the Cruzan case, the U.S. Supreme Court issued its first decision about the "right to die" (4–7). The ruling sparked state and federal legislation to encourage the use of advance directives.

The Case

Nancy Cruzan was a 33-year-old woman who was in a PVS following an automobile accident in 1983. A month after the accident, a feeding gastrostomy tube was inserted. In 1986, realizing that her condition would not improve, her parents asked that the tube feedings be discontinued. Because the state hospital caring for Cruzan insisted on a court order, the case entered the legal system.

A year before her accident, Cruzan told her housemate that she "didn't want to live" as a "vegetable." If she "couldn't do for herself things even halfway, alone not at all, she wouldn't want to live that way and she hoped that her family would know that" (8). Cruzan's parents asked that tube feedings be discontinued because they knew "in our hearts" that she would not want to continue living in her condition (8).

The Missouri Ruling

The 1988 Missouri Supreme Court ruling severely restricted family decision-making on behalf of incompetent patients (4). Life-sustaining interventions could be withheld only with "the most rigid of formalities," such as a living will or a clear and convincing statement that the patient *would not want the specific intervention in that situation.* The court found no reliable evidence that Nancy Cruzan would have specifically refused artificial feedings. It asserted that Missouri's "unqualified" interest in preserving life, regardless of the patient's prognosis, outweighed any rights an incompetent patient might have to refuse treatment.

The U.S. Supreme Court Ruling

By a 5 to 4 vote, the U.S. Supreme Court affirmed the Missouri ruling in 1990 (5). Although competent patients may have a "constitutionally protected liberty interest in refusing unwanted medical treatment," the Court declared that incompetent patients do not have the same right because they cannot exercise it directly. Thus, states may establish "procedural safeguards" governing medical decisions for incompetent patients that are more stringent than requirements for competent patients.

The majority opinion declared that the individual's right to refuse treatment must be balanced against relevant state interests. The Court held that the Constitution allows states to assert an unqualified interest in "the protection and preservation of human life." It ruled that the Constitution also allows states to establish procedures to prevent abuses, to exclude quality of life as a consideration in treatment decisions, and to err on the side of continuing life-sustaining treatment. In short, states may require life-sustaining interventions when there is no clear and convincing evidence that the incompetent patient would refuse it.

The Court also held that, although the Constitution permits states to rely on family decision-making for incompetent patients, it does not mandate that they do so. The decision acknowledged the reasons for turning to close family members in cases like Cruzan's. The majority opinion, however, found "no automatic assurance" that the family's views "will necessarily be the same as the patient's would have been had she been confronted with the prospect of her situation while competent" (5).

The Court recognized that Cruzan's condition would not improve and that the evidence about her preferences suggested that she would not want further tube feedings. "Missouri's requirement of proof in this case may have frustrated the effectuation of the not-fully-expressed desires of Nancy Cruzan," the majority acknowledged. "But the Constitution does not require general rules to work faultlessly; no general rule can" (5).

In dissent, Justice Brennan, joined by justices Marshall and Blackmun, declared that being free of unwanted medical treatment is a fundamental constitutional right that extends to incompetent as well as competent patients and includes refusal of artificial fluid and nutrition. For someone like Nancy Cruzan, no state interest could outweigh this right to refuse treatment. Families or patient-designated surrogates should generally make decisions for incompetent patients. In a separate dissent, Justice Stevens went further, declaring that the Constitution requires that the best interests of the incompetent patient be followed.

The Death of Nancy Cruzan

After the Supreme Court ruling, the Cruzans petitioned the trial court in Missouri to rehear their request to discontinue tube feedings because new witnesses had come forward. One women who worked with Cruzan testified that Cruzan had said that if she were a "vegetable," she would not want to be fed by force or kept alive by machines. Cruzan's attending physician testified that he had changed his mind and was now in favor of stopping her feedings. The state of Missouri withdrew from further court proceedings. In December, the judge authorized removal of Cruzan's tube feedings (9). Pro-life demonstrators kept a vigil outside Cruzan's nursing home. The tube feedings were stopped, and Cruzan died 12 days later.

Implications of the Cruzan Case

State by State Variation

The Supreme Court allows states to impose procedural requirements on decisions about life-sustaining interventions. Physicians therefore need to be familiar with the legal requirements in their states. Unlike Missouri, most states allow family decision-making.

Evidence of Patient Refusal

According to the Cruzan ruling, states may insist on "clear and convincing" evidence that an incompetent patient would refuse life-sustaining treatment. Such standards can be met by written directives or by oral statements that specifically mention the particular intervention and clinical situation being considered. This clear and convincing standard may be so strict that few directives will satisfy it.

The Role of Families

The Supreme Court allowed Missouri to exclude families from decisions regarding life-sustaining interventions for incompetent patients. However, as Chapter 13 discusses, such family decision-making is generally accepted as standard medical practice.

Legislative Responses

The Cruzan ruling spurred legislation to facilitate the use of advance directives. Many states adopted laws specifically allowing patients to appoint health care proxies. The federal Patient Self Determination Act was enacted and took effect in December 1991. Under this law, virtually all hospitals, nursing homes, and health maintenance organizations must give patients written information at the time of admission regarding their right to provide advance directives.

THE PHYSICIAN-ASSISTED SUICIDE CASES

The Cases

Two court cases were brought by competent, terminally ill patients in New York and Washington who wanted to end their lives by taking a lethal dose of medications and by physicians who were willing to write such a prescription. These patients had various terminal illnesses, including cancer, the acquired immunodeficiency syndrome, and emphysema. The plaintiffs asserted that the prohibitions on physician-assisted suicide by these states were unconstitutional.

The Lower Court Rulings

The Second Circuit federal court of appeals ruled that New York State violated the Fourteenth Amendment's guarantee of equal protection by allowing terminally ill patients to hasten death by foregoing life-sustaining treatments, while forbidding other terminally ill patients to hasten death using a prescription for a lethal dose of medication (10). In the Washington case, the Ninth Circuit appeals court decided that physician-assisted suicide was part of a fundamental right to determine the time and manner of one's death, protected by the Fourteenth Amendment's guarantee of liberty (11). In asserting a constitutional right to physician-assisted suicide, these appellate courts equated physician-assisted suicide with refusal of life-sustaining treatment and rejected the double effect rationale for aggressive palliative care (12).

The U.S. Supreme Court Rulings

In 1997, the Supreme Court issued a pair of unanimous rulings, which held that there is no constitutional right to physician-assisted suicide (13,14). Thus the Washington and New York laws prohibiting physician-assisted suicide did not violate the Constitution.

The Supreme Court rejected the conclusion that terminally ill patients had a "fundamental liberty interest" in obtaining physician-assisted suicide. According to the Court, states have legitimate reasons for prohibiting assisted suicide (13). These include preserving human life, preventing suicide, protecting vulnerable groups, protecting the integrity of the medical profession, and avoiding a slippery slope to euthanasia. The Court also ruled that under the Constitution states may permit patients to forego life-sustaining treatment, while prohibiting physician-assisted suicide (14). The Court declared that the distinction between physician-assisted suicide and withdrawal of life-sustaining treatment is important and logical. When the physician withdraws treatment, he intends only to respect the patient's wishes, not to end the patient's life. Moreover, the cause of death is the underlying fatal disease, not the physician's action.

The Court further declared that the Constitution allowed states to prohibit physician-assisted suicide, which intentionally hastens death, while permitting palliative care that may hasten death but is intended to relieve pain (15). According to the Court, the rationale of double effect distinguished the use of high-dose narcotics from euthanasia or assisted suicide. The Court noted that "painkilling drugs may hasten a patient's death, but the physician's purpose and intent is, or may be, only to ease his patient's pain. . . . The law has long used actors' intent or purpose to distinguish between two acts that may have the same result" (15).

Implications of the Cases

These two Supreme Court rulings have important implications for physicians and nurses who care for dying patients (16–18).

The Right to Refuse Life-Sustaining Interventions

While not dealing specifically with this issue, the Court did not question the right of a competent patient to refuse life-prolonging interventions. Thus, these cases illustrate how the ethical and legal debate has moved beyond the right to refuse unwanted interventions.

Improved Access to Palliative Care

The majority opinion concludes that the double effect doctrine provides a rational and constitutional basis for states to allow high-dose narcotics for pain relief in terminally ill patients, while prohibiting assisted suicide. Thus, the majority opinion offers a justification for aggressive palliative care. Three concurring justices go further, suggesting that states are obligated by the Constitution to permit physicians to provide adequate pain relief at the end of life, even if such care leads to unconsciousness or hastens death.

The opinions may help lift legal barriers to palliative care. Many states have laws that restrict the amount of narcotics that can be prescribed or dispensed or sanction investigations of physicians who prescribe high doses of narcotics to terminally ill patients. These measures may conflict with a putative constitutional right to palliative care (16). Such conflicts might be resolved through state legislation. A proposed Model Pain Relief Act protects health care professionals from legal liability if they substantially comply with accepted guidelines for treatment of pain (19). Legislation based on this model could provide a safe harbor for physicians who provide intensive palliative care to their terminally ill patients in accordance with appropriate clinical guidelines.

Support for the Doctrine of Double Effect

The Court strongly supported the doctrine of double effect and emphasized the importance of the physician's intention in evaluating the appropriateness of end-of-life care. As Chapter 14 discusses, the Court's reasoning can provide support for the practice of terminal sedation.

Physicians need to obtain informed consent of patients or surrogates to terminal sedation, and the dose of sedation should be increased only if there is clinical evidence that the patient is suffering. Increasing sedation if the patient appears comfortable and does not have restlessness, tachycardia, tachypnea, or other findings that could reasonably be interpreted as suffering would imply that the physician intended to hasten death and would cross the line from terminal sedation to active euthanasia (16).

The Physician-Assisted Suicide Debate

The Supreme Court noted that "Americans are engaged in an earnest and profound debate about the morality, legality, and practicality of physician-assisted suicide (13)." The Court implied that these issues needed to be resolved through the legislative process, not by the courts. In the meantime, these two important rulings will help shift the focus of the debate from physician-assisted suicide to palliative care.

In summary, landmark court cases have helped shape public policy regarding life-sustaining interventions. Physicians need to know enough about these court rulings to correct misunderstandings by patients and colleagues.

REFERENCES

1. In the matter of Karen Quinlan, 70 N.J. 10, 335 A. 2d 647 (1976).
2. Lo B. The death of Clarence Herbert: withdrawing care is not murder. *Ann Intern Med* 1984;101:248–251.
3. Barber *v.* Superior Court, 195 Cal Rptr. 484, 147 Cal. App. 3d 1054 (1983).
4. Cruzan *v.* Harmon, 760 S.W.2d 408.
5. Cruzan *v.* Missouri Department of Health, 497 U.S. 261, 110 S.Ct. 2841 (1990).
6. Lo B, Rouse F, Dornbrand L. Family decision-making on trial: who decides for incompetent patients? *N Engl J Med* 1990;322:1228–1231.
7. Lo B, Steinbrook R. Beyond the Cruzan case: the U.S. Supreme Court and medical practice. *Ann Intern Med* 1991;114:895–901.
8. Brief for petitioners, Cruzan *v.* Missouri Department of Health.
9. Cruzan *v.* Harmon, No. CV384–9P, Circuit court of Missouri (Mo. Cir. Ct. Jasper County Dec 14, 1990) (Teel, J.).
10. Quill *v.* Vacco, 830 F3d 716 (2nd Cir 1966).
11. Compassion in Dying *v.* Washington, 79 F3d 790 (9th Cir 1966) (en banc).
12. Annas GJ. The promised end—constitutional aspects of physician-assisted suicide. *N Engl J Med* 1996; 335:683–687.
13. Washington *v.* Glucksberg, 117 S.Ct. 2258 (1997).
14. Vacco *v.* Quill, 117 S.Ct. 2293 (1997).
15. Quill *v.* Vacco, 117 S.Ct. 2293 (1997).
16. Alpers A, Lo B. The Supreme Court addresses physician-assisted suicide: can its decisions improve palliative care? *Arch Fam Pract* 1999;8:200–205.
17. Burt RA. The Supreme Court speaks: not assisted suicide but a constitutional right to palliative care. *N Engl J Med* 1997;337:1234–1236.
18. Gostin LO. Deciding life and death in the courtroom. *JAMA* 1997;278:1523–1528.
19. Johnson S. Disciplinary actions and pain relief: analysis of the Pain Relief Act. *J Law Med Ethics* 1996; 24:319–327.

ANNOTATED BIBLIOGRAPHY

1. Meisel A. *The right to die*, 2nd ed. New York: John Wiley & Sons, 1995.
   Comprehensive and lucid treatise on legal rulings on decisions about life-sustaining interventions.
2. Meisel A. A retrospective on Cruzan. *Law Med Health Care* 1992;20:340–353.
   Reviews legal developments after the 1990 Cruzan decision.
3. Burt RA. The Supreme Court speaks: not assisted suicide but a constitutional right to palliative care. *N Engl J Med* 1997;337:1234–1236.
4. Alpers A, Lo B. The Supreme Court addresses physician-assisted suicide: can its decisions improve palliative care? *Arch Fam Pract* 1999;8:200–205.
   These articles discuss the important Supreme Court rulings in the two 1997 physician-assisted suicide cases.

24

Myths About the Law
on Life-Sustaining Interventions

Physicians and laypeople may misunderstand the law regarding life-sustaining interventions. Acting on such misunderstandings, doctors may impose interventions that are medically and ethically inappropriate.

HOW THE LAW WORKS

The law regarding health care comprises statutes, regulations, the U.S. and state constitutions, and rulings by courts on cases brought before them.

Sources of Law

Statutes (or legislation) passed by state legislatures or by the U.S. Congress may regulate issues in medical ethics. For example, states may pass legislation authorizing advance directives, family decision-making for incompetent patients, or confidentiality of medical information. Federal statutes require hospitalized patients to receive information about advance directives, require hospitals to provide emergency care to uninsured patients, and prohibit discrimination based on disability.

Regulations may be issued by governmental agencies. The federal Centers for Disease Control and state departments of health mandate reporting of persons with certain contagious diseases. State agencies may issue regulations regarding the withholding of life-sustaining interventions from nursing home residents. On a local level, municipal or county agencies may issue policies regarding the withholding of cardiopulmonary resuscitation by emergency medical personnel.

State constitutions and the *U.S. Constitution* are also sources of law. For example, some state constitutions explicitly guarantee a right of privacy. Such provisions have been used by courts to overturn legislative restrictions on withholding life-sustaining interventions (1).

Case law, also called common law, is an important source of law regarding life-sustaining interventions. We now discuss case law in more detail.

CASE LAW

The Nature of Case Law

Case law consists of decisions by appellate courts that set legal precedent for similar cases in the future. Strictly speaking, the precedent is only binding in the jurisdiction of the court. For example, a decision by a state supreme court is binding only in that state. In reality, a thoughtful and well-written opinion influences rulings in other jurisdictions as well.

Courts can rule only on cases that are brought to them for trial or appeal. Their decisions depend heavily on the facts and issues in the particular cases that reach them. Thus some issues in clinical ethics have received much more attention by the courts than others. Because many more cases on feeding tubes have reached appellate courts than cases on Do Not Resuscitate (DNR) orders, case law on feeding tubes is far more developed than case law on DNR orders.

In many states, several cases regarding life-sustaining interventions have reached the appellate level, and the common law rules are fairly clear. On the other hand, physicians and their legal advisors may be uncertain about how the courts might rule on some issues.

Uncertainty in Case Law

It is impossible to predict with certainty how the courts will decide a particular case.

The Current Case May Be Distinguished from Precedents

No two cases are identical. The case under consideration may differ from previously decided cases in numerous ways. If the court considers the difference from a previous case to be legally significant, it is said to distinguish the previous cases, and the previous case is therefore not a relevant precedent. For example, a court may distinguish a previous case because the patient's prognosis was different or because evidence of the incompetent patient's previous wishes was different.

There May Be No Precedents

In a given situation, a state may have no previous rulings at that appellate level on the issues raised by the current case. It may be difficult to predict how a court will rule on a "case of first impression."

Legal Precedents May Be Overturned

Although courts pay great respect to legal precedent, they can also overrule precedents that they currently consider erroneous. For example, in New Jersey parts of the 1976 Quinlan decision have subsequently been overturned.

Individual Judges May Have Different Views

Judges exercise discretion and judgment and cannot eliminate their own values from their decisions. Different judges, working from similar facts and legal precedents, may therefore arrive at conflicting legal conclusions.

Absolute certainty is as unrealistic in the law as it is in clinical medicine. Physicians learn to manage uncertainty in clinical medicine. Similarly, doctors must learn to live with legal uncertainty, to take effective steps to reduce it, and to recognize when it may be counterproductive to try to reduce it. For instance, physicians or hospitals may ask the courts to give them legal immunity before they limit life-sustaining interventions. However, the courts are understandably reluctant to give immunity in advance because they cannot know the specifics of care (2).

State by State Variation

The law on life-sustaining interventions differs from state to state. For instance, states have different statutes regarding advance directives and family decision-making for incompetent patients (3,4). In the absence of relevant federal law, state courts may hand down conflicting rulings in similar cases. Indeed, the courts praise such state by state variation, referring to the "laboratory of the states" as a way of "crafting appropriate procedures" for decisions for incompetent patients (5).

It may be difficult for physicians to accept the idea that state laws regarding life-sustaining intervention may differ markedly. The medical profession aims to provide one standard of care to all patients, regardless of where they live (6). Scientific journals and conferences transcend state boundaries. Medical schools, training programs, specialists, and hospitals are accredited nationally.

SPECIFIC MYTHS ABOUT THE LAW ON LIFE-SUSTAINING INTERVENTIONS

Physicians commonly have misconceptions regarding the law on life-sustaining interventions (7,8). Other chapters discussed legal misconceptions regarding advance directives, surrogate decision-making for incompetent patients, artificial nutrition, and high-dose narcotics (*see* Chapters 12 to 14). In this chapter we discuss other misconceptions about the law.

Myth 1: Courts Must Be Involved in Decisions Regarding Incompetent Patients

Some physicians fear that unless they seek court approval, they risk legal liability for withholding life-sustaining treatment. Such fears are particularly strong when patients lack decision-making capacity and have not provided written advance directives. A legal expert notes, ". . . Most courts continually make clear that judicial review [of decisions about life-sustaining treatment] is not routinely required and that review should occur, if at all, in the clinical setting (3)." The courts generally accept determinations by physicians that a patient lacks decision-making capacity and subsequent decisions made by physicians and surrogates (3).

Myth 2: Life-Sustaining Treatment May Be Withheld Only if Patients Are Terminally Ill or Permanently Unconscious

Many appellate cases have involved terminally ill patients or persons in persistent vegetative states (3). Often decisions cite the patient's prognosis as a reason for withholding treatment. For example, the Quinlan ruling commented that "the State's interest contra [withdrawing treatment] weakens and the individual's right to privacy grows as the degree of bodily invasion increases and the prognosis dims" (9).

Some physicians extrapolate this line of reasoning, mistakenly believing that courts will allow life-sustaining treatment to be withheld *only* if the patient is terminally ill or in a persistent vegetative state. However, this interpretation of the law is inaccurate. Courts have allowed treatment to be withheld in numerous cases in which the patient was neither terminally ill nor unconscious (3). These situations include such diverse conditions as bleeding from trauma, gangrene, ventilatory failure, renal failure, cancer, dementia, quadriplegia, and amyotrophic lateral sclerosis.

Myth 3: Physicians May Face Criminal Charges for Providing Appropriate Palliative Care

Courts have repeatedly stated that withholding or withdrawing life-sustaining treatment is not murder or assisted suicide (3,8), yet a handful of physicians have faced criminal charges and served jail sentences as a result of providing end-of-life care. Cases have involved withdrawing life-sustaining interventions, providing opioids to terminally ill patients, and injecting potassium chloride. These cases involved such atypical features as falsification of medical records, severe disagreements with nurses or family members, and withdrawal of mechanical ventilation in a patient receiving neuromuscular blockade (10,11).

Physicians can take several steps to minimize their risk of legal liability in end-of-life care (11). First, they should obtain the concurrence of family members of incompetent patients and the nursing staff to the plan of care. Second, doctors need to document in the medical record the reasons for their decisions. Third, injections of potassium chloride cannot be justified as palliative care and suggest that the physician's intent is to hasten death, rather than to palliate suffering.

The legal system may fail to appreciate the wide range of appropriate doses of opioids in palliative care because of individual patient variation and tolerance (11,12). No dosage can be categorized as inappropriate without consideration of the clinical situation. The ineffectiveness of lower doses of opioids should be clearly documented.

Myth 4: The Most Prudent Legal Advice Is to Continue Treatment

Some physicians and lawyers believe that although there may be some legal risk in withholding life-sustaining interventions, there is no legal risk for continuing them. However, the courts have allowed suits to be brought against physicians who have imposed treatment against the wishes of the patient or surrogate (13).

In summary, physicians may hold misconceptions about the law that make them reluctant to withhold life-sustaining interventions. In reality, the law presents few barriers to physicians doing what is ethically and medically appropriate regarding such interventions.

REFERENCES

1. Corbett *v.* D'Allesandro, 498 So. 2d 368 (Fla. App. 2d Dist, 1986).
2. Annas GJ. Asking the courts to set the standard of emergency care—the case of Baby K. *N Engl J Med* 1994; 330:1542–1545.
3. Meisel A. *The right to die*, 2nd ed. New York: John Wiley & Sons, 1995:218;216–271.
4. Areen J. Advance directives under state law and judicial decisions. *Law Med Health Care* 1991;19:91–100.
5. Cruzan *v.* Missouri Department of Health, 497 U.S. 261, 110 S.Ct. 2841 (1990).
6. Lo B, Steinbrook R. Beyond the Cruzan case: the U.S. Supreme Court and medical practice. *Ann Intern Med* 1991; 114:895–901.
7. Kapp M, Lo B. Legal perceptions and their influence on medical decision making. *Milbank Memorial Q* 1986;64[Suppl]:163–202.
8. Meisel A. Legal myths about terminating life support. *Arch Intern Med* 1991;1551:1497–1502.
9. In the matter of Karen Quinlan, 70 N.J. 10, 335 A. 2d 647 (1976).
10. Lo B. The death of Clarence Herbert: withdrawing care is not murder. *Ann Intern Med* 1984;101:248–251.
11. Alpers A. Criminal act or palliative care: prosecutions involving the care of the dying. *J Law Med Ethics* 1998;26:308–331.
12. Johnson S. Disciplinary actions and pain relief: analysis of the Pain Relief Act. *J Law Med Ethics* 1996; 24:319–327.
13. Annas GJ. Adding injustice to injury: compulsory payment for unwanted treatment. *N Engl J Med* 1992; 327:1885–1887.

SECTION IV

The Doctor–Patient Relationship

25

Overview of the Doctor–Patient Relationship

A strong doctor–patient relationship has many dimensions. Physicians have a fiduciary obligation to act in the best interests of their patients. To this end, technical expertise and sound clinical judgment are essential. Physicians also should help patients make informed decisions about their care by providing clear information and helping them weigh the pros and cons of different alternatives. Physicians should also maintain confidentiality, avoid misrepresentation, and keep promises. Beyond that, patients also want caregivers who have compassion and empathy, who make them feel listened to and cared for. In addition, patients want a primary care physician to guide them through the complicated health care system, coordinating recommendations from different specialists. In addition, patients want access to care and continuity of care. They want to be able to see their physician when they need to, and they want a single physician to help them make crucial decisions over the course of an illness.

In modern medicine, many incentives encourage physicians to adopt an entrepreneurial approach to their work. The danger of regarding medicine as a business is that many standard business practices may conflict with the goals and ideals of medicine (1). Businesspeople can greatly increase their net income through targeting profitable markets, dropping unprofitable services, and using advertising to increase demand for their product (2). These practices are considered acceptable for people who are selling computers or running a restaurant. However, should physicians or health care organizations offer services only to well-insured patients, drop unprofitable services such as primary care, or increase demand for profitable services that offer little or no benefit to patients? To the extent that health care is considered a need or a right, rather than a commodity, such a commercial approach is ethically disturbing.

The chapters in this section discuss specific situations in which the doctor–patient relationship is problematical or difficult. Chapter 26 discusses situations in which physicians refuse to care for patients. Doctors may fear that their own health or safety is jeopardized or consider a patient difficult or obnoxious. Chapter 27 discusses the ethical issues that may arise when patients give gifts to their physicians. Chapter 28 analyzes sexual relationships between physicians and patients and discusses how patients may be harmed by such contact. Chapter 29 suggests how physicians should respond when family members or friends provide unsolicited information about a patient and ask that it be kept secret. Chapter 30 analyzes how clinical research, which is essential for medical progress, also presents risks to patients who participate in studies. The physician who also is a clinical investigator has additional responsibilities to ensure that the potential benefits of research are proportionate to the risks, to inform patients about the study, and to avoid conflicts of interest.

REFERENCES

1. Kassirer JP. Managed care and the morality of the marketplace. *N Engl J Med* 1995;333:50–52.
2. Jonsen AR. Ethics remain at the heart of medicine: physicians and entrepreurship. *West J Med* 1986;144:480–483.

26

Refusal to Care for Patients

Physicians may refuse to care for persons because they believe the threat to their personal safety or economic security is unacceptable. In other situations, physicians may seek to terminate a counterproductive or adversarial doctor–patient relationship. The following case illustrates such a refusal to care for a patient.

CASE 26.1. SURGERY IN AN HIV-INFECTED PATIENT. *A 43-year-old man with asymptomatic human immunodeficiency virus (HIV) infection has fever, right upper quadrant pain, and jaundice and is found to have acute cholecystitis. The surgeons decline to operate, saying that cholecystectomy is not indicated because the patient can be managed medically and because operating on seropositive patients subjects health care workers to an unacceptable risk of lethal illness.*

In Case 26.1, standard treatment for acute cholecystitis is cholecystectomy. Without an operation the patient is likely to experience recurrent episodes of gallbladder disease. The law generally permits physicians to decide which individuals to accept as patients, but it may seem inhumane if sick persons are denied needed medical care because no physician will provide them services. This chapter analyzes whether physicians have an ethical obligation to care for patients who are contagious, violent, uninsured, or uncooperative.

THE CONTEXT OF THE DOCTOR–PATIENT RELATIONSHIP

Ethical Obligations to Care for Patients

Physicians present themselves to the public as helpers of the sick and needy. Doctors have special expertise about illness, which they profess to use for the benefit of patients. The ethical ideal is that patients will receive needed care, even though the physician may find it risky, difficult, or inconvenient. In the beginning of the HIV epidemic, the Surgeon General declared, "Health care in this country has always been predicated on the assumption that somehow, everyone will be cared for, and no one will be turned away. As a physician and an American, I'm proud to be part of a tradition of care that will not abandon the sick or disabled, whoever they are" (1).

In the doctor–patient relationship, the best interests of the patient should take priority over the self-interest of the doctor (*see* Chapter 4). The guideline of beneficence has several important implications for refusals to care for patients. Physicians should not refuse care to patients whom they dislike or find unpleasant. They are urged to continue caring for patients whose actions make treatment more difficult, such as smoking, abusing alcohol, or not taking medications. It would also be ethically objectionable for physicians to refuse care to patients on the basis of social class, ethnic background, lifestyle, or political or religious views. Even in war, physicians are expected to attend to the sick and injured, regardless of which side they are on. Furthermore, physicians are exhorted to provide needed medical care even to patients whom they find morally objectionable. Doctors are expected to provide care to the perpetrator of a violent assault as well as to the victim and to be nonjudgmental about a patient's substance abuse or sexual practices.

This ethical ideal of altruism has limits. In providing care, physicians are not expected to compromise their own moral or religious beliefs. For example, Catholic physicians are not required to perform abortions. Although physicians are urged to tolerate patient behavior they personally consider immoral, they are not obligated to carry out an immoral action requested by the patient. One philosopher has cautioned physicians to distinguish deeply held moral objections from "personal distaste or prejudice" (2). In addition, the physician's own interests and needs cannot be ignored. In Case 26.1, the physicians claim that their ethical obligation to provide care is overridden by serious personal risks.

Legal Definition of the Doctor–Patient Relationship

Society as a whole and individual physicians have a moral obligation to care for sick persons, yet doctors generally have no legal duty to provide care. The law generally characterizes the doctor–patient relationship as a contract between autonomous individuals who are free to enter into or break off the relationship, provided that the patient is not abandoned (3). In the absence of an agreement to provide medical care, such as a contract with a health maintenance organization, there is no doctor–patient relationship. Courts have ruled that generally there is no legal duty for physicians to treat all patients who seek care. For example, it is legal for physicians to have their receptionist schedule new patient appointments only for those people with adequate health insurance. Similarly, physicians may restrict the scope of their practice to a particular specialty or range of problems. Thus an internist would not be expected to perform surgery, and a psychiatrist would not be expected to treat meningitis.

The legal right to decline to care for patients, however, is limited in many important ways. Employment contracts, as with hospitals or health maintenance organizations, may oblige physicians to care for all qualified persons who seek treatment. Similarly, physicians who are on call for a hospital may be required as a condition of staff privileges to provide care to persons who present there. As discussed later in the chapter, emergency departments are required to provide indicated emergency care to patients who seek it.

Antidiscrimination laws may also limit the physician's right to decline to care for patients on the basis of race, sex, national origin, religion, or disability. The Americans with Disabilities Act of 1990 states, "No individual shall be discriminated against on the basis of disability in the full and equal enjoyment of the . . . services [or] facilities" of a hospital or physician's office (4). Physicians and hospitals are not required to provide care when an "individual poses a direct threat to the health or safety of others that cannot be eliminated or reduced by reasonable accommodation" (5). Direct threat means "a significant risk of substantial harm," not merely a "slightly increased risk" or a "speculative or remote risk" (6). The determination of risk must be made according to objective, scientific evidence, not on the subjective judgment of the health care worker. Caring for HIV-infected persons is not considered a "direct threat" to health care workers (6).

OCCUPATIONAL RISKS TO PHYSICIANS

Health care workers may contract serious contagious diseases on the job. They may contract HIV infection if they injure themselves with a needle or other sharp instrument contaminated with the blood of a seropositive patient. Similarly, they may be infected with multidrug-resistant tuberculosis through caring for patients. In addition, angry or psychotic patients may physically threaten or harm health care workers. In one survey, 20% of residents reported that they had been physically assaulted during their training (7). Fearful of these serious occupational risks, physicians may be reluctant to provide care to patients they regard as contagious or violent. Avoiding such patients, however, may conflict with their needs for medical care.

The Risk of Occupational HIV Infection

Epidemiological Studies

The risk of seroconversion after a single percutaneous exposure to the blood of a seropositive patient is 0.3% (8). The transmission rate is lower after mucocutaneous exposures. After mucocutaneous exposure, a few cases of seroconversion in health care workers have been documented, but no such cases have been found in several large prospective studies.

Surgeons and operating room staff are at higher risk for occupational HIV infection than office-based physicians who do not perform invasive procedures. Surgical personnel sustain percutaneous injuries in 1.7% to 6.9% of operations (9,10). If percutaneous exposure occurs, postexposure prophylaxis reduces transmission by 79% (11). It has been estimated that one surgeon or operating room nurse every 8 years will acquire occupational HIV infection in a hospital with a heavy HIV caseload (9).

Perceptions of Risk

The magnitude of a risk is only one component of a person's perception of the risk. People regard familiar and voluntary risks as more acceptable than unfamiliar, involuntary, and uncertain risks, even if the latter are far less likely (12). For example, the risk of death in an automobile accident usually causes less concern than the risk of death in an earthquake or nuclear accident, even though people are more likely to be killed in automobile accidents. The risk of occupational HIV infection seems especially ominous. HIV infection is fatal and can be transmitted to loved ones. Physicians believe that they have no control over the risk because percutaneous exposure can occur despite precautions. The stigma of HIV infection makes the occupational risk even more threatening (13).

Universal Body Fluid Precautions

The Centers for Disease Control and Prevention recommends universal precautions, such as gloves, masks, goggles, and gowns, whenever there is a risk that a health care worker will be exposed to a patient's body fluids (14). Although universal precautions reduce the risk of occupational infection with blood-borne pathogens, such as HIV, hepatitis B, and hepatitis C, they do not eliminate the risk. Gowns and gloves, even double gloves, do not protect against needlesticks and scalpel cuts.

Responding to Occupational Risks

Moral Exhortation

Moral exhortations to provide care in risky situations may go unheeded. In previous epidemics, many physicians, including Galen and Sydenham, fled from patients with fatal contagious diseases (15). Practically speaking, moral exhortation is unlikely to convince health care workers to care for HIV-infected patients. Health care workers may be outraged at the suggestion that it is unethical to worry about their personal safety.

Give Reassurance That the Risk Is Small

A natural response to fears of personal safety is to reassure health care workers that the risk is small. However, reassurance that a risk is low or comparisons with other risks generally do not change people's perceptions of risk (12,16,17). In particular, comparisons that appear to trivialize a risk are counterproductive. People reject the suggestion that because they accept risks of greater magnitude, such as the risk of automobile accidents, they should also accept the risk in question (12).

Although moral exhortation and reassurance are ineffective, the following strategies may be helpful (Table 26-1).

Acknowledge Fears

As physicians, we must acknowledge our human fears and limitations; only then are reflection, discussion, and constructive action possible. Fears about safety need to be acknowledged as an understandable human reaction, not condemned as irrational hysteria (18). Health care workers will benefit from having their concerns addressed in a nonjudgmental way.

Reduce the Occupational Risks

Once fears are acknowledged, health care workers can discuss specific aspects of occupational risk and infection. Hospitals are required to provide a safe working environment, which includes protective equipment and instruments to reduce the risk of blood-borne infections. Health care workers need to learn how to identify potentially violent patients and to take precautions. If health care workers feel threatened, they should keep the door to the examining room open and stay between the patient and the door. If the threat seems more serious, they can ask security guards to stand outside the door.

Balance Risks to Health Care Workers and Benefits to Patients

Health care workers should provide care if the medical benefit to the patient is clearly established, highly probable, and substantial, provided that appropriate precautions have been taken to reduce risk. On the other hand, severe risks to health care workers may justify delaying or denying interventions whose benefits are unproved, uncertain, or marginal.

Judgments about the benefits and risks of treatment need to be scientifically sound. In Case 26.1, it would be misleading for physicians to say that cholecystectomy for acute cholecystitis is not indicated in seropositive persons who have no signs or symptoms of HIV infection. HIV-infected patients generally survive for many years, and the operation would be expected to cure the episodes of biliary pain. In addition, such surgery is routinely performed for this indication in patients who have other diseases, such as cancer, with poor prognoses. If physicians bias

---

TABLE 26-1. *Strategies for dealing with risk to health care workers*

Acknowledge fears.
Reduce the occupational risks.
Balance risks to health care workers and benefits to patients.

their medical judgments in order to avoid caring for seropositive persons, then patients and the public will justifiably question their recommendations on other policy issues.

OBLIGATIONS TO PROVIDE EMERGENCY CARE

Forty-three million Americans lack adequate health insurance. They may be denied medical care, even in life-threatening emergencies. Some emergency departments have transferred uninsured patients to public hospitals in circumstances that endangered the patients (19–21). Critics have called this practice "patient dumping."

CASE 26.2. THE CRITICALLY ILL PATIENT WITH NO HEALTH INSURANCE. *A 23-year-old man presents to the emergency room with fever, headache, photophobia, stiff neck, and skin rash. He does not have health insurance. The hospital administrator in charge of the emergency room tells the physician to transfer the patient to the county hospital, because he has no insurance. "We lose thousands of dollars on patients like him. This hospital won't survive if we keep losing money this way."*

In Case 26.2, the patient may have meningococcal meningitis, a life-threatening emergency. Standard care is an immediate lumbar puncture, followed by antibiotics while awaiting laboratory results. Without timely care, the patient will die.

Objections to Patient Transfers

Financially motivated transfers of emergency patients violate the ethical principle that physicians should act in the best interests of patients. When patients need immediate life-saving emergency care, the economic self-interest of the hospital should be subordinated to the well-being of patients. One physician declared, "All of us need to reconsider why we are practicing medicine, and if the bottom line is not to provide good care to all who need it regardless of the situation, then a change in profession is indicated (22)."

The public relies on emergency departments and physicians to provide proper emergency treatment and expects them to do so. In an emergency, delays caused by refusal of care may seriously harm patients. Furthermore, once emergency departments begin a medical evaluation, patients justifiably rely on them to provide proper ongoing care (19).

Guidelines for Patient Transfer

Both professional standards and federal law now condemn transfers that endanger emergency patients (23). The Emergency Medical Treatment and Labor Act prohibits emergency departments from transferring patients in unstable condition who need emergency care as well as pregnant women in active labor (24). Every person seeking treatment in an emergency department must receive a screening examination. If the patient is determined to have an emergency condition, the hospital must provide treatment to stabilize the patient's condition, within the constraints of the available staff and facilities. If the hospital has done what it can to minimize the risks to the patient, transfer is appropriate provided that the receiving hospital accepts the patient, that all medical records accompany the patient, and that appropriate personnel and equipment are used during transport. A patient whose condition has not been stabilized may not be transferred unless the patient consents to transfer or unless a physician certifies that the benefits of transfer outweigh the risks to the patient, for example, when the receiving hospital has superior facilities.

Economically motivated refusals to care for patients will continue as long as so many people lack adequate health insurance. Substandard care resulting from such transfers should motivate doctors to press for access to health care for all Americans.

DIFFICULT DOCTOR–PATIENT RELATIONSHIPS

Ideally, the doctor–patient relationship is a partnership whose goal is the well-being of the patient. In some cases, however, the relationship may be unproductive or adversarial, and the physician may consider the patient a "problem" or "difficult" patient (25,26).

CASE 26.3. DISRUPTIVE AND UNCOOPERATIVE PATIENT. *Ms. W. is 35-year-old woman with end-stage renal disease who repeatedly misses dialysis appointments and requires emergency dialysis. She also does not take her medications regularly or follow her diet, is frequently intoxicated, and disrupts the dialysis unit with her obscene language and threats of violence. Her nephrologist negotiates a contract with her; he agrees to continue to provide dialysis, while she agrees keep scheduled appointments, enter substance abuse treatment, follow her diet, take her medications, and seek psychological counseling. When Ms. W. does not change her behavior, he notifies her that he will no longer provide chronic dialysis and gives her a list of other nephrologists in the area. When she presents to the emergency department with hyperkalemia and congestive heart failure, the nephrologist considers refusing dialysis (27).*

In Case 26.3, Ms. W. undermines her care by repeatedly missing appointments and failing to take her medications. In addition, she insists on emergency care after missing scheduled appointments. Health care workers are understandably frustrated when the patient's own actions bring about or exacerbate her medical problems. They question why they should spend great effort trying to help Ms. W., only to have her irresponsibility and personal problems undermine their efforts. Furthermore, health care workers resent her anger and hostility.

Disruptive patients may subject staff and other patients to verbal abuse, physical threats, or actual violence. It seems fair to require patients to refrain from threatening health care workers and other patients. In addition, health care workers may have to spend so much time and energy on a difficult patient that they provide insufficient attention to other patients.

Improving Difficult Doctor–Patient Relationships

In most cases, physicians can find ways to improve a difficult doctor–patient relationship (Table 26-2).

Acknowledge That Problems Exist

The first step is for physicians and patients alike to acknowledge problems. The physician might say, "I sense that both of us are disappointed with how your care is turning out." Once problems are acknowledged, physicians and patients can to try to resolve them. Furthermore, it may be therapeutic for health care providers to vent their feelings to colleagues.

TABLE 26-2. *Improving difficult doctor–patient relationships*

Acknowledge that problems exist.
Try to understand the patient's perspective.
Try to understand your own responses.
Try to negotiate mutually acceptable grounds for continued care.

Try to Understand the Patient's Perspective

Physicians may feel that some patients intentionally vex them and make medical care more difficult. From the patient's perspective, however, there may be sound reasons for missing appointments, such as difficulties with insurance coverage, transportation, or child care. Illness may cause patients to feel angry, frustrated, helpless, or out of control. Patients may not be able to control some behaviors, because of addiction to alcohol and drugs or psychiatric conditions.

Physicians can elicit patients' perspectives through open-ended questions about the impact of their illness, competing demands in their life, and barriers to care. Acknowledging a patient's emotions also encourages further discussion. Once their problems and frustration are acknowledged, patients may be better able to appreciate how their behavior is disrupting their care or the care of other patients. The physician might say, "We're trying our best to help you, but it's hard for us if you shout and don't keep appointments."

Try to Understand Your Own Responses

Physicians need to understand how their own actions might exacerbate the patient's behavior. The problem is not simply a difficult patient; it is a difficult relationship, for which the physician shares responsibility. Physicians and nurses who are frustrated and angry at having to provide emergency dialysis may vent their anger on the patient or treat her curtly. Differences in ethnic background, social class, and lifestyle often exacerbate tensions.

Try to Negotiate Mutually Acceptable Grounds for Continued Care

Physicians can try to set limits on disruptive behaviors and find mutually acceptable conditions for the doctor–patient relationship (28). Often a psychiatric or social work consultation can help health care workers resolve interpersonal conflicts with patients. For example, patients might be given more control over some aspects of their care. As in Case 26.3, physicians can warn patients that certain behaviors will lead to termination of the doctor–patient relationship. Doctors can negotiate a formal "contract" that explicitly describes the conditions under which the patient and physician will continue the relationship. A family member may be required to accompany the patient to dialysis sessions (27). Agreement can also be sought on treatments for substance abuse and mental illness, which may be causing the disruptive actions.

Terminating the Doctor–Patient Relationship

The doctor–patient relationship can be terminated in several ways that present no ethical problems. The patient's medical problem may be resolved, so that care is no longer required. The patient may withdraw from the physician's care. The patient and physician may agree that the care of the patient should be transferred to another physician. Physicians may also unilaterally terminate the doctor–patient relationship in certain situations, for example, the patient described in Case 26.3 broke her agreement about subsequent behavior and continued to be disruptive and violent. Because termination is a drastic measure, it should be used only as a last resort after attempts to find common ground for ongoing care have failed.

Patient Abandonment

Legally and ethically, physicians may not abandon patients with whom they have established a doctor–patient relationship (27). Abrupt termination of the relationship might seriously harm patients who are not able to obtain needed care in a timely manner. When terminating a relationship, physicians need to give patients reasonable notice, so that patients have time to find another physician. It is prudent to provide such notice in written form. To help patients find another physician, doctors can give patients a list of other qualified physicians in the area or refer them to the county medical society.

Need to Provide Emergency Care

Although physicians may withdraw from a long-term doctor–patient relationship, an emergency department is required to provide emergency care to patients who seek it. Thus if the dialysis patient in Case 26.3 presents to the emergency department with life-threatening hyperkalemia and congestive heart failure, emergency dialysis must be provided. This requires the help of a nephrologist and dialysis nurse. Thus the health care workers who refuse to provide chronic dialysis may still have to perform emergency dialysis. Sometimes the emergency care of such patients can be shared among different individuals or institutions. When providing such emergency care, health care workers do not have to suffer verbal or physical abuse. Having a hospital security guard stand outside the room usually allows care to be given in a peaceful manner.

In summary, physicians have an ethical obligation to care for patients even at some annoyance or personal risk. Before unilaterally terminating a difficult doctor–patient relationship, physicians should try both to understand the patient's perspective and to find some mutually acceptable arrangement for continuing care.

REFERENCES

1. Koop CE. Testimony before Presidential Commission on AIDS. Washington, DC, September 8, 1987.
2. Jonsen A, Siegler M, Winslade W. *Clinical ethics*, 3rd ed. New York: Macmillan, 1991:73–74.
3. Annas GJ. Not saints, but healers: the legal duties of health care professionals in the AIDS epidemic. *Am J Public Health* 1988;78:844–849.
4. Americans with Disabilities Act of 1990, 42 USC §§12181,12182.
5. Americans with Disabilities Act Public Accommodation Regulations, 28 CFR § 36.201.
6. Gostin LO, Feldbaum C, Webber DW. Disability discrimination in America: HIV/AIDS and other health conditions. *JAMA* 1999;281:745–752.
7. Cook DJ, Liutkus JF, Risdon CL, et al. Residents' experiences of abuse, discrimination and sexual harassment during residency training. McMaster University Residency Training Programs. *CMAJ* 1996;154:1657–1665.
8. CDC. Public health service guidelines for management of health care worker exposures to HIV and recommendations for postexposure prophylaxis. *MMWR* 1998:1–33.
9. Gerberding JL, Littell C, Tarkington A, et al. Risk of exposure of surgical personnel to patients' blood during surgery at San Francisco General Hospital. *N Engl J Med* 1990;322:1788–1793.
10. Tokars JI, Bell DM, Culver DH, et al. Percutaneous injuries during surgical procedures. *JAMA* 1992;267:2899–2904.
11. CDC. Case-control study of HIV seroconversion in health-care workers after exposures to HIV-infected blood—France, United Kingdom and United States, January 1988–August 1994. *MMWR* 1995:929–933.
12. National Research Council. *Improving risk communication*. Washington, DC: National Academy Press, 1989.
13. Aoun H. When a house officer gets AIDS. *N Engl J Med* 1989;321:693–696.
14. CDC. Update: universal precautions for prevention of transmission of human immunodeficiency virus, hepatitis B virus, and other bloodborne pathogens in health-care settings. *MMWR* 1988;37:377–382, 387–388.
15. Zuger A, Miles SH. Physicians, AIDS, and occupational risk. Historic traditions and ethical obligations. *JAMA* 1987;258:1924–1928.
16. Nelkin D. Communicating technological risk: the social construction of risk perception. *Ann Rev Public Health* 1989;10:95–113.
17. Slovic P. Perception of risk. *Science* 1987;236:280–285.
18. Gerbert B, Maguire B, Badmer V, et al. Why fear persists: health care professionals and AIDS. *JAMA* 1988;260:3481–3483.

19. Kellermann AL, Ackerman TF. Interhospital patient transfer: the case for informed consent. *N Engl J Med* 1988; 319:643–647.
20. Schiff RL, Ansell DA, Schlosser JE, et al. Transfers to a public hospital: a prospective study of 467 patients. *N Engl J Med* 1986;314:552–557.
21. Reed WG, Cawley KA, Anderson RJ. The effect of a public hospital's transfer policy on patient care. *N Engl J Med* 1986;315:1428–1432.
22. Wrenn K. No insurance, no admission. *N Engl J Med* 1985;312:373–374.
23. Beitsch LM. Economic patient dumping: whose life is it anyway? *J Legal Med* 1989;10:433–478.
24. 42 U.S.C. § 1395dd.
25. Groves JE. Taking care of the hateful patient. *N Engl J Med* 1978;298:883–887.
26. Drossman DR. The problem patient: evaluation and care of medical patients with psychosocial disturbances. *Ann Intern Med* 1978;88:366–372.
27. Orentlicher D. Denying treatment to the noncompliant patient. *JAMA* 1991;265:1579–1582.
28. Quill TE. Partnerships in patient care: a contractual approach. *Ann Intern Med* 1983;98:228–234.

ANNOTATED BIBLIOGRAPHY

1. Annas GJ. Not saints, but healers: the legal duties of health care professionals in the AIDS epidemic. *Am J Public Health* 1988;78:844–849.
   Discusses how physicians have no legal duty to treat patients in most situations, despite a strong moral duty to do so.
2. Quill TE. Partnerships in patient care: a contractual approach. *Ann Intern Med* 1983;98:228–234.
   Practical suggestions on improving difficult doctor–patient relationships.
3. Orentlicher D. Denying treatment to the noncompliant patient. *JAMA* 1991;265:1579–1582.
   Discusses legal and ethical aspects of denying treatment to noncompliant, abusive patients.
4. Gostin LO, Feldbaum C, Webber DW. Disability discrimination in America: HIV/AIDS and other health conditions. *JAMA* 1999;281:745–752.
   Summary of disability law; physicians may decline to care for infectious patients only if there is a significant risk of substantial harm.

27

Gifts from Patients to Physicians

Gifts from patients are gratifying to physicians. Holiday cards, cookies or candy, flowers, and toys for children allow patients to express their appreciation. Some gifts, however, may cause discomfort, either because they are expensive and might compromise the physician's judgment, or because they are too personal and imply more than a professional relationship. Physicians may find that a gift from a patient makes them uncomfortable, and they may be uncertain as to how to respond.

Gifts from patients are often considered a matter of etiquette and manners, not ethics. This chapter points out how gifts from patients may raise ethical issues because they may change the doctor–patient relationship, impair clinical judgment, or erode public trust. Because physicians often find it embarrassing to discuss gifts, the chapter also suggests how to respond to problematical gifts from patients.

REASONS FOR PATIENTS TO GIVE GIFTS TO PHYSICIANS

To Thank Physicians

Patients commonly send gifts to express appreciation to physicians for their care. Patients who have recovered from serious illness are understandably grateful to their physicians, particularly if the diagnosis was difficult, the treatment was complicated, or the physician was particularly supportive or involved.

To Satisfy Their Own Needs

Gifts may also reflect the psychological needs of the patient.

CASE 27.1. COOKIES FROM A LONELY ELDERLY PATIENT. *A 74-year-old widow has hypertension, osteoarthritis, and mild depression. She has no surviving relatives, few friends, and few social activities. A new resident takes over her care. She talks about her sadness and emptiness, and he encourages her to attend a senior center. On the next visit, she brings him a box of home-baked cookies.*

This lonely patient may feel that her physician is one of the few people who listens or pays attention to her. Bringing a gift may give her a sense of purpose or alleviate her loneliness. Taking initiative and showing concern for other people may be therapeutic for her. For other patients, giving physicians gifts on holidays or at the birth of a child allows them to make personal connection to an otherwise impersonal medical care system.

To Enhance Future Care

In a few cases, gifts may represent expectations for future care rather than thanks for past efforts. Patients may feel that if they give the physician a gift, they will receive special consideration. For instance, some patients may want to have the last appointment of the day because of difficulties getting off from work. Other patients may hope that gifts will gain them timely appointments or prompt responses to phone calls.

In rare cases, patients who give gifts may subsequently ask physicians to do something that is ethically questionable.

CASE 27.2. REQUEST FOR DISABILITY CERTIFICATION. *A patient with mild asthma gives his physician a toy for his son at Christmas. The next month, he asks the physician to complete a form for a disability parking sticker. The patient does not meet the objective criteria for hypoxemia or dyspnea listed on the form.*

In Case 27.2, the timing of the gift and the request are disturbing. The physician may feel manipulated because an apparently thoughtful gift may have had hidden strings attached. Deceving third parties about a patient's condition is ethically problematical (*see* Chapter 6). To do so after receiving a gift would appear to be accepting a bribe.

To Meet Cultural Expectations

In some cultures, gifts to physicians or other healers are routinely expected. Such gifts may show respect or be considered an essential aspect of the healing process. In some societies, bribery may be necessary to ensure that a patient is scheduled promptly or seen by senior physicians. Physicians need to consider whether gifts may have special cultural significance for patients and correct any misconceptions about the U.S. medical care system.

PROBLEMS WITH GIFTS

It is human nature for patients who have given gifts to expect some consideration in return, either consciously or unconsciously (1). Most patients have the understandable expectation of a more personal connection with the medical care system. However, gifts may create ethical problems if they lead to inappropriate expectations by patients.

Expectations for Personal Treatment

As mentioned above, some patients might believe that gifts entitle them to special treatment, such as more convenient or prompter appointments. Other patients might expect freedom to call the physician at home or to have medications refilled over the telephone without an office visit. Even apparently small gifts may be problematical if such expectations become burdensome to physicians. For example, physicians understandably want to limit add-on appointments and after-hours phone calls in order to reduce personal stress and to protect their family life, yet they might find it difficult to refuse a request from a patient who has given a gift.

Changes in the Doctor–Patient Relationship

Some gifts may change the doctor–patient relationship inappropriately.

CASE 27.1, continued. FOCUS ON THE PHYSICIAN'S PROBLEMS, RATHER THAN THE PATIENT'S. *The lonely, elderly patient starts to bring cookies or other gifts of food at every visit. Moreover, visits now focus on the physician rather than on the patient. The patient inquires about what foods the physician likes so that she can plan her next gift. She also expresses concern about whether he is getting enough sleep and has enough time off.*

In Case 27.1, an overworked and underappreciated house officer may be delighted that someone takes a personal interest in him, but it is problematical if the physician assumes the role of a surrogate grandchild. Patient visits should focus on the patient's problems, not the physician's. The physician may miss opportunities to encourage and reinforce the patient's efforts to become more socially active in the community. In the long run, it is counterproductive and unrealistic for lonely patients to depend totally on the medical system for their emotional and social needs.

In other circumstances, gifts violate the boundaries of the professional relationship. An extreme example might be the gift of lingerie or other intimate apparel. Such gifts imply a personal relationship, not a professional one. Patients who overstep the boundaries of a professional relationship are acting out their own needs or fantasies. Not only should such gifts be refused, but appropriate boundaries need to be promptly and firmly reestablished. In many cases, the physician may not feel comfortable continuing the doctor–patient relationship after such an episode and will need to arrange to transfer care to another physician.

Impairment of Clinical Judgment

Gifts can create or strengthen personal ties, but too close a relationship may be undesirable. It is difficult to provide care to a close relative because emotional ties may cloud clinical judgment (2). In a similar way, gifts that establish or imply a very close personal relationship may compromise the physician's judgment. Expectations of special treatment may compromise care, as when a patient expects the physician to diagnose and treat a complicated problem on the basis of a telephone call rather than an office visit. Psychologically, it is difficult to say no to patients who have given gifts, even if they request interventions that are unsound medical practice or not in their best interests. Similarly, a gift from a seriously ill patient may be problematical if it leads the physician to misrepresent bad news or causes the patient to develop unrealistic expectations.

Erosion of Public Trust

The doctor–patient relationship may be weakened if other patients believe that they will receive second-class care unless they offer gifts. Physicians serve as gatekeepers, allocating appointments, their time and attention, and, in managed care systems, health care resources. Generally phone calls or appointments are allocated primarily on the basis of patient need. It would damage both the individual physician and the profession as a whole if patients believed that the best way to get the physician's attention is through a gift. Even a perception that physicians are allocating their efforts on the basis of favoritism would erode public trust.

Soliciting Gifts

This chapter has focused on gifts that patients offer to physicians. Solicitation of gifts by physicians also merits attention. It is unethical for physicians to solicit personal gifts in return for services rendered because physicians' fees should be adequate compensation for their services. It may also be problematical for physicians to solicit contributions for some cause, such as a hospital or a political movement. Such solicitations may seem a natural way for physicians to work for causes they believe in, but patients may not feel free to decline the solicitation if their physician solicits it personally and knows whether they have responded. They may fear that the physician will not render prompt or meticulous care in the future if they refuse.

HOW TO RESPOND TO GIFTS FROM PATIENTS

In responding to gifts, physicians need to take into account the nature of the gift and the circumstances.

Accept Appropriate Gifts Graciously

In the vast majority of cases, gifts from patients are well intentioned and appropriate and should be accepted graciously. Indeed patients would rightly feel insulted if physicians did not accept home-made cookies, toys at Christmas, or clothes for a new baby. Similarly, it would be unfeeling not to accept a small gift after the physician has devoted a great deal of effort in helping a patient recover from a difficult illness.

Don't Let Gifts Go to Your Head

Physicians should not allow gifts from patients to give them an exaggerated sense of their importance or their skill. Many patients, because they are sick and dependent, are extremely grateful for competent, humane care. It is gratifying that such qualities in physicians are recognized and reinforced, but physicians should appreciate that they may not have done anything extraordinary, just provided standard care.

Appreciate That Some Gifts are Problematical

Some gifts may seem disproportionate to the services rendered (3).

CASE 27.3. TICKETS TO THE OPERA. *A 52-year-old businessman establishes care with a new physician. At the first visit, they discuss preventive measures such as exercise and diet. The next week the businessman offers the physician opera tickets to the opening night gala.*

Intuitively, some gifts seem out of proportion to what the physician has done. Most physicians would feel comfortable accepting gifts worth less than $20, but many would feel uncomfortable accepting $300 tickets to the opening night of the opera after a routine new patient visit. Even if a wealthy patient considers this a small gift, it might give the wrong impression to other patients. Furthermore, the physician might wonder whether such a lavish gift reflects unrealistic expectations for care. Finally, many physicians feel uncomfortable accepting cash gifts because they seem associated with commerce and profits.

Get Advice about the Gift

Most physicians, even if they are uncomfortable about gifts, hesitate to discuss them with colleagues. Physicians may not appreciate that many colleagues also feel awkward and uncertain about gifts. Other people, however, can help the physician interpret the significance of gifts and understand the patient's possible expectations. Physicians need to be aware that the patient's interpretation may be radically different from their own. In judging the appropriateness of a gift, physicians can apply a practical rule of thumb: how would colleagues and other patients react if they knew about the gift? If other patients would question the gift, it is best not to accept it.

Consider Sharing the Gift with Others

Concerns about gifts can often be prevented or resolved by sharing the gift with other people and letting the patient know. For example, the physician might share the gift with other staff who care for the patient or donate the gift to charity. Home-made cookies and cakes can be shared with office staff. Monetary gifts can be given to a house staff fund for refreshments or books, to the hospital volunteer fund, or to a medical charity. The physician should let the patient know how the gift was distributed and explain why this was done. Such sharing acknowledges the thoughtfulness of the patient, while making it less likely that patients feel they are entitled to special care from the individual physician.

Decline Gifts without Rejecting the Patient

Even when physicians believe that declining the gift is appropriate, they may find it awkward to do so. Several strategies may allow the physician to decline the gift while respecting the patient's feelings. In each approach, physicians should start by saying that they are grateful and touched. One approach is to explain that accepting such a gift might compromise the physician's ability to give high-quality care in the future. Although this approach is straightforward, patients often protest that they would never ask for special consideration. A second approach is to decline the gift politely but firmly without giving more specific reasons. The physician might simply say that she could not possibly accept the gift and that her policy is not to accept such gifts, even though she is touched by the thoughtfulness. Often this strategy works in conjunction with telling the patient that the gift will be shared with others.

If the physician suspects that gifts reflect the patient's social isolation or other needs, as in Case 27.1, these issues should be addressed separately during patient visits.

What if the Patient Later Requests Special Treatment?

After a gift, the patient may later request special treatment. The physician needs to distinguish different types of requests. A good rule of thumb is for physicians to ask what they would do if the same request had come from a patient who had not given a gift.

Personal Favors

The patient may ask to have an appointment a little earlier or later than usual office hours, because such times are more convenient.

Inappropriate Medical Care

Some patients may request the physician to diagnose or treat complicated problems over the telephone, or may want to call the physician at home rather than at the office. Such requests may lead to substandard care as well as disrupt the physician's personal life.

Unethical Actions

In rare cases, the patient may request the physician to do something ethically problematical, such as completing a disability form in a deceptive manner as in Case 27.3. A previous gift from the patient should not sway the physician. Indeed, it would be worse to do something unethical after receiving a gift, because the physician would appear to be influenced by a bribe.

In all these situations, the physician should respond to the patient's request as if no gift had been given (3). In explaining the refusal, physicians may find it more tactful not to refer to the previous gift but instead to focus on their general policy regarding such requests.

In conclusion, gifts from patients strengthen social relationships and expectations. Usually gifts are thoughtful gestures of appreciation that should be accepted graciously. Some gifts, however, may be problematical. Discussing gifts with colleagues as well as the giver may help physicians respond to them appropriately.

REFERENCES

1. Murray TH. Gifts of the body and the needs of strangers. *Hastings Center Rep* 1987;17:30–38.
2. LaPuma J, Priest ER. Is there a doctor in the house? An analysis of the practice of physicians' treating their own families. *JAMA* 1992;267:1810–1812.
3. Lyckholm LJ. Should physicians accept gifts from patients? *JAMA* 1998;280:1944–1946.

ANNOTATED BIBLIOGRAPHY

1. Lyckholm LJ. Should physicians accept gifts from patients? *JAMA* 1998;280:1944–1946.
   Brief, thoughtful review of topic.

28

Sexual Contact Between Physicians and Patients

The Hippocratic Oath forbids sexual relationships between physicians and patients. Some people believe that this prohibition is no longer appropriate: sexual mores have changed, and sexual relationships between consenting adults should be considered private. This chapter discusses ethical issues regarding sexual contact between physicians and current or former patients. It argues that such relationships are unethical if they take advantage of the trust, dependency, and vulnerability of patients.

PREVALENCE OF SEXUAL RELATIONSHIPS BETWEEN PHYSICIANS AND PATIENTS

In a national survey, 9% of physicians reported at least one sexual contact with a patient or former patient (1). The vast majority of cases involved male physicians and female patients. This study excluded cases in which the sexual relationship preceded the medical care, such as the provision of medical care to a spouse. Twenty-three percent of respondents reported that one or more of their patients had revealed sexual contact with a previous physician. In other studies, between 5% and 10% of psychiatrists and other mental health professionals admitted to sexual contact with patients (2).

JUSTIFICATIONS FOR SEXUAL CONTACT BETWEEN PHYSICIANS AND PATIENTS

Several justifications are commonly offered for relaxing the traditional prohibition on sexual contacts between physicians and patients (3).

Respect for Privacy

Generally, sexual relationships between consenting adults are considered private matters, with which other people and society have no right to interfere. For many persons, it makes no difference that the partners are physician and patient. In this view, it is demeaning and unrealistic to view patients as so vulnerable that they must be protected from physicians. Most patients are fully capable of making their own decisions about their private lives. Accordingly, restricting freedom to enter into sexual relationships would be paternalistic and intrusive.

Lack of Harm to Patients

Many people believe that patients are no more likely to be harmed in sexual relationships with their physicians than in other sexual relationships. In the United States, short-term relationships and divorces are common. Anecdotally, many people know of happy marriages between physicians and former patients. In this view, even if some sexual relationships with physicians harm patients, there is no reason to prohibit all such relationships.

Lack of Social Opportunities for Physicians

In small towns and rural areas, a physician may care for a large proportion of the community. Social opportunities for physicians would be very limited if romantic and sexual relationships with patients were barred.

OBJECTIONS TO SEXUAL RELATIONSHIPS WITH CURRENT PATIENTS

Professional codes of ethics consider sexual relationships with current patients unethical. The American Medical Association recently declared, "Sexual conduct or a romantic relationship with a patient concurrent with the physician-patient relationship is unethical" (2). Patients may feel "angry, abandoned, humiliated, mistreated, or exploited by their physicians. Victims [sic] have been reported to experience guilt, severe mistrust of their own judgment, and mistrust of both men and physicians" (2). There are several reasons for such role-specific restrictions on physicians (Table 28-1).

Physicians Should Not Take Advantage of the Doctor–Patient Relationship

It may be difficult for patients to make truly autonomous decisions regarding sexual relationships with physicians. The physician–patient relationship arises from the patient's illness, which can cause patients to be vulnerable and dependent (4). Patients usually place great weight on their physicians' advice and judgment and naturally develop feelings of trust, gratitude, and admiration toward physicians. Unconsciously, the patient may mistake such feelings for romantic or sexual attraction. Patients as well as physicians may not appreciate how such positive feelings result from the doctor's role as well as the doctor's personal attributes. Although such transference has been most clearly described in patients undergoing psychotherapy, similar feelings may occur in all physician–patient relationships. Physicians may also misinterpret their own feelings of caring and concern for patients, which are a natural part of the doctor–patient relationship, as romantic or sexual attraction.

In the course of a professional relationship, patients make intimate revelations to physicians, as in the following case.

CASE 28.1. CURRENT PATIENT RECEIVING ACTIVE THERAPY. *A 45-year-old male physician is treating a 32-year-old woman for depression and peptic ulcer disease. The woman reveals that*

TABLE 28-1. *Objections to sexual relationships with current patients*

Physicians should not take advantage of the doctor-patient relationship.
Physicians have power over patients.
Trust in the profession will be undermined.
Some patients are particularly vulnerable.

she was sexually abused as a child. The physician, who is going through a divorce, finds her attractive and considers initiating a romantic and sexual relationship with her.

In Case 28.1, a depressed patient discloses private information, which she may not have told anyone else. In their professional role, physicians are privy to intimate personal information. During the medical history, physicians may take a detailed sexual history. Patients may reveal their innermost fantasies and fears. Patients undress for examinations and allow physicians to touch them and even invade their bodies during medical or surgical procedures. Such intimacy within the doctor–patient relationship is one-sided. Physicians do not ordinarily reveal their personal feelings, thoughts, or bodies to patients. Thus physicians know much more personal information about patients than patients know about them. Physicians may betray the patient's trust if they take advantage of such intimate information, either consciously or unconsciously, in pursing sexual relationships with patients.

Physicians Have Power Over Patients

Physicians have power over patients that they can use to their advantage in sexual relationships. Because physicians order tests and treatments and schedule appointments, they control patients' access to medical care. There may be an implied or inferred threat that if the patient does not agree to sexual contact, the doctor–patient relationship will be terminated (5). Physicians may also provide false reassurance to patients that an effective therapeutic relationship can continue even if a sexual liaison is initiated (5). In egregious cases, the physician may portray a sexual liaison as part of medical therapy. Inequalities in power may make it more difficult for patients to decline sexual relationships with their physicians than with other people. In Case 28.1, the very framing of the issues implies unequal power: the physician considers initiating a sexual liaison, as if it were inconceivable that the patient would refuse.

Trust in the Profession Will Be Undermined

If the profession were to condone sexual relationships with patients, the public might begin to believe that physicians are motivated by self-interest and are willing to take advantage of patients. Patients might be reluctant to visit physicians or discuss intimate matters. Patients with psychiatric or gynecological problems may be particularly deterred from seeking care.

Some Patients Are Particularly Vulnerable

Some patients may be especially harmed in sexual relationships with physicians. In Case 28.1, the patient's depression might compromise her ability to consent freely to a sexual relationship. Furthermore, patients who have suffered incest or rape may find it difficult to refuse sexual relationships with authority figures and may feel particularly betrayed if the current relationship repeats previous traumatic experiences. Such persons may not even be aware that they are repeating a previous pattern of behavior.

The Patient's Medical Care May Be Compromised

Just as being the physician for a spouse is unwise (6), providing medical care to a sexual partner may lead to suboptimal care. When physicians are having a sexual relationship with the patient, their clinical judgment is likely to be compromised (7). They may be less thorough in taking a history, conducting an examination, or ordering diagnostic tests.

Legal Issues

In several states, sexual relationships between physicians and current patients may lead to criminal charges or to disciplinary action by licensing boards (8). Physicians may also face civil suits for malpractice. Malpractice insurers may exclude coverage for civil claims relating to sexual misconduct, asserting that such behavior is not part of providing medical care.

Comparisons with Other Professions

In other professions, sexual relationships with clients are also condemned. Churches are criticized for covering up sexual relationships between clergy and parishioners and transferring offending priests or ministers without appropriate disciplinary action (9). Similarly, lawyers have been criticized for sexual relationships with clients, particularly clients in divorce cases (10). As in medicine, the charge is that these professionals abuse their trust and power in sexual relationships with clients.

SEXUAL RELATIONSHIPS WITH FORMER PATIENTS

Although sexual relationships with current patients are generally considered inappropriate, there is less agreement regarding relationships with previous patients. In the previously cited survey, although 94% of physicians considered it unethical to have sexual relationships with current patients, only 36% of physicians considered it unethical to have sexual relationships with former patients (1).

CASE 28.2. FORMER PATIENT, WITH NO ONGOING RELATIONSHIP. *A female emergency physician cares for a 28-year-old man who requires a tetanus shot for a foot injury. Several years later, they meet again as single parents whose children are in the same school. They discover that they share many common interests. The physician wonders if a romantic relationship would be unacceptable because of their previous professional relationship.*

In Case 28.2, it is unlikely that the former patient feels dependent on the physician. Furthermore, the patient revealed little personal information during the doctor–patient relationship and is not particularly vulnerable on that basis. A relationship between equals seems as possible for them as for any other couple.

Feelings of dependency, however, may persist after care is terminated, as in the following case.

CASE 28.3. RECENT SURGICAL PATIENT. *A male surgeon performs an emergency laparotomy on a woman with appendicitis. During postoperative visits, he finds himself spending much more time with her than he usually does with patients. She is appreciative of his attention and solicitous about his long hours and fatigue. A month after her final postoperative visit, he invites her to dinner.*

In Case 28.3, the patient may have strong feelings of gratitude and dependency soon after emergency surgery. Unlike Case 28.2, it may be more difficult for the patient to make an independent judgment about a relationship or to decline invitations from the surgeon, compared with other men she knows.

Regarding former patients, the American Medical Association (AMA) states, "Sexual or romantic relationships with former patients are also unethical if the physician uses or exploits trust, knowledge, emotions, or influence derived from the previous professional relationship" (2). Thus it is important to identify situations in which the doctor–patient relationship has been terminated before the sexual relationship is initiated. Several factors should be considered.

Termination of Medical Care

Termination of care and absence of contact should be complete, including cessation of office visits, telephone consultations, prescriptions, and reminder postcards about appointments or screening tests. In addition, a new physician should be identified, so that the patient no longer regards the partner as his or her physician. The intent of terminating care should not be the initiation of a sexual relationship.

Nature of the Doctor–Patient Relationship

Some types of medical care are so intimate that the doctor–patient relationship may never be completely ended. Counseling and therapy evoke powerful feelings of transference that may last for years. Patients report intense feelings of dependency and gratitude toward physicians years after therapy has been terminated. The American Psychiatric Association considers any sexual contact with a former psychiatric patient unethical. As already noted, some patients may be particularly vulnerable because of past victimization (11). In specialties such as surgery or gynecology, which involve unique and intimate physical contact, the patient may still regard the physician as being in that role years later. In contrast, in Case 28.2, tetanus immunization is so routine that any feelings of dependency in the patient are likely to be transient and weak. In that situation, the patient's dependence on the physician may be similar to dependence on a librarian.

Time Since Last Medical Care

In Case 28.3, during the immediate postoperative period the patient's feelings of vulnerability and dependency undoubtedly continue. Amorous advances by the physician may take advantage of these feelings in the patient. The passage of time helps to extinguish feelings of dependency toward physicians and reduces the risk that physicians will abuse their power in initiating sexual relationships with patients (5). To prevent abuse, the Ontario College of Physicians and Surgeons Task Force recommends a waiting period of 2 years since the last episode of patient care, with no contact in the interim (12). The crucial issue, however, is not simply the amount of time but rather the lack of a continuous relationship and the "potential for misuse of emotions derived from the former professional relationship" (2).

Circumstances of Renewal of Contact

If the doctor and former patient renew their acquaintance in a medical context, the patient may resume his or her previous role as dependent patient. On the other hand, the physician and former patient may meet again in a nonmedical context, as in Case 28.2. Being reacquainted in a nonmedical setting makes it more likely that the relationship is not colored by the previous doctor–patient relationship.

SUGGESTIONS

Physicians who are considering sexual relationships with current or former patients might consider the following suggestions.

Recognize Early Signs of Romantic Interest

Rarely are sexual or romantic feelings so overwhelming that the physician is literally swept away by uncontrollable passion. Physicians should be alert to early signs of romantic feelings for a patient. For example, they might look forward to the next visit or pay particular attention to their appearance the day of the patient's visit. Sexual misconduct often begins with seemingly minor violations of the boundaries of the doctor–patient relationship, such as talking about the physician's problems rather than the patient's or scheduling appointments outside office hours (7). Recognizing these early symptoms gives physicians time to act thoughtfully and to consider the potential problems.

Seek Advice

It is hard to think critically about romantic or sexual interests. The AMA recommends that "it would be advisable for a physician to seek consultation with a colleague before initiating a relationship with a former patient" (2). Confidential advice can provide an honest appraisal of the potential harm to the patient, the physician, and the medical profession. Such counsel may be a safeguard for physicians who might otherwise act impulsively. Discussing such an intimate decision with other people may seem intrusive. However, such sexual relationships are not completely private if they harm patients or undermine public trust in the medical profession.

Responding to Advances by Patients

In some cases, the patient, not the physician, takes the initiative in pursuing a romantic or sexual liaison. However, physicians are in a better position than patients to recognize the potential harms of such relationships. In medical decisions, physicians do not simply accede to a patient's requests or demands. Physicians have an ethical duty to act in the best interests of patients, even if it clashes with their own self-interest. Thus it is reasonable to consider the physician responsible for sexual relationships with a patient; the patient's initiative or agreement does not in itself justify the relationship.

In summary, patients naturally feel trust, dependency, and gratitude toward their physicians. Sexual relationships with current patients exploit such feelings and are unethical. Sexual relationships with former patients are also unethical to the extent that the physician takes advantage of emotions and influence deriving from the doctor–patient relationship.

REFERENCES

1. Gartrell NG, Milliken N, Goodson WH, et al. Physician-patient sexual contact: prevalence and problems. *West J Med* 1992;157:139–143.
2. Council on Ethical and Judicial Affairs of the American Medical Association. Sexual misconduct and the practice of medicine. *JAMA* 1991;266:2741–2745.
3. Appelbaum PS, Jorgenson LM, Sutherland PK. Sexual contact between physicians and patients. *Arch Intern Med* 1994;154:2561–2565.
4. Pellegrino ED, Thomasma DG. *For the patient's good: the restoration of beneficence in health care.* New York: Oxford University Press, 1988.
5. Appelbaum PS, Jorgenson L. Psychotherapist-patient sexual contact after termination of treatment: an analysis and proposal. *Am J Psychiatry* 1991;148:1466–1473.
6. LaPuma J, Priest ER. Is there a doctor in the house? An analysis of the practice of physicians' treating their own families. *JAMA* 1992;267:1810–1812.
7. Gabbard GO, Nadelson C. Professional boundaries in the physician-patient relationship. *JAMA* 1995;273: 1445–1449.
8. Johnson SH. Judicial review of disciplinary action for sexual misconduct in the practice of medicine. *JAMA* 1993;270:1596–1600.
9. Steinfels P. The Church faces the trespasses of priests: messages on sexual misconduct. *New York Times*, June 27, 1993:D1.
10. Margolick D. On lawyerly lasciviousness and new efforts to deal with a "dirty little secret." *New York Times*, May 22, 1992:B10.
11. Schoener G. Psychotherapist-patient sexual contact after termination of treatment [Letter]. *Am J Psychiatry* 1992;149:981.

12. An Independent Task Force Commissioned by the College of Physicians and Surgeons of Ontario. The final report of the Task Force on Sexual Abuse of Patients. Toronto: College of Physicians and Surgeons, 1991.

ANNOTATED BIBLIOGRAPHY

1. Council on Ethical and Judicial Affairs of the American Medical Association. Sexual misconduct and the practice of medicine. *JAMA* 1991;266:2741–2745.

Thoughtful discussion of the topic, proposing that all sexual contact during the physician–patient relationship is unethical.

2. Gabbard GO, Nadelson C. Professional boundaries in the physician-patient relationship. *JAMA* 1995;273: 1445–1449.

Discusses how sexual misconduct with patients usually begins with apparently minor violations of the therapeutic relationship.

29

Secret Information about Patients

Physicians may receive information about a patient from family members or friends who ask that their role be kept secret (1). Such unsolicited information is disconcerting to doctors. Telling the patient the secret may pass on inaccurate or unhelpful information, while keeping the secret may involve the physician in deception. This chapter discusses the ethical issues posed by such secret information and how physicians can respond to them.

TYPES OF SECRETS

Most commonly, a family member tells the doctor about deleterious personal habits of the patient, such as alcohol use or smoking (1). Often the family member tells a member of the physician's staff, rather than telling the physician directly. The informer hopes that the physician will make the patient stop these unhealthy behaviors. Another type of secret involves mental or physical incapacity. The family member may tell the physician that the patient is demented, depressed, or psychotic. Similarly, the family may be concerned that an elderly patient can no longer drive safely or live independently. The confider also may seek to draw the physician into family disputes over money, marital problems, or the lifestyles of grown children. Finally, family members may alert the physician to hidden physical symptoms, such as chest pain, that the patient might choose not to discuss.

PROBLEMS WITH SUCH INFORMATION

Secret information may be problematic in many ways. The information may be inaccurate. The informer may have ulterior motives, such as gaining an advantage in a family dispute. Secrets are disrespectful to the patient, because they involve deception rather than open discussions. Finally, such secret disclosures trap the physician in a bind because both disclosing and keeping the secret are objectionable.

APPROACHES TO SECRETS

When presented with such a secret, the physician has several options, some of which involve deception or undermine patient trust.

Reveal the Secret to the Patient

There are several ethical objections to keeping such a secret. Patients may consider it a violation of trust if physicians talk to other people about them behind their backs (2). Patients may question the physician's allegiance. It is also deceptive for physicians to base their recommendations and plans on secret information from third parties, not on the history obtained from the patient. Chapter 6 discusses why deception is ethically problematical for physicians.

Keeping secrets from patients also is impractical. Like all forms of deception, it may require additional, increasingly elaborate deception. Patients may ask why the physician is posing a particular question or ordering a particular test. In that case, physicians will either have to reveal the secret information or else deceive the patient.

Do not Disclose to the Patient

One physician who was philosophically opposed to keeping such secrets found that he did not tell the patient in about one-half of cases (1). First, there may be no point in doing so because the information is obvious or trivial. For example, a family member's report that the patient was a heavy smoker provides no new information if the patient smells of cigarettes. Second, the physician does not disclose the information because it is not relevant to the patient's medical care. For example, few physicians want to get involved in a parent's concerns about the patient's marriage. Third, disclosure may do more harm than good in the short run. Revealing the mother's objections to the patient's marriage may well precipitate or intensify a family argument. Fourth, the physician may intend to tell the patient but find no opportunity to bring it up naturally in the conversation. Physicians must appreciate that the right moment to disclose the secret may never occur.

In some cases, the physician promised to keep the secret. The physician is then caught between conflicting obligations to be forthright with patients and to keep promises. Physicians can avoid this dilemma and maintain their primary obligation to the patient by rejecting the informer's initial request to keep the information secret. Family members often preface their revelations with phrases such as, "I don't want my husband to know I told you, but . . . ." It would be prudent for the physician to interrupt at this point, before the information is revealed, and explain her policy of disclosing such information and its source to patients.

Ask Informers to Disclose Their Role

Ethically, the best approach is for the physician to convince the informer to tell the patient about the information presented to the physician or to allow the physician to disclose the source of the information. If this is done, the physician can discuss the issue freely with the patient.

In summary, physicians face dilemmas when family members or friends give information about patients that they ask to be kept secret. Acquiescence with such secrets, even if well intentioned, may undermine the patient's trust. Such situations are best prevented by telling the family member or friend that the information needs to be shared with the patient.

REFERENCES

1. Burnham JF. Secrets about patients. *N Engl J Med* 1991;324:1130–1133.
2. Bok S. *Secrets*. New York: Pantheon Books, 1982.

ANNOTATED BIBLIOGRAPHY

1. Burnham JF. Secrets about patients. *N Engl J Med* 1991;324:1130–1133.
   Thoughtful discussion of the topic based on the author's clinical experience.

30

Clinical Research

Clinical research is essential for medical progress. Physicians may be involved in research in various roles, from referring patients to a clinical study to serving as an investigator. In these roles, physicians need to understand the ethical issues raised at each stage of clinical research.

ETHICAL ISSUES AT VARIOUS STAGES OF RESEARCH

When patients consider entering a research project, their primary physicians should make a recommendation regarding participation. Even if an institutional review board (IRB) or a funding agency has approved the project, the primary physician needs to assess independently whether the research study is appropriate for the particular patient. Among the relevant considerations are the importance of the research question, the rigor of the study design, the selection of participants, and the risks and benefits of the study. Because of the social utility of clinical research, physicians should encourage their patients to participate in well-designed studies.

Traditionally, clinical research has been regarded as risky, and potential subjects were considered guinea pigs who might be subjected to dangerous interventions that would confer little or no benefit and who therefore needed to be protected. Increasingly, however, clinical research is regarded as beneficial, rather than risky, because it provides access to potentially life-saving new therapies in such conditions as human immunodeficiency virus (HIV) infection, cancer, and organ transplantation. Patients who are eager to obtain promising new drugs for fatal conditions want increased access to clinical research, not greater protection (1).

Clinical research should be distinguished from innovative clinical practice, in which a physician goes beyond the usual standards of practice to try to benefit a particular patient. For example, a surgeon may modify a technique, or an internist may use a drug for an indication not approved by the Food and Drug Administration (FDA).

Design of the Research Protocol

According to the ethical guideline of beneficence, research protocols should aim to provide valid and generalizable knowledge, and the prospective benefits of the research should be proportional to the risks to participants. Thus if the research question has already been settled or is trivial, or if the design of the study is so weak that valid conclusions are impossible, even slight risk to subjects cannot be justified.

Randomized Controlled Trials

Although randomized controlled trials are the most rigorous design for evaluating interventions, they may present special ethical concerns because treatment is determined by chance.

The ethical basis for assigning treatment by randomization is the judgment that both arms of the protocol are in equipoise. In other words, current evidence does not prove that either arm is superior. Some experts believe that one arm offers more effective treatment, whereas others believe the opposite (2). Furthermore, individual patients and their physicians must find randomization acceptable. If physicians believe strongly that one arm of the trial is superior and can provide treatment offered in that arm outside the study, they cannot in good faith recommend that patients enter the trial. Similarly, a particular patient may not consider the alternatives equivalent, as when medical and surgical interventions are compared.

Selection of Participants in Research

CASE 30.1. RESEARCH ON PATIENTS WITH DEMENTIA. *A new urinary catheter has been devised. A clinical trial is proposed to evaluate whether the new catheter is clinically more effective than the conventional catheter. Nursing home residents with Alzheimer's disease and incontinence will be recruited as subjects because enrollment and follow-up will be easier than in ambulatory patients.*

Participants in research assume risks in order to gain potential benefits for themselves and for society as a whole. The potential benefits and harms of participation in research should be distributed equitably among groups eligible for the study. Vulnerable, disadvantaged, or minority groups should be neither overrepresented in dangerous studies nor underrepresented in trials of promising new therapies.

Patients Who Lack Decision-Making Capacity

As in Case 30.1, patients who lack decision-making capacity cannot give informed consent to research studies, yet, research is essential to improve therapies for their conditions. It seems reasonable to allow surrogates to consent for research that presents minimal risks and offers the prospect of direct therapeutic benefits to participants (3). One study cautions, however, that surrogate decisions regarding research for mentally incapacitated persons often are not based on the patients' wishes or best interests (4). In that study, 31% of surrogates who believed that the patient would refuse to participate nonetheless gave consent, apparently contradicting the patient's preferences. Furthermore, 20% of surrogates who would not themselves agree to the study nevertheless allowed the patient to participate in the research, perhaps acting in a manner contrary to what they consider the best interests of the patient.

Patients Whose Consent May Not Be Free

Potential participants in research may be vulnerable because their consent may be constrained. Subjects may depend on physician-researchers for ongoing medical care, as in nursing homes, Veterans Affairs hospitals, or public hospitals and clinics. As in Case 30.1, such dependent populations are sometimes recruited as research subjects because access for recruitment is easier and follow-up more complete than with more autonomous individuals. However, such patients may not feel free to refuse to participate. They or their surrogates may fear that their physicians will be upset if they do not enroll in research studies, in which case they could not readily transfer their care to another physician or institution.

Fairness requires that vulnerable populations not be used as a source of research subjects primarily for the convenience of investigators, if other populations would also be suitable subjects for the study. The use of vulnerable subjects for research is more justifiable if the research addresses the condition that makes the subjects vulnerable, if the research offers the prospect of direct therapeutic benefit, or if advocates for the vulnerable population have given approval to the project.

Informed Consent

The guideline of respect for persons and their autonomy requires that adult subjects give informed consent to participate in research. Participants in research should be regarded not as sources of data, but as individuals whose welfare and rights must be respected. The primary physician plays an important ethical and clinical role in helping the patient make an informed decision, as in the following case.

CASE 30.2. INVASIVE HEMODYNAMIC MONITORING. *A 70-year-old woman develops congestive heart failure after a myocardial infarction. She is eligible to participate in a study of the dose–response properties of a new angiotensin-coverting enzyme inhibitor in patients with congestive heart failure. The study involves Swan-Ganz catheterization and hemodynamic monitoring in the coronary care unit when the drug is started and again 6 months later. The patient has always been reluctant to be hospitalized and to undergo invasive cardiac procedures.*

In this case, participation in the study offers little direct benefit to the patient. Numerous effective standard therapies exist. Although patients should be encouraged to enter clinical studies for altruistic motives, this patient may well react adversely to a prolonged stay in intensive care or to invasive procedures. The primary physician should raise these concerns with the patient and try to ensure that she is informed about the research study. Table 30-1 lists pertinent issues that the prospective subject needs to understand (5).

The Nature of the Research Project

The prospective subject should be told explicitly that research is being conducted, what the purpose of the research is, and how subjects are being recruited. Any financial interest of the investigators in the drug or device being studied needs to be disclosed (6).

The Procedures of the Study

Subjects need to know what they will be asked to do in the research project. On a practical level, they should be told how much time will be required and how often. The fact that blood will be drawn may mean more to subjects than the names of the tests that will be conducted. Procedures that are not standard care should be identified as such. Alternative procedures or treatments that may be available outside the study should be discussed. If the study involves blinding or randomization, these concepts should be explained in terms the patient can understand. In interview or questionnaire research, the subject should be informed of the topics to be addressed and the length of time required.

TABLE 30-1. *Informed consent in research projects*

The nature of the research project
The procedures of the study
The potential harms and benefits of the study
Assurances that participation in the research is voluntary
Misconceptions about research
Protection of confidentiality

The Potential Harms and Benefits of the Study

Medical, psychosocial, and economic harms and benefits should be described in lay terms. These include physical harm from complications of tests or treatments, as well as psychosocial harm such as loss of privacy and inconvenience.

Economic risks may also be important. Participants should appreciate that insurance companies may deny reimbursement for procedures that are not standard clinical care. In Case 30.2, for example, the patient needs to understand that she may need to pay for the costs of hemodynamic monitoring in the cardiac care unit, which would not ordinarily be carried out.

Assurances That Participation in the Research Is Voluntary

Subjects must be told that declining to participate in the study will not compromise their medical care and that they may withdraw from the project at any time.

Misconceptions About Research

A common misconception is that research will provide direct therapeutic benefits to the subjects. This has been termed the "therapeutic misconception" (7). Most promising new interventions, despite encouraging preliminary results, fail to show significant advantages over standard therapy. Patients may downplay the risks and be unrealistically optimistic regarding the benefits.

The primary physician plays a crucial role in helping the patient make an informed decision. After talking with an enthusiastic clinical investigator, patients may have an unrealistic impression of the study. The primary physician can elicit and correct any misunderstandings and encourage the patient to ask questions. Finally, the primary doctor should make a recommendation based on the patient's values. In Case 30.2, given the patient's reluctance about invasive procedures, the physician should recommend against participating in the protocol.

Protection of Confidentiality

Confidentiality is important for its own sake (*see* Chapter 5) and also promotes participation in research. For example, concerns about breaches of confidentiality may deter potential subjects from participating in research regarding HIV infection, mental illness, or genetics. Investigators need to take appropriate steps to protect the confidentiality of research data. During the informed consent process, potential subjects need to be told about possible risks to confidentiality and the steps that will be taken to avoid them.

In some studies, identification of child abuse, elder abuse, or contagious diseases can be anticipated. In clinical practice, such cases must be reported to appropriate officials. Investigators need to determine in advance whether cases identified during the research project will be reported and, if so, inform patients during the informed consent process.

Review by an Institutional Review Board

Approval from an IRB is required for most federally funded research, for research that will be submitted to the FDA to gain approval for new therapies, and for all researchers at many universities. The function of IRB review is to protect research subjects. The best intentioned researchers, in their eagerness to conduct important research, may not pay sufficient attention to potential ethical problems.

COMPETING AND CONFLICTING INTERESTS

Physician-researchers may have competing or conflicting interests that might compromise the integrity of their research. These other interests may impair researchers' objectivity and undermine public trust in research (8). Even the most scrupulous and well-intentioned investigators may subconsciously introduce bias into the research design, data collection, or analysis (8,9).

Competing Interests

Researchers may have other incentives that may compete with the goal of finding scientific truth.

Academic Rewards

Research publications lead to academic prestige, grants, and promotions.

Dual Roles for Clinician-Investigators

The investigator may also be the primary physician for an eligible research subject. As already discussed, such patients may fear that their future care will be jeopardized if they decline to participate in research. Furthermore, what is best for a particular patient's medical care may not be what is best for the research project. It may be better for the patient to drop out of the study and receive individualized care that differs from the research protocol. As an investigator, however, the physician wants study participants to continue to the end of the trial. If many subjects drop out, the power of the study to answer the research question will be compromised.

Such role conflicts should be explained to subjects in advance. Whenever possible, the patient should have the opportunity to receive care from a personal physician who is not associated with the study. Because the welfare of the patient should be paramount, the role of personal physician should take priority over the role of clinical researcher.

Research Funded by Drug Manufacturers

Clinical investigators are increasingly turning to drug companies for funding (10). The company manufacturing the drug has an obvious interest in having the drug proved effective. Thus the bias against publishing negative studies may be particularly strong in studies sponsored by drug companies (11). Another problem is that reimbursement from the drug company to investigators may greatly exceed the actual costs of the research. This excess reimbursement may offer researchers perverse incentives both to suggest experimental therapy for a patient when conventional therapy is in the patient's best interests and also to interpret findings in the most favorable light (12).

Finder's Fees for Research Subjects

In some situations, physicians may receive a finder's fee for referring patients to a research project.

CASE 30.3. FINDER'S FEES. *To encourage enrollment in a clinical trial of a new antibiotic, physicians are offered $350 for referring patients who subsequently enroll in the study (13). The referring physician needs to make a phone call to the coordinating research nurse, who will explain the study to the patient.*

Enrollment is often the rate-limiting step in clinical trials. Finder's fees facilitate the completion of clinical trials. Several objections to finders fees have been raised. They give the appearance that physicians refer patients to clinical trials for their own interest, rather than the patient's (13). Critics of finders fees also point out that the analogous situation of kickbacks for referring patients to a another physician for clinical care are considered unethical. Furthermore, the physicians reward may seem excessive for the services rendered.

Conflicting Interests

In some situations, investigators may face conflicts of interest (*see* Chapter 31). To further one interest, the investigator must hinder the other interest, and *vice versa.*

Financial Interest in the Drug Manufacturer

Investigators may hold stock or stock options in the company making the drug under study. Stock or stock options reward researchers for their work and create long-term relationships that may lead to future projects. Clinical researchers who hold options may reap huge financial rewards if the treatment is shown to be effective, in addition to their compensation for conducting the study. However, if the drug proves ineffective, investigators face an inevitable conflict of interest: fostering scientific progress will unavoidably harm their personal financial interests.

Fee-for-Service Research

Some clinical investigators may support their research through patient fees.

CASE 30.4. CHARGING PATIENTS FOR RESEARCH. *A for-profit corporation offers monoclonal antibody therapy to cancer patients on a research protocol. Patients will pay $35,000 for the costs of producing individualized antibodies to their tumor (14). The principal investigator is the president of the corporation.*

Advocates of such fee-for-service research argue that it will expand access to experimental therapies and expedite the process of clinical research (15). In this view, such research promotes patient autonomy by providing more alternatives for care. Serious concerns have been raised, however, about this practice (14). The investigator has a powerful financial incentive to continue to administer the therapy under study, rather than to determine whether or not the therapy is effective. Because of this incentive, early stopping rules may not be included in the protocol, negative results may not be published promptly, or results may be presented as inappropriately encouraging. If the therapy proves ineffective, there is an unavoidable conflict of interest between the promotion of scientific truth and the financial interests of the researcher and company.

Responding to Competing and Conflicting Interests

Investigators must respond to competing and conflicting interests. Researchers can respond to competing interests in ways that substantially eliminate the potential for bias. With conflicting interests, however, the potential for bias may be so great that physicians need to avoid placing themselves in such situations.

Minimize Competing or Conflicting Interests

In well-designed clinical trials, several standard precautions help keep competing interests in check. Investigators in clinical trials can be *blinded* to the intervention a subject is receiving, to prevent unconscious bias from influencing how clinical outcomes for patients are evaluated. An independent *data review committee* can review interim data and terminate the study if the data provide convincing evidence of benefit or harm. The *peer review* process for grants, abstracts, manuscripts, and promotion also serves as a check against biased or falsified research.

If research is funded by a pharmaceutical company, investigators need to ensure that they have *control over the primary data and statistical analysis* and will have the *freedom to publish findings* whether or not the drug is found to be effective (9). The sponsor should be able to review the manuscripts, make suggestions, and ensure that patent applications have been filed before submission. However, the drug company should have no power to veto or censor publication (16).

Problems with finders fees can be eliminated if the amount of the fee is commensurate with the services performed. If a physician is simply making a phone call to refer the patient, $350, as in Case 30.2, seems excessive.

If fee-for-service research is contemplated, the project is best conducted by independent investigators under contract, rather than by persons with stock or equity holdings in the company.

Disclose Competing and Conflicting Interests

Conflicts of interest need to be disclosed to potential participants in research. In a landmark court case, a patient sued a physician-researcher who had patented a cell line derived from the patient's cells without his knowledge or permission (6). The patient alleged that the physician-researcher had failed to disclose his personal financial stake in the research and had recommended several procedures without disclosing that they were for research, not clinical care. The California Supreme Court declared that physicians need to "disclose personal interests unrelated to the patient's health, whether research or economic, that may affect the physician's professional judgment" (6). This ruling implies that patients must be told if referring physicians receive a finder's fee or if the investigators have a financial stake in the product being studied.

Although disclosure is necessary to protect patients, it may be a halfway and inadequate response to potential conflicts of interest (8). Laypeople cannot adequately evaluate how research might be biased. Physicians reading a publication may not have enough information about the study to judge whether bias actually occurred. For example, readers may not be told how well blinding of investigators was maintained. Because disclosure alone may not adequately safeguard patients, additional safeguards may be needed.

Ban Certain Situations that Give Rise to Conflicts of Interest

Clinical investigators should avoid direct financial stakes in the therapies under evaluation. As one writer has noted, "It is difficult enough for the most conscientious researchers to be totally unbiased about their own work, but when an investigator has an economic interest in the outcome of the work, objectivity is even more difficult" (8). Many productive investigators support such prohibitions (17,18).

In conclusion, rigorous clinical research is essential to evaluate promising new therapies. Physicians should encourage patients to participate in appropriate clinical research. Investigators should ensure that the potential benefits of research are proportionate to the risks and that participants give informed consent. Conflicts of interest, which may impair objectivity and erode public trust in research, should be avoided.

REFERENCES

1. Levine C, Dubler NN, Levine RJ. Building a new consensus: ethical principles and policies for clinical research on HIV/AIDS. *IRB* 1991;13:1–17.
2. Freedman B. Equipoise and the ethics of clinical research. *N Engl J Med* 1987;317:141–145.
3. National Bioethics Advisory Commission. *Research involving persons with mental disorders that may affect decisionmaking capacity.* Rockville, MD: National Bioethics Advisory Commission, 1998.
4. Warren JW, Sobal J, Denney JH, et al. Informed consent by proxy: an issue in research with elderly patients. *N Engl J Med* 1986;315:1125–1128.
5. Lo B, Feigal D, Cummins S, et al. Addressing ethical issues. In: Hulley SB, et al. *Designing clinical research*, 2nd ed. Philadelphia: Lippincott Williams & Wilkins, (in press).
6. Moore *v.* Regents of University of California, 51 Cal.3d 120; Cal. Rptr. 146, 793 P.2d 479 (1990).
7. Appelbaum PS. False hopes and best data: consent to research and the therapeutic misconception. *Hastings Center Rep* 1987;17:20–24.
8. Relman AS. Economic incentives in clinical investigation. *N Engl J Med* 1989;320:933–934.
9. Hillman AL, Eisenberg JM, Pauly MV, et al. Avoiding bias in the conduct and reporting of cost-effectiveness research sponsored by pharmaceutical companies. *N Engl J Med* 1991;324:1362–1365.
10. American Federation for Clinical Research guidelines for avoiding conflict of interest. *Clin Res* 1990;38:239–240.
11. Davidson DA. Source of funding and outcome of clinical trials. *J Gen Intern Med* 1986;1:155–158.
12. Shimm DS, Spece RG. Industry reimbursement for entering patients into clinical trials: ethical issues. *Ann Intern Med* 1991;115:148–151.
13. Lind S. Finder's fees for research subjects. *N Engl J Med* 1990;323:192–194.
14. Lind SE. Fee-for-service research. *N Engl J Med* 1986;314:312–315.
15. Oldham RK. Patient-funded cancer research. *N Engl J Med* 1987;316:46–47.
16. Rennie D, Flanagin A. Thyroid storm. *JAMA* 1997;277:1238–1243.
17. Healy B, Campeau L, Gray R, et al. Conflict-of-interest guidelines for a multicenter clinical trial of treatment after coronary-artery bypass-graft surgery. *N Engl J Med* 1989;320:949–951.
18. Topol EJ, Armstrong P, Van de Werf F, et al. Confronting the issues of patient safety and investigator conflict of interest in an international trial of myocardial reperfusion. *J Am Coll Cardiol* 1992;19:1123–1128.

ANNOTATED BIBLIOGRAPHY

1. Levine RJ. *Ethics and regulation of clinical research.* Baltimore, MD: Urban & Schwarzenberg, 1986.
   Comprehensive and thoughtful book on all aspects of designing and conducting clinical research.
2. Brody BA. *The ethics of biomedical research.* New York: Oxford University Press, 1998.
   Clear, up-to-date monograph, with excellent discussion of international perspective.
3. National Bioethics Advisory Commission. *Research involving persons with mental disorders that may affect decisionmaking capacity.* Rockville, MD: National Bioethics Advisory Commission, 1998.
   Analyzes ethical dilemmas that occur when research subjects lack the capacity to make informed decisions.

SECTION V

Conflicts of Interest

31

Overview of Conflicts of Interest

In *The Doctor's Dilemma,* George Bernard Shaw questioned whether people can be "impartial where they have a strong pecuniary interest on one side" (1). He wrote, "Nobody supposes that doctors are less virtuous than judges; but a judge whose salary and reputation depended on whether the verdict was for plaintiff or defendant, prosecutor or prisoner, should be as little trusted as a general in the pay of the enemy. To offer me a doctor as my judge, and then weight his decision with a bribe of a large sum of money. . . is to go wildly beyond . . . [what] human nature will bear" (1). Shaw's words have particular relevance to contemporary U.S. medicine because of increasing concerns over conflicts of interest in managed care.

A conflict of interest exists when a person entrusted with the interests of a client, dependent, or the public violates that trust. Rather than acting in the patient's best interests, physicians may promote their own self-interest or the interests of third parties, such as a hospital, physician group, or insurance plan. Some conflicts of interest are financial, such as those resulting from reimbursement incentives or personal investments in medical facilities. Other conflicts of interest involve personal or professional roles, as when physicians respond to mistakes, deal with impaired colleagues, or need to learn invasive procedures. Chapters 32 to 38 analyze specific conflicts of interest. This chapter discusses how to define conflicts of interest, who should decide what constitutes an unacceptable conflict of interest, and how physicians can manage conflicts of interest.

CONFLICTS OF INTEREST IN NONMEDICAL SITUATIONS

Conflicts of interest occur in all professions and in public service (2). For example, a trustee may use the trust fund of an elderly person or child for his own profit. A public official may accept expensive gifts or trips from a company whose business he oversees.

Consider a judge who presides over a case involving a relative or a former law partner or in which she has a personal financial stake in the outcome (3). In such a situation, the decisions of the judge may favor her relative, her former partner, or her self-interest. Even if the outcome of the legal proceedings is fair, the process by which the decision was reached may be biased. For instance, the judge may take into account inappropriate factors or make rulings about motions and objections that no impartial decision-maker would make. These procedural errors would be disturbing even if the outcome seemed fair. Public trust in the judicial system may be undermined. Simply the appearance of a conflict of interest may be unacceptable.

The judge may honestly believe that she will be impartial and may even consciously try to compensate for her ties to a litigant. However, the opposing party and the public may still suspect that another judge would have decided the case differently. People naturally tend to believe that they are acting with integrity, even when this may not be the case. Thus, even if the individual judge believes that she can be impartial, she may be required to withdraw from the case. Society decides when judges or officials must recuse themselves, through legislation, regulation, and case law (3). There is no implication that she is immoral or unprofessional. Instead, the idea is that it would be untenable to place anyone in such a situation.

WHY ARE CONFLICTS OF INTEREST ETHICALLY PROBLEMATICAL FOR PHYSICIANS?

Conflicts of interest may be ethically problematical for physicians for several reasons. First, patients may suffer physical harm if physicians base clinical decisions on what is best for themselves or third parties, rather than on what is best for patients. Second, the integrity of medical judgment may be violated even though the patient suffers no clinical harm. If physicians violate standards of good practice to foster their own self-interest or the interest of third parties, future patients may suffer adverse clinical outcomes. Third, conflicts of interest undercut patient trust. Patients may fear that physicians are not acting on their behalf in other situations.

HOW ARE CONFLICTS OF INTEREST DEFINED?

Different criteria for conflicts of interest have been used. Often people use the term "conflict of interest" without clarifying how they define it.

Detrimental Patient Outcomes

The narrowest definition of conflict of interests is that the patient's outcome is worse because the physician has subordinated the best interests of the patient (4,5). The physician may do so either intentionally or subconsciously.

Compromise of Physicians' Judgment or the Decision-Making Process

A broader definition is that the physician's judgment or decision-making process is compromised, even though clinical outcomes are not impaired. Failure to order an indicated test or therapy because of a conflict of interest must be distinguished from a mistake or incompetence.

Potential for Detrimental Outcomes or Compromised Judgment

A still broader definition of conflicts of interest includes the *potential* for detrimental outcomes or for compromised judgment, without evidence of *actual* harm or compromised judgment (6). For example, personal investments in medical facilities provide physicians financial incentives for ordering more services, even when they are not medically necessary for the patient (*see* Chapter 34). In any particular case, however, it may be difficult to show that a physician's decisions are inappropriate or that the patient suffered harm.

Perceived Conflicts of Interest

Some situations present only *perceived* conflicts of interest, without actual harm or even significant potential for harm. For example, many physicians claim that small gifts from drug companies, such as pens and writing pads, are harmless (*see* Chapter 35), yet the perception of a conflict of interest may be damaging even though the actual or potential compromise of patient well-being is small. If the public believes that physicians are serving the interests of drug companies rather than those of their patients, trust in the individual doctor or the profession as a whole may be undermined.

Physicians may be offended because concerns about potential or perceived conflicts of interest seem to impugn their integrity. Doctors need to understand that the public is not singling them out for censure, but simply treating them as human and therefore fallible. The situation is viewed as problematical, not the person; it would be untenable to place anyone in such a situation.

Competing versus Conflicting Interests

The interests of the patient and physician never coincide completely. *Conflicting* interests cannot both be fulfilled. The physician literally cannot advance one interest without setting back the other. *Competing* interests, in contrast, are not congruent with the patient's best interests, but can be furthered without harm to the patient. Conversely, the patient's interests can be achieved without gravely setting back the competing interests. For example, time devoted to patient care cannot be spent on continuing medical education, teaching, clinical research, personal hobbies, or family activities. Such competing interests can usually be accommodated.

Situations That Are Not Conflicts of Interest

The term *conflict of interest* is often used loosely. A conflict of interest, in the senses defined above, needs to be distinguished from conflicts between ethical guidelines, disagreements among health care professionals, or disagreements between patients and physicians.

REIMBURSEMENT INCENTIVES

Medicine is regarded as an altruistic profession because its primary goal is to benefit the patient, not to maximize physicians' income. However, no one expects physicians to work for free or begrudges them a comfortable income. Helping the sick is commendable and difficult work and requires extensive training. This tension between altruism and self-interest is unavoidable in medicine (7). Ideally, financial rewards to the doctor should be secondary to fostering patients' well-being.

Any reimbursement system may provide incentives to physicians to act contrary to patients' best interests. Traditional fee-for-service reimbursement provides incentives to increase services and to give services of little or no benefit, thereby raising the cost of health care (*see* Chapter 33). Managed care systems, which use capitation and prospective payment, may provide incentives to decrease health care services and withhold beneficial care (*see* Chapter 34).

The concern about financial incentives is not simply that unscrupulous physicians will deliberately subordinate the patient's interests to their own self-interest or the interests of hospitals or insurance plans (8). Subtle incentives may also exert unconscious influence on physician decisions. When several management options are plausible, "financial incentives may influence even the best, most highly principled doctors to overlook subtle clues that suggest an optimal approach" (8).

MANAGING CONFLICTS OF INTEREST

Often it is difficult to draw a clear line between improper conflicts of interest and situations in which the interests of the patient are adequately protected. When conflicting interests are identified, how can sick and vulnerable patients be protected? In general, physicians should consider the following steps (Table 31-1), which are discussed in more detail in subsequent chapters dealing with specific conflicts of interest.

Reaffirm That the Patient's Interests Are Paramount

Given the increasing public concern over conflicts of interest, individual physicians and the medical profession need to reaffirm their fiduciary responsibility to their patients. The doctor's primary responsibility is to foster the well-being of patients, not their own self-interest or the interests of third parties.

To check whether they are acting in the patient's best interest, doctors might ask what they would recommend if they were working under the opposite reimbursement system. Physicians in managed care might ask whether they would recommend the intervention under fee-for-service. Similarly, fee-for-service physicians might ask what they would recommend if they or the hospital would lose money doing the procedure. The answer is simple: physicians should recommend care that is in the patient's best interests, no more and no less. The goal of economic incentives should be to "prompt the physician to consider costs appropriately—to remind him pointedly that economics really does matter—but not to distort his reasoning. A well-designed incentive should prompt the physician to consider more carefully what he does with clinical uncertainties and borderline options; it should not induce him to forego what he believes is clearly in the patient's interest" (9).

Although reaffirmation of ethical guidelines is a necessary first step, additional steps may also need to be taken.

Disclose Conflicts of Interest

Disclosure is salutary for several reasons. First, the requirement to disclose incentives may prevent physicians and organizations from making some unacceptable arrangements. If the physician would find it hard or awkward to justify a situation, it probably presents an unacceptable conflict of interest. In controversial situations, it is prudent for physicians to err on the side of the patient's interests, rather than their own self-interest. Second, patients who know about a conflict of interests may be able to make more informed decisions by placing the physician's recommendations in context and compensating for any bias. However, it may be unrealistic to expect patients to assess whether a situation has biased the physician's judgment. Thus in some situations, disclosure alone may be inadequate to protect patients.

Take Precautions to Protect Patients

In some circumstances, society may determine that additional steps must be taken to safeguard patients or the public. Physicians' actions may be regulated and their discretion limited (5). For example, in clinical research, informed consent of subjects and review by an institutional review board are required (*see* Chapter 30).

TABLE 31-1. *Managing conflicts of interest*

Reaffirm that the patient's interests are paramount.
Disclose conflicts of interest.
Take precautions to protect patients.
Prohibit certain actions and situations.

Prohibit Certain Actions and Situations

Although disclosure and precautions are necessary steps, they still may be insufficient to protect patients. Some actions and situations present such strong and direct conflicts of interest that they should be prohibited. Because "it is difficult if not impossible to distinguish cases in which financial gain does have improper influence from those in which it does not," it may be prudent to prohibit certain actions and situations (6). For example, continuing education programs controlled by drug companies may provide biased or incomplete coverage of topics. To avoid this, programs should not accept support from drug companies that attempt to influence the choice of topics or speakers (*see* Chapter 35).

In summary, conflicts of interest are ethically perilous because they may harm patients, impair physicians' judgments, and undermine trust in physicians. The ethical ideal is that patients' interests should take priority over the self-interest of physicians or the interests of third parties, such as hospitals or insurers.

REFERENCES

1. Shaw GB. *The doctor's dilemma.* London: Penguin Books, 1946.
2. Wells P, Jones H, Davis M. *Conflicts of interest in engineering.* Dubuque, IA: Kendall/Hunt Publishing Company, 1986.
3. Gillers S, Dorsen N. *Regulation of lawyers: problems of law and ethics.* Boston: Little, Brown, 1989:790–808.
4. Rothman KJ. Conflicts of interest: the new McCarthyism in science. *JAMA* 1993;269:2782–2784.
5. Rodwin MA. *Medicine, money, and morals: physicians' conflicts of interest.* New York: Oxford University Press, 1993:179–211.
6. Thompson DF. Understanding financial conflicts of interest. *N Engl J Med* 1993;329:573–576.
7. Jonsen AR. Watching the doctor. *N Engl J Med* 1983;308:1531–1535.
8. Hillman AL. Health maintenance organizations, financial incentives, and physicians' judgments. *Ann Intern Med* 1990:112:891–893.
9. Morreim EH. *Balancing act: the new medical ethics of medicine's new economics.* Boston: Kluwer Academic Publishers, 1991:124.

32

Bedside Rationing of Health Care

Physicians are ethically obligated to act in the best interests of patients (*see* Chapter 4). However, acting in the best interests of one patient may sometimes make it impossible for physicians to act on behalf of another patient who is likely to benefit more from care. Dilemmas arise because resources such as physician time and medical supplies are in limited supply and people have different priorities for limited resources (1,2).

CASE 32.1. LIMITED CORONARY CARE BEDS. *Mr. H. presents to the emergency department with substernal chest pain. An electrocardiogram (EKG) shows an acute anterior myocardial infarction, multifocal ventricular premature beats, and some couplets. The cardiac care unit (CCU) and intensive care unit (ICU) are full. One of the patients in the CCU is a 73-year-old man who had an emergency operation for a ruptured aortic aneurysm. A week after the operation, he is comatose, in ventilatory failure, and has hypotension despite vasopressors. Another patient in the CCU experienced chest pain after an angioplasty earlier in the day but has no persistent EKG changes and has normal cardiac enzymes. The physicians consider whether to transfer one of these patients out of the CCU to free a bed for Mr. H.*

In Case 32.1, the patient with multisystem failure is so sick that he is highly unlikely to survive even if CCU care is continued. The postangioplasty patient is receiving only monitoring, not active treatment, and is highly likely to have a good outcome even if he is transferred out of the unit. In contrast, Mr. H. will benefit greatly from thrombolytic and antiarrhythmic therapy, which can be administered only in an intensive care setting. If CCU beds are allocated on a strictly first-come, first-served basis, Mr. H. would be denied substantial benefits.

This chapter discusses the ethical considerations that arise when the interests of one patient conflict directly with the interests of other patients. In addition, the chapter analyzes whether the scarcity of financial resources justifies limiting the care of an individual patient. Chapter 34 deals with conflicts of interest between the health care provider and patient, rather than conflicts of interest between patients.

The terms used to discuss these issues are hard to define precisely, are often used inconsistently, and commonly evoke strong emotions (3–5). In this book, "allocation" refers to decisions that set levels of funding for programs, rather than determining care for individual patients. For example, funds must be allocated between Medicaid and other social programs such as education and transportation and, within Medicaid, between inpatient services and prenatal care. Sometimes these policy-level choices are termed "macroallocation." Allocation choices are unavoidable because resources are limited and because people have different priorities for using them. In contrast, this book uses the term "rationing" to refer to decisions at the bedside or in the office to limit care for individual patients because of limited resources. Often the term *rationing* connotes limiting beneficial care because it is too expensive. The term "microallocation" is also used in this context. The term rationing excludes clinical decisions that are straightforward implementation of macroallocation policies, such as health plans' decisions not to cover cosmetic surgery. Unlike other countries such as Great Britain, the United States has not developed coherent societal allocation policies (6,7). The ethical issue is whether, in the absence of a fair social agreement on allocation, physicians can ethically carry out rationing at the bedside.

ARGUMENTS AGAINST BEDSIDE RATIONING

Traditionally, bedside rationing by physicians has been considered unethical (8,9). Opponents of bedside rationing argue that doctors should act as fiduciaries and patient advocates, helping patients receive all beneficial care that the system allows. One eminent physician wrote, "Physicians are required to do everything that they believe may benefit each patient without regard to costs or other societal considerations. In caring for an individual patient, the doctor must act solely as the patient's advocate, against the apparent interests of society as a whole" (10). This fiduciary role is deemed essential for maintaining patient trust. In their roles as citizens and civic leaders, physicians should help determine how resources should be allocated. At the bedside, however, physicians should not limit care to one patient primarily to benefit other patients or to save money for society.

ARGUMENTS SUPPORTING BEDSIDE RATIONING

An absolute prohibition against bedside rationing, however, is ethically problematical (Table 32-1).

Acting in the Patient's Best Interests Is Not an Absolute Duty

The physician's ethical obligation to act in the best interests of the individual patient is not absolute. Under several circumstances, physicians are ethically or legally required to act against the best interests of the patient in order to benefit third parties. For example, although maintaining confidentiality of medical information is in a patient's best interest, it is overridden when third parties may be harmed by infectious diseases, threats of physical violence, or the patient's inability to drive safely (*see* Chapter 5). Furthermore, the guideline of beneficence is not without limit. The physician is not obliged to do literally everything that might benefit the patient. One philosopher writes that the traditional ethic of advocacy needs to be redefined to "proportional advocacy": the advocate "argues not for 'everything possible' but for everything 'probably beneficial'" (11). Similarly, the American Medical Association declares that "physicians must advocate for any care they believe will materially benefit their patients" (12). Other advocates of the fiduciary role enjoin physicians to practice "parsimonious" or "efficient" medicine (8,9). These views acknowledge that if physicians ordered all tests and drugs that provided any benefit, costs would soar out of control. In other words, all these views allow some

TABLE 32-1. *Arguments in favor of bedside rationing*

Acting in the patient's best interests is not an absolute duty.
Leaving physicians out of microallocation decisions will harm patients.
Other patients may be seriously harmed if resources are not rationed.

forms of rationing, without calling it such. It is more honest to call rationing by name (5) and to proceed to the constructive debates over when it is justified (4).

Leaving Physicians Out of Microallocation Decisions Would Harm Patients

If physicians were not involved in microallocation, clinical decisions would be made according to practice guidelines or utilization review guidelines, or by administrators in health care organizations. Centralized allocation decisions, through guidelines or rules, fail to take into account meaningful differences in individual patient circumstances (13–16). Individual patient cases are too complex to be captured in simple guidelines or rules. Physicians can often bring to bear pertinent clinical information to justify an exception to a general rule (17). Treating everyone with a clinical condition the same is unfair if there are clinically and ethically pertinent differences among patients.

Other Patients May Be Seriously Harmed if Resources Are Not Rationed

Providing care to one patient may deny care to another patient who would receive much greater medical benefit. Two patients may be competing for such limited resources as physician time or ICU beds. In this situation, informal rationing is standard medical practice that has strong ethical justification.

CASE 32.2. LIMITED PHYSICIAN TIME. *Mr. M., a 48-year-old man, comes to the physician's office after 40 minutes of crushing substernal chest pain and shortness of breath. At the same time, a 21-year-old woman with asthma comes to the office with worsening shortness of breath for the past day, despite increasing use of inhaled bronchodilators. These patients do not have appointments, and the physician's schedule is already full.*

Because their time is limited, physicians must decide which patients deserve higher priority. In a life-threatening situation such as a probable myocardial infarction in Case 32.2, the priority of the emergency case over other patients is clear. Mr. M. needs to be stabilized and transported to the emergency department. Regularly scheduled patients presumably would agree to wait because they would want similar priority if they should suffer such a serious emergency. However, how is an emergency defined? If care is instituted promptly for the woman with a severe asthma attack, her symptoms of shortness of breath will be relieved more rapidly and a hospitalization may be avoided. However, how much benefit or potential harm to the asthma patient justifies asking regularly scheduled patients to wait? Referring the asthma patient to the emergency department would not resolve the dilemma, but only push it back a step. Physicians there would need to decide which patient presenting for care deserves first priority.

Physicians routinely make decisions to allocate their time, and indeed patients and society expect them to do so. It is difficult to imagine anyone other than the individual physician making ultimate decisions on who should wait. General rules can be set; for example, patients with serious emergencies should take priority, and patients with minor or self-limited illnesses should wait. However, physicians will still need to interpret those general rules in a particular case, for example, by deciding whether a patient's asthma attack is severe enough to warrant asking other patients to wait.

In Case 32.1, involving a patient with a heart attack, essential medical resources—CCU beds—are in short supply. Some ethicists assert that physicians have an ethical obligation to ration scarce intensive care beds by transferring out of the CCU patients who are either too sick or too healthy to benefit significantly from intensive care (18). In clinical practice, physicians frequently transfer patients in order to allow others to receive intensive care. When the CCU or ICU is full, physicians identify patients who are too sick to benefit from continued intensive care and set more restrictive standards for admission to the unit. Several empirical studies have shown that such transfers occur commonly and that, under moderate constraints, physicians can make such transfers without adversely affecting overall patient outcomes (19).

Increasing the supply of CCU beds will not resolve the problem of rationing but only postpone the dilemma of the last bed. Transferring patients to other hospitals with open CCU beds is also not a solution, because Mr. H. needs immediate treatment.

In Case 32.1, an identified patient would be seriously harmed if care was not rationed. In the following case, a future patient will predictably be harmed unless care is rationed.

CASE 32.3. SHORTAGE OF BLOOD PRODUCTS. *A 36-year-old man with alcoholic cirrhosis is admitted for severe variceal bleeding and encephalopathy. He is not a candidate for liver transplantation because of his active alcohol and amphetamine use. The surgeons do not believe he will survive a portacaval shunt operation. After 3 days, he has consumed 42 units of blood and continues to bleed briskly despite endoscopic sclerotherapy and percutaneous placement of a therapeutic portal-systemic shunt (TIPS). The regional blood bank has only 3 more units of his type of blood, despite appeals for more donations. It is New Year's Eve, when many victims of automobile accidents will need blood transfusions.*

In Case 32.3, there is no identified individual who will be harmed if blood products are not rationed, but the existence of such an individual can be predicted with virtual certainty. Many trauma victims can recover completely with vigorous emergency care. Thus a future trauma victim may be seriously harmed if all available blood were given to the patient in Case 32.3, who has not improved despite maximal care.

Physicians may be reluctant to ration interventions to patients who are already receiving care. Doctors may believe that they have made an implied promise to the patient to provide ongoing care and not to curtail it to benefit other patients, that is, physicians feel that they owe loyalty or fidelity to their current patients. The emotional appeal of this position is clear, and keeping promises is an important ethical guideline. However, fidelity should refer to appropriate ongoing care, not unlimited care regardless of the benefits to the patient or the harms to others.

Although limitations on transfusions are justified in Case 32.3, there are problems implementing such limits in a fair manner. Various physicians may set different limits in practice. Some physicians might stop after 40 units, others after 60 units. More specific practice standards would make such decisions more consistent and therefore more fair.

RATIONING ON THE BASIS OF FINANCIAL RESOURCES

We have argued that compelling ethical arguments exist in some situations for limiting care to one patient in order to provide much more beneficial clinical services to other patients. However, when rationing is done primarily to save money rather than to benefit other patients directly, the reasons are often weaker. The following case illustrates these issues.

CASE 32.4. EXPENSIVE CARE FOR A PATIENT WITH POOR PROGNOSIS AND QUALITY OF LIFE. *Mrs. D. is a 76-year-old woman with severe dementia. She recognizes her family only occasionally and does not respond to questions or requests by health care workers. She develops chronic renal failure and symptoms of uremia. While competent, she had never expressed her preferences regarding renal dialysis. Although her primary physician and the nephrologist strongly recommend that renal dialysis not be performed, her family insists on it. They believe that as long as she recognizes them and smiles, her life should be prolonged. They un-*

derstand that dialysis would not improve her mental functioning or mobility. The family seems informed and caring.

At the time, the public hospital in the community is considering closing obstetrical and substance abuse services because of budget deficits. The physicians feel they are accomplices with an unjust health care system if they use resources on this patient when more pressing health needs lack funding. A vascular surgery consultant writes in the medical record, "In the current climate of out-of-control medical costs, it is unconscionable to provide expensive care for this patient."

Under the guidelines regarding life-sustaining treatment discussed in Chapter 14, it would be appropriate to provide renal dialysis to Mrs. D. Dialysis would achieve the family's goal of prolonging her life at a quality they consider acceptable. The physicians, however, believe that Mrs. D.'s quality of life is so poor that the cost of dialysis is not justified.

Everyone agrees that physicians should support more enlightened policies regarding allocation, but in most circumstances, attempts by physicians to ration care on the basis of costs at the level of the individual patient, although well intentioned, are not justified.

No Public Policy Authorizes Physicians to Ration Based on Costs

The physicians caring for Mrs. D. felt partly responsible for the soaring cost of health care. However, no public policy authorizes physicians to limit the care of patients on renal dialysis to save resources for other patients. On the contrary, U.S. public policy pays for dialysis to all patients with end-stage renal failure. In the 1960's, selecting patients for a limited number of renal dialysis machines on the basis of prognosis or quality of life proved so controversial that Congress singled out end-stage renal disease for universal coverage under the Medicare program.

Bedside Rationing Based on Costs Would Be Inconsistent and Unfair

Physicians at one hospital might withhold dialysis from Mrs. D., whereas physicians at another hospital might provide it. Indeed, the public nursing home in the area provided chronic dialysis to numerous patients with severe Alzheimer's disease. Such inconsistency would be arbitrary and unfair. It violates the ethical guideline of justice to treat similar patients unequally. Whether Mrs. D. receives dialysis should not be based on choice of hospital.

Bedside rationing may also be unfair if certain patients or certain interventions are singled out for review. It makes little sense to limit one health care intervention as not cost-effective without looking at the cost-effectiveness of other interventions as well. Many people would object to limiting dialysis for Mrs. D. if other interventions, such as intensive care for patients with extremely poor prognoses, were not similarly scrutinized.

Money Saved by Rationing Cannot Be Reallocated

Physicians in the United States who save money on the care of an individual patient generally cannot redirect those resources to patients or projects that have higher priority (20). If physicians terminated dialysis on Mrs. D., they could not redirect funds to more pressing medical or social needs, such as prenatal care or childhood immunizations. Furthermore, in managed care organizations, savings from limiting care to patients may be directed toward higher salaries for administrators or greater profits for investors in for-profit organizations (21). In the absence of broader health care reform, attempts to limit health care costs at the bedside are ineffective gestures.

Opponents of bedside rationing would argue that physicians in Case 32.4 fulfilled their ethical obligations by discussing dialysis with Mrs. D.'s family and making a strong recommendation against it.

An Example of Ethically Acceptable Bedside Rationing: Tiered Formulary Benefits

In some situations, it is ethically acceptable for physicians to limit services to one patient in order to conserve a pool of money that pays for services to a population of patients. Formulary restrictions are one common example. Because drug expenditures are the most rapidly growing part of health care costs, many managed care plans have established restricted formularies and tiered copayments. For example, patients may have a $5 copayment for preferred drugs on the formulary, a $10 copayment for nonpreferred formulary drugs, and a still higher copayment for nonformulary drugs. Alternatively, nonformulary drugs may not be covered at all without physician authorization. Typically preferred drugs are cheaper than other drugs in the same class because a discount from the manufacturer has been negotiated.

In some situations, there are no meaningful clinical differences among drugs in a class, but significant differences in cost. Examples are different statin-class drugs for hypercholesterolemia or different angiotensin converting-enzyme inhibitors for congestive heart failure. In these situations, it is ethical for the physician to start with the presumption that preferred formulary drugs are appropriate. For instance, the physician can recommend that the patient try a preferred drug rather than an equivalent nonpreferred drug. For a stable chronic conditon, the risk to the patient of using a preferred medication within the same class of drugs is small, provided the patient receives close follow-up care.

This presumption in favor of a preferred drug may be overridden in some situations. For example, if a patient is already on a nonpreferred drug, it may be continued if it was very difficult to titrate the proper dose or if the patient is confused by changes in the drug regimen. Furthermore, if the patient develops unacceptable side effects, an unsatisfactory clinical outcome, or poor adherence, it would be appropriate for the physician to authorize a nonpreferred or nonformulary drug. The physician may need to provide guidance to patients as to whether a nonpreferred drug is worth the higher out-of-pocket cost.

SUGGESTIONS FOR PHYSICIANS

Physicians who are considering rationing care at the bedside should take several actions (Table 32-2).

Try to Get More Resources for the Patient Within the System

Physicians should try to obtain more resources within the system. For example, beds in the postoperative recovery room might be used as temporary ICU beds in Case 32.1. Such efforts, however, may lead to other problems, such as disruption of operating room schedules.

TABLE 32-2. *Suggestions for physicians considering bedside rationing*

Try to get more resources for the patient within the system.
Make decisions openly.
Get a second opinion.
Notify patients or surrogates when care is rationed.

Make Decisions Openly

Discussing rationing dilemmas explicitly may prevent inconsistent and unfair decisions. In such emotionally charged decisions, unquestioned assumptions and hidden value judgments are a concern. When people must make their arguments and values explicit, others can present rebuttals or disagreements.

Get a Second Opinion

A second opinion from another attending physician or from a hospital ethics committee or consultant may improve decision-making. For example, such review may clarify the prognosis of the patients or point out unwarranted value judgments.

Notify Patients or Surrogates When Care Is Rationed

Patients or their surrogates should be notified when beneficial care will be rationed. It is disrespectful to transfer patients out of intensive care or stop transfusions without explaining to them or their families what is happening. If possible, it is preferable to make such explanations before a clinical crisis occurs.

In summary, bedside rationing may be ethically appropriate if providing services to one patient would directly deprive another patient of services that will provide much greater medical benefits. However, decisions to ration in order to save money may be problematical. Physicians facing such bedside rationing decisions should take steps to help ensure that these decisions are consistent and fair.

REFERENCES

1. Thurow LC. Learning to say "no." *N Engl J Med* 1984;311:1569–1572.
2. Fuchs VR. The "rationing" of medical care. *N Engl J Med* 1984;311:1572–1573.
3. Eddy DM. Rationing by patient choice. *JAMA* 1991;265:105–108.
4. Asch DA, Ubel PA. Rationing by any other name. *N Engl J Med* 1997;336:1668–1671.
5. Ubel PA, Goold S. Recognizing bedside rationing: clear cases and tough calls. *Ann Intern Med* 1997;126:74–80.
6. Schwartz WB. The inevitable failure of current cost-containment strategies. Why they can provide only temporary relief. *JAMA* 1987;257:220–224.
7. Boren SD. I had a tough day today, Hillary. *N Engl J Med* 1994;330:500–502.
8. Pellegrino ED, Thomasma DG. *For the patient's good: the restoration of beneficence in health care.* New York: Oxford University Press, 1988.
9. Kassirer JP. Managing care—should we adopt a new ethic? *N Engl J Med* 1998;339:397–398.
10. Levinsky NG. The doctor's master. *N Engl J Med* 1984;311:1573–1575.
11. Jonsen AR. *The new medicine and the old ethics.* Cambridge: Harvard University Press, 1990:59.
12. Council on Ethical and Judicial Affairs. *Code of medical ethics: current opinions with annotations.* Chicago: American Medical Association, 1998:143.
13. Hillman AL. Managing the physician: rules versus incentives. *Health Aff (Millwood)* 1991;10:138–146.
14. Hall MA. *Making medical spending decisions.* New York: Oxford University Press, 1997.
15. Morreim EH. Fiscal scarcity and the inevitability of bedside budget balancing. *Arch Intern Med* 1989;149:1012–1015.
16. Morreim EH. *Balancing act: the new medical ethics of medicine's new economics.* Boston: Kluwer Academic Publishers, 1991.
17. Ellrodt AG, Conner L, Riedinger M, et al. Measuring and improving physician compliance with clinical practice guidelines. *Ann Intern Med* 1995;122:277–282.
18. Engelhardt HT, Rie MA. Intensive care units, scarce resources, and conflicting principles of justice. *JAMA* 1986;255:1159–1164.
19. Strauss MJ, LoGerfo JP, Yeltatzie JA, et al. Rationing of intensive care unit services: an everyday occurrence. *JAMA* 1986;255:1143–1146.
20. Daniels N. Why saying no to patients in the United States is so hard. *N Engl J Med* 1986;314:1380–1383.
21. Woolhandler S, Himmelstein DU. Costs of care and administration at for-profit and other hospitals in the United States. *N Engl J Med* 1997;336:769–774.

ANNOTATED BIBLIOGRAPHY

1. Levinsky NG. The doctor's master. *N Engl J Med* 1984;311:1573–1575.
   Argues eloquently that the physician's primary responsibility is to the individual patient, not to society.
2. Daniels N. Why saying no to patients in the United States is so hard. *N Engl J Med* 1986;314:1380–1383.
   Points out that in the U.S. system, there is no way to direct money saved on one patient to more cost-effective purposes.
3. Asch DA, Ubel PA. Rationing by any other name. *N Engl J Med* 1997;336:1668–1671.
   Clarifies the range of situations in which physicians limit beneficial services because they are too costly.
4. Boren SD. I had a tough day today, Hillary. *N Engl J Med* 1994;330:500–502.
   First-person account by medical director of a managed care plan, describing the types of expensive interventions that insurers are asked to cover.

33

Incentives for Physicians
to Increase Services

Under fee-for-service reimbursement, physicians and health care organizations can increase their incomes by providing more services. They can see more patients, see them more frequently, perform more interventions per patient, or raise their charges for services (1).

PROBLEMS WITH FEE-FOR-SERVICE REIMBURSEMENT

Provides Services of Little or No Benefit

Fee-for-service reimbursement offers incentives to increase all services, not only those services that are effective or cost-effective. When fee-for-service reimbursement was dominant, many older studies found extensive overuse of expensive interventions. Thirty-two percent of carotid endarterectomies performed between 1979 and 1982 did not have any medical indication, as determined by a panel of experts (2). Similarly, 22% of coronary artery bypass operations, and 70% of pacemakers were not medically indicated (3–5). In some situations, physicians have been reported to order tests and therapies that clearly are not medically indicated, solely to increase their own income or the profit of the health care organization (6). Economic studies suggest that physicians increase demand for medical services in order to achieve a target income (7). For example, when fees for procedures are reduced, physicians may increase the number of procedures they perform. When patients receive interventions that are unnecessary or only of marginal benefit, they are exposed to unwarranted risks.

Drives Up the Cost of Health Care

In the aggregate, fee-for-service incentives drive up the cost of health care. Because of unacceptable increases in the cost of health care, employers, insurers, and policy makers have increasingly turned to alternative reimbursement systems that offer incentives to limit health care expenditures.

Encourages Invasive Rather Than Cognitive Procedures

Fee-for-service reimbursement currently encourages invasive procedures rather than spending time talking with patients about decisions or counseling them about preventive care (8). For example, Medicare reimburses a cardiologist a professional fee of $445 for inserting a temporary pacemaker, a procedure that takes about 30 minutes. In contrast, Medicare reimbursement for a 1-hour family meeting about withdrawing life-sustaining procedures is $100.

SELF-REFERRAL BY PHYSICIANS

During the 1980's, many physicians invested in medical facilities to which they referred patients. In 1992, virtually all diagnostic imaging centers in Florida, almost 80% of radiation therapy centers, and 75% of ambulatory surgical facilities were owned by physicians (9). At least 40% of physicians in the state had invested in a health care business to which they refer patients (9). Such so-called physician self-referral has been criticized as a conflict of interest. Physicians who profit from referrals may send patients for services that are unnecessary or overpriced.

Justification for Self-Referral

Benefits to Patients

Proponents argue that such physician investment increases access to care because state-of-the-art technology may not be available otherwise, particularly in rural areas (10). The evidence, however, does not support these claims. For example, none of the physician-owned radiation therapy centers in Florida are located in rural areas or inner cities (11).

Fair Rewards for Financial Risks

Advocates argue that if physicians take financial risks when investing in free-standing facilities, they should be able to share in any profits. Physicians may be more willing than other investors to take such risks because they better appreciate the promise of new technologies (10).

Problems With Self-Referral

Potential Conflicts of Interest

A conflict of interest may exist when physicians recommend services from which they profit financially. According to the American Medical Association (AMA), self-referral may "undermine the commitment of physicians to professionalism" (10).

Ownership of medical facilities has been shown to increase physician use of services under fee-for-service reimbursement (10,12). When physicians invest in ambulatory clinical laboratories, imaging centers, and radiation therapy facilities, they order more services than physicians who do not have such a financial stake (10,13). There is no direct evidence that such increased services are inappropriate. However, many studies show that, in general, greater use of medical services is not associated with better patient outcomes (14).

Increased Cost of Care

Physician self-referral increases the cost of care (10,12). Given the soaring health care costs in the United States, it is difficult to justify arrangements that increase costs without clear evidence that patient outcomes are improved.

Undermining of Public Trust in the Profession

Even the appearance that physicians are trying to increase profits may erode trust in the profession. The AMA has stated, "There are some activities regarding their patients that physicians should avoid whether or not there is evidence of abuse" (10). Financial reward for physicians is traditionally regarded as a consequence of serving patients, not as a goal to be pursued for its own sake.

Distinguishing Self-Referral from Other Practices

Traditional professional ethics does not allow physicians to refer patients to pharmacies that they own. The concern is that physicians may overprescribe when it is in their self-interest to do so, and patients may not check whether prices at the physician-owned pharmacy are competitive. Pragmatically, banning referrals to physician-owned pharmacies is justified because it is difficult to monitor for cases of abuse.

Physicians are permitted recommend services that they personally perform, such as endoscopy, angiography, or surgery. Physicians who directly provide services are responsible for assuring the quality of care. In addition, quality assurance programs in hospitals monitor the use of such procedures. Free-standing facilities, however, may not have comparable quality assurance programs.

Regarding physician-owned office laboratory or imaging equipment, the traditional view is that professional responsibility to ensure appropriate quality of care will prevail over self-interest. Given heightened concern over conflicts of interest, however, physicians will need to look afresh at such practices (15,16).

How Can Dilemmas Be Resolved?

Disclosure to Patients

Disclosure is a necessary step because otherwise patients, insurers, and the public would not suspect physician investments. However, disclosure alone may not sufficiently safeguard patients. Even if patients know that the physician has a financial incentive to increase referrals, they may not be able to judge whether recommendations for testing or treatment are sound. In addition, patients may be afraid of offending physicians if they do not go to the facility in question. Furthermore, disclosure does not diminish referrals by physician-investors (17).

Standards by Professional Organizations

The AMA has published guidelines to curb abuses but still allow physician investments that would benefit patients (10). The AMA guidelines permit investment and self-referral only when adequate alternative facilities do not exist and when alternative financing is not available. Physicians may not receive special consideration as investors. In addition, the AMA requires such physician-owned facilities to set up utilization review programs. The guidelines also require disclosure to patients when a referral is made.

Banning Certain Practices

The federal government has banned self-referral in the Medicare program. Physicians who own, invest in, or have certain compensation arrangements with clinical laboratories may not refer Medicare patients to them (12). Exceptions are made for office laboratories; group medical practices, health maintenance organizations, and hospitals; rural areas; and investment in facilities whose stock is publicly traded (12). Some states have also banned self-referrals (18).

NONFINANCIAL INCENTIVES TO PROVIDE MORE SERVICES

Social and psychological factors reinforce financial incentives in fee-for-service medicine to provide more services. First, both the public and physicians regard high-technology procedures such as magnetic resonance imaging, angioplasty, and endoscopy as the epitome of excellent medical care. The prestige that hospitals and physicians gain by providing these services encourages their wider use. Second, the inherent uncertainty in clinical medicine encourages the use of additional interventions. Every case varies from the textbook presentation of illness, and the course of a patient's illness is difficult to predict. One response to such uncertainty is doing an additional test or trying a new drug. Faced with an individual patient, physicians may recommend interventions that they would not recommend as a general clinical guideline (19). Finally, the malpractice system encourages "defensive medicine," the ordering of interventions of small marginal benefit to patients in order to prevent potential lawsuits.

In summary, the fee-for-service reimbursement system encourages physicians to provide more services and in some instances to overuse services. Both health care organizations and individuals need to ensure that clinical decisions are based on the best interests of patients, not on their own self-interest.

REFERENCES

1. Roe RB. The UCR boondoggle: a death knell for private practice? *N Engl J Med* 1981;305:41–45.
2. Franks P, Clancy CM, Nutting PA. Gatekeeping revisited—protecting patients from overtreatment. *N Engl J Med* 1992;327:424–429.
3. Brook RH, Park RE, Chassin MR, et al. Predicting the appropriate use of carotid endarterectomy, upper gastrointestinal endoscopy, and coronary angiography. *N Engl J Med* 1990;323:1173–1177.
4. Greenspan AM, Kay HR, Berger BC, et al. Incidence of unwarranted implantation of permanent cardiac pacemakers in a large medical population. *N Engl J Med* 1988;318:158–163.
5. Winslow CM, Josecoff JB, Chassin M, et al. The appropriateness of performing coronary artery bypass surgery. *JAMA* 1989;260:505–509.
6. Bock RS. The pressure to keep prices high at a walk-in clinic: a personal experience. *N Engl J Med* 1988;319:785–787.
7. Rodwin MA. *Medicine, money, and morals: physicians' conflicts of interest.* New York: Oxford University Press, 1993:339.
8. Hsiao WC, Verrilli DK. Assessing the implementation of physician payment reform. *N Engl J Med* 1993;328:928–933.
9. Mitchell JM, Scott E. New evidence of the prevalence and scope of physician joint ventures. *JAMA* 1992;268:80–84.
10. Council on Ethical and Judicial Affairs, AMA. Conflicts of interest: physician ownership of medical facilities. *JAMA* 1992;267:2366–2369.
11. Mitchell JM, Sunshine JH. Consequences of physician ownership of health care facilities—joint ventures in radiation therapy. *N Engl J Med* 1992;327:1497–1501.
12. Iglehart JK. Efforts to address the problem of physician self-referral. *N Engl J Med* 1991;325:1820–1824.
13. Hillman BJ, Joseph CA, Mabry MR, et al. Frequency and costs of diagnostic imaging in office practice—a comparison of self-referring and radiologist-referring physicians. *N Engl J Med* 1990;323:1604–1608.
14. Wennberg JE, Freeman JL, Shelton RM, et al. Hospital use and mortality among Medicare beneficiaries in Boston and New Haven. *N Engl J Med* 1989;321:1168–1173.
15. Morreim EH. Unholy alliances: physician investment for self-referral. *Radiology* 1993;186:67–72.
16. Evens RG. What to do about self-referral? *Radiology* 1993;186:75–76.
17. *Financial arrangements between physicians and health care businesses.* Washington, DC: Office of the Inspector General, U.S. Department of Health and Human Services, 1989.
18. Pear R. Health care costs up sharply again, posing new threat. *New York Times*, January 5, 1992:A1.
19. Redelmeier DA, Tversky A. The discrepancy between medical decisions for individuals and for groups. *N Engl J Med* 1990;322:1162–1164.

= 34 =

Incentives for Physicians
to Decrease Services

During a recent open-enrollment period for health insurance, my employer completely covered premiums for several health maintenance organization (HMO) plans. Other plans required an employee contribution to premiums. For a point-of-service (POS) plan, the employee contribution was $48 a month for a family of four, or $576 annually. For a fee-for-service plan, the contribution was $1791 a month, or over $21,000 a year. Few patients can afford fee-for-service plans. As consumers choosing health care plans, people want low costs. Dilemmas occur because a person's perspective shifts when he becomes a sick patient seeking medical care rather than a consumer choosing plans (1–3). As patients, people do not want to forego potentially beneficial interventions in order to save money (4). Less expensive insurance plans, however, have financial and organizational arrangements that raise ethical concerns about the role of physicians and their relationship to patients.

The soaring cost of U.S. health care has led to pressures to control expenditures and to allocate resources more efficiently. The United States spent 14% of its gross domestic product on health care in 1997, more than any other nation (5). Despite these huge expenditures, quality of care and access to care are problematical. Infant mortality and life expectancy are worse in the United States than in such countries as Great Britain and Canada that spend less per capita on health care. Given this context, it is hard to argue for increasing health expenditures for insured persons rather than addressing other pressing social needs, such as education, the environment, or public transportation. Eliminating inefficiency and waste will not solve the problem of rising costs because new medical technologies and an aging population will continue to drive up costs (6,7). Neither employers, taxpayers, nor individual patients are willing to pay higher premiums for health insurance.

Managed care systems try to restrain the cost of health care by offering financial incentives to physicians to practice cost-effective medicine, allowing patients to see only selected physicians, and imposing administrative controls (8). The Appendix discusses incentives to decrease costs, which include:

- Gatekeeping requirements on primary care physicians
- Financial incentives to physicians, including capitation, salary, bonus, and withhold
- Administrative measures, such as utilization review, practice guidelines, and direct limitation on services
- Deselection

Managed care reverses fee-for-service financial incentives to provide more services. Ideally, the new incentives cause physicians to eliminate services that offer little or no benefit to patients. However, physicians may also be encouraged to withhold interventions that provide substantial benefit (9,10).

In many situations, incentives and administrative arrangements in managed care are ethically acceptable. This chapter focuses on situations in which the self-interest of physicians and health care organizations may conflict with the best of interests of the patient. Chapter 32 analyzes the related issue of conflicts of interest between different patients.

ETHICAL CONCERNS ABOUT INCENTIVES TO DECREASE SERVICES

Beneficial Care May Be Withheld

Empirical evidence on how managed care impacts on the quality of care and health outcomes is inconclusive. Some studies have identified conditions in which the quality of care is lower in managed care than in fee-for-service care. Overall, however, outcomes seem similar (11).

There is a widespread perception among both physicians and the public that some forms of managed care compromise the quality of care (12,13). In one study, physicians reported that they were less satisfied with the quality of care they provided to capitated patients, compared with their overall practice (14). In particular, they were less satisfied with their ability to follow their best judgment and to obtain specialty referrals. In another study, 20% of physicians believed that gatekeeping has a negative effect on the overall quality of care, compared with 6% who believe that it has a positive effect (15). More specifically, 40% of physicians believed that gatekeeping has a negative effect on the appropriate use of specialist care, compared with 14% who believe that it has a positive effect (15). However, these physicians also reported that gatekeeping improves coordination of care and preventive care (15). Finally, physicians rate various managed care plans differently regarding overall quality of care and specific aspects of care, such as access to specialists and identification of underused preventive services (12).

Trust in Physicians May Be Undermined

Managed care may exacerbate the vulnerability and uncertainty that sick people inherently feel. In one survey, 61% of persons in heavily managed plans were worried that if they became sick, the plan would be more concerned about saving money than providing the best medical treatment (13). In comparison, 51% of persons in less tightly managed plans and 34% of patients in traditional plans had such worries. Capitated patients have lower levels of trust than fee-for-service patients (16). The reduction in trust is associated with a doubling of the odds that patients had considered changing physicians. Patient trust in health plans was significantly lower than trust in their physicians.

It is understandable how financial and organizational arrangements in managed care may undermine patient trust. Capitation, withholds, and bonuses may create conflicts of interest: physicians may act in their own self-interest or in the interest of third parties, rather than in the best interests of patients. Because of utilization review and practice guidelines, patients may no longer regard physicians as professionals who exercise independent clinical judgment, but rather as bureaucrats carrying out policies set by administrators. Patients are particularly vulnerable if they have few options to change physicians or plans if they are dissatisfied or receive poor care.

Such Incentives Undermine Professional Ethics

Critics charge that some financial incentives create conflicts of interest and undermine the physician's fiduciary role. Many physicians contend that doctors cannot serve two masters and that responsibilities to patients should be paramount (17). Furthermore, critics charge that an emphasis on cost containment and efficiency leads physicians to become entrepreneurs focused on profits instead of healers focused on the well-being of patients (18).

RESPONSIBILITY OF HEALTH CARE ORGANIZATIONS FOR INCENTIVES TO DECREASE SERVICES

Health care organizations can reduce or mitigate conflicts of interest in several ways.

Use Acceptable Financial Incentives

Given the need to reduce costs and enhance efficiency, incentives to physicians have advantages over guidelines or rules (19,20). Incentives allow physicians to exercise discretion and take into account the circumstances of an individual case. Incentives also avoid micromanagement and bureaucratic requirements for documentation.

Some financial arrangements, however, offer such direct and strong incentives to decrease services as to create an unacceptable risk that physicians will act contrary to patients' interests (21–24). The income at risk for physicians may be so great that their economic survival seems jeopardized. For example, the rates of withholding may be very high, there may be penalties beyond the withheld amounts, or a large percentage of the physician's base income may be at risk (10,22,24). If the risk pool is very small, a single complicated, sick patient may lead to severe economic losses for the physician. Some of these problems can be addressed through reinsurance or stop-loss arrangements that limit risk.

Increasingly, managed care organizations are using a blend of incentives. Physicians may receive a base salary, with adjustments for productivity, utilization, quality of care, and patient satisfaction (25). For instance, physicians may receive a bonus for ensuring that patients receive indicated preventive measures, such as screening mammography. Such combined reimbursement systems may promote a strong doctor–patient relationship and quality of care as well as cost containment.

Allow Justified Exceptions to Guidelines

Even the best clinical guidelines or utilization review system cannot cover all cases appropriately. There may be circumstances that the guidelines did not anticipate or capture, or a case may have particular features that justify an exception (26). The physician is in a unique position to articulate why a particular case is a justified exception to general guidelines. Organizations need to acknowledge that such advocacy is essential because of variations among cases and the limitations of guidelines and utilization review. Also, organizations need to encourage physicians to provide information as to why an intervention should be authorized for a particular patient. The procedure for physicians to provide such information should not be unduly burdensome.

Structure the Delivery of Care to Strengthen the Doctor–Patient Relationship

Continuity of care is likely to enhance trust and mitigate concerns about conflicts of interest. Managed care organizations should arrange physician schedules so that ambulatory visits are not too brief and timely return visits can be scheduled. Health care organizations should identify and compensate physicians who care for complicated, sicker patients.

Some managed care plans discourage physicians from discussing certain options for care with patients. So-called gag rules are clauses in physician contracts with managed care organizations that forbid doctors from discussing with patients interventions that are not covered or still under utilization review. Such restrictions on communication are unethical because they violate the physician's duty to inform patients of medically reasonable options. Many states have outlawed such restrictions on physician–patient discussions (27).

Disclose Economic Incentives to Patients

Managed care systems should disclose to enrollees their financial arrangements with physicians (28). Such disclosure is required by federal Medicare and Medicaid regulations, as well as by some state laws (22,29,30). Disclosure may benefit patients in several ways. Disclosure may help patients choose a physician, physician group, or plan because some patients may prefer to avoid certain types of reimbursement arrangements. Knowing how physicians are reimbursed may help patients put physicians' recommendations into context and decide whether to appeal or pay out of pocket when coverage is denied. In addition, disclosure and adverse publicity may deter problematic financial arrangements.

RESPONSES BY PHYSICIANS TO INCENTIVES TO DECREASE SERVICES

The concept of the physician as fiduciary stresses that patients are vulnerable and that they trust physicians to act in their best interests. How can physicians act appropriately in an environment where controlling costs is also important? See Table 34-1 for a summary.

Inform Patients When Standard Care is Not Available

In some situations, care available within a managed care system may be significantly worse than standard care outside the system.

CASE 34.1. STANDARD CARE NOT AVAILABLE IN THE SYSTEM. *A 64-year-old business executive has ongoing angina on medical management. Her medications are causing unacceptable side effects such as fatigue and decreased ability to concentrate. The physician recommends angiography and revascularization. The cardiologists and cardiac surgeons available under the patient's insurance plan have poorer outcomes than elsewhere in the community. Both the hospital and the cardiovascular surgery group have mortality rates for coronary bypass surgery that are higher than 99% of providers in the state. The hospital mortality rate is over 5%, while the state average is under 2%. Moreover, with this plan, approval for invasive cardiology procedures is more difficult and often delayed, compared with other plans.*

Several states collect and publish surgeon-specific and hospital-specific mortality rates for coronary bypass surgery (31). Although the adequacy of risk adjustment can always be criticized, such data are as rigorous as can be expected. The variation in Case 34.1 is clinically as well as statistically significant.

In Case 34.1, should the physician discuss services that are available outside the system, even if the plan will not cover them? On the one hand, physicians may fear that such disclosure will only make the patient angry or confused. The physician also may be reluctant to disparage col-

TABLE 34-1. *Responses by physicians to ethical problems regarding reimbursement*

Inform patients when standard care is not available.
Recommend out-of-plan interventions that provide significant clinical benefits.
Serve as a patient advocate.
Avoid deception.

leagues with whom he works in other cases. In addition, referring to a more distant hospital may disrupt continuity of care.

On the other hand, the ethical guidelines of autonomy and beneficence require physicians to discuss such alternatives. A reasonable patient probably would want to know that a provider has a mortality rate of 5% rather than 2%. If the patient is not informed of alternatives outside the managed care system, she cannot make informed decisions about her care. Furthermore, she cannot try to obtain services if she does not know about them. The patient might pay out of pocket for care, postpone care until she can change insurance plans, or try to convince the plan to pay for care outside the system.

Recommend Out-of-Plan Interventions That Provide Significant Clinical Benefits

In addition to discussing options that are not covered by the plan, the physician should order or recommend out-of-plan options that provide clinically significant benefits over care available in the plan. Such actions are required by the ethical guideline of beneficence. Recommendations should take into account both published evidence and clinical judgment about the individual patient's circumstances and values.

Acting for the patient's benefit is not an absolute duty. Physicians have no ethical obligation to order interventions that provide little or no clinical benefit. Although the term "clinically significant" is ambiguous and needs to be interpreted, under any reimbursement system physicians should recommend only those interventions whose risks are proportionate to the benefits. The term "benefits" needs to be interpreted broadly, to include psychosocial variables as well as biomedical outcomes. For some patients, convenience in taking medications, reassurance about not missing a serious diagnosis, or speedy recovery to full function are extremely important. For such patients, a strategy that involves inconvenience, delay, or a small risk is not in their best interests. In Case 34.1, the benefits are clearly substantial.

It is ethical for physicians to take into account the cost of care in recommending an approach whose expected outcome does not differ in clinically significant ways from a considerably more costly approach. In many situations, it is appropriate to use preferred drugs on health plan formularies. Physicians may prescribe a preferred statin for cholesterol reduction or a preferred angiotensin-converting enzyme inhibitor for congestive heart failure and reserve more expensive drugs in that class for patients who have an unsatisfactory outcome, unacceptable side effects, or poor adherence. Similarly, physicians would be ethically justified in withholding imaging studies for headache, back pain, and ankle injuries when the clinical examination suggests a very low likelihood of serious pathology. Physicians and patients alike need to acknowledge that such decisions are a form of bedside rationing (32) but recognize that they are ethically appropriate.

Serve as a Patient Advocate

The guideline of beneficence also urges physicians to act as advocates to intercede for or speak on behalf of patients (33,34). Advocacy should be based on sound clinical judgment and evidence-based medicine. It is not equivalent to doing whatever the patient requests. Advocating for a patient is fair only if it would also be appropriate for other physicians to advocate for their patients in similar situations. In addition to ordering interventions that provide significant clinical benefits, physicians should make reasonable efforts to help patients obtain such care (35). As in Case 34.1, such efforts include filling out forms and making phone calls to obtain authorizations or make appeals.

Being a patient advocate may entail personal and professional hassles. It will take time and may be emotionally grueling. Furthermore, it may be awkward for the physician in Case 34.1

to continue to work with the HMO specialists on other cases. Ideally, the physician's fiduciary duty to patients should be paramount when the clinical benefits are substantial.

Physicians may be legally liable if, against their medical judgment, they withhold beneficial care at the behest of the insurer. One court declared, "the physician who complies without protest with the limitations imposed by a third-party payer, when his medical judgment dictates otherwise, cannot avoid his ultimate responsibility for his patient's care" (36).

Avoid Deception

In a survey, 48% of physicians reported that during the previous 2 years they had exaggerated the severity of a patient's condition to get the patient care that they thought was medically necessary, and 5% said they did so often (37). However, the ethical duty to avoid deception limits the duty to serve as patient advocates (33). Chapter 6 argues that deception is difficult to justify, even when physicians believe that it is unfair for the plan not to cover the intervention.

PATIENTS' REQUESTS FOR INTERVENTIONS THAT PHYSICIANS BELIEVE ARE INAPPROPRIATE

Such requests may occur in any system of health care but may be more acrimonious in managed care.

CASE 34.2. PATIENT REQUESTS MEDICALLY UNWARRANTED DIAGNOSTIC TESTS. *A 26-year-old man receiving care in an HMO has mild occipital headaches without any other symptoms. His headaches are relieved with heat or acetaminophen. His examination is remarkable only for mild trapezius spasm. His neurological examination is normal. He insists on a magnetic resonance imaging (MRI) scan to be sure that he does not have a brain tumor. He also wants a referral to a neurologist. The physician believes that the patient has tension headaches and that further workup would not be indicated. The patient exclaims, "You're just trying to save money for the HMO!"*

The key ethical issue in this case is whether the MRI scan or neurology referral would benefit the patient. The likelihood of finding a serious intracranial lesion is so low in this case that an MRI or referral would not be recommended, even under fee-for-service reimbursement. The mere possibility that the headaches might be caused by a serious intracerebral lesion does not justify scanning or referral at this time. Anecdotal reports of patients who had a brain tumor discovered on an MRI for headaches should be regarded simply as anecdotes, not as persuasive evidence of effectiveness. It is ethically appropriate for the physician to follow practice guidelines or utilization review restrictions that would disallow the test or referral.

Physicians should interpret "benefit" broadly to include psychosocial factors. Reassurance may be crucial to some patients. If a patient is so worried about having a brain tumor that his everyday activities are compromised, it would be appropriate to order an imaging study for reassurance and to appeal a utilization review denial. However, the test should be part of a comprehensive plan of care that also explores the patient's concerns and provides counseling.

How can the physician respond to patient concerns that physicians are trying to save money for the system, rather than providing high-quality care (38)? First, the physician should explore the patient's concerns and acknowledge the uncertainty of the situation. Also, the doctor should explain to the patient why these interventions are not recommended at this time. The physician should arrange to see the patient again in case the headaches do not resolve satisfactorily. If both parties know that the doctor will see the patient again if there is no improvement, the physician has an incentive to do what is reasonable to help the patient. This social incentive may counterbalance financial incentives to provide fewer services. In addition, the doctor should leave open the possibility of further evaluation in the future if the headaches do not resolve satisfactorily.

In summary, some reimbursement systems present ethical dilemmas to physicians. Within the constraints of health care plans, physicians need to act as patient advocates when the patient could receive significant clinical benefit from a referral, test, or therapy that the plan disallows. In addition, financial incentives that are highly likely to lead physicians to medically inappropriate care need to be identified and limited.

APPENDIX: COST-CONTAINMENT MEASURES IN MANAGED CARE

Managed care systems include health maintenance organizations (HMOs) and preferred provider organizations (PPOs) (39). Patients in HMOs select a primary physician or physician group and must obtain covered services through them. HMO physicians contract to provide comprehensive medical care for capitated payments, which are a fixed amount per patient, regardless of the actual costs of care. A few HMOs are staff or group model HMOs, with a closed panel of physicians working exclusively for the HMO. Other HMOs are less tightly organized independent practice associations (IPAs), which contract with physicians or physician groups to provide services. A physician or group may belong to several competing IPAs.

In PPOs, "preferred" physicians and hospitals accept discounted fee-for-service reimbursement rates and administrative controls in exchange for a flow of patients. PPO patients may also visit nonpreferred providers in the network, but at additional cost.

Point of service (POS) plans allow still greater choice of physicians or hospitals. Out-of-network care is still covered, but less completely and with higher copayments. Typically premiums for POS plans are about 10% higher than HMO premiums. POS plans are the fastest growing type of plan.

We discuss here how managed care systems try to control health care expenditures through gatekeeping, financial incentives, and administrative measures.

The Physician as Gatekeeper

In most managed care systems, primary care physicians serve as gatekeepers who must approve diagnostic tests, referrals to subspecialists, or hospitalizations in order for them to be reimbursed (9,21). Gatekeepers may be financially at risk for the costs of care for their panel of patients.

Gatekeeping restrictions are unpopular with patients and physicians alike (40). Demands for "freedom of choice" of physicians have led many plans to modify strict gatekeeping. Direct access to some specialists, such as gynecologists, is common and even mandated in some states. Some insurers are offering plans that provide unrestricted access to specialists (40).

Financial Incentives to Physicians

Managed care plans may offer physicians a range of incentives to practice cost-effective medicine (24).

Capitation

Plans may pay primary physicians or physician groups on a capitated basis. The provider receives a fixed amount per patient enrolled, regardless of how often the patient visits.

Salary

Salary is common as a base reimbursement in staff-model HMOs and in large physician groups. Because the physician receives the same income regardless of how much time and resources are spent on patients, salary, like capitation, provides a financial incentive to limit the amount of health care provided and to avoid more complicated patients.

Bonus and Withhold

Primary care physicians may also be financially liable for excessive expenditures (9,21,24). The managed care plan may withhold part of the primary care physician's capitated payments, and, if expenditures are high, the plan may keep the withheld funds. Alternatively, some plans give gatekeepers a bonus if expenditures for specialty care or hospitalizations fall below a target level.

Balanced Incentives

Increasingly, physicians also receive bonuses for patient satisfaction, adherence to prevention and chronic care guidelines, and other measures of quality of care (25,39). These quality incentives counterbalance incentives to provide fewer services.

Typical bonuses range from 5% to 10% of net income (26). When more of the physician's income is at stake, concerns about conflicts of interest intensify. When a withhold exceeds 16% of payments, 79% of managed care leaders are concerned that physician judgments would be compromised (41).

Financial arrangements are complicated because the incentives a managed care plan presents to a physician group may differ from the incentives the group presents to the individual physician. Physicians also commonly face various incentives from different insurance plans and may not know the details of reimbursement for any particular patient.

Administrative Measures to Control Costs

In addition to financial incentives, managed care systems use a variety of administrative measures to control costs. Most fee-for-service plans also use some of these techniques.

Utilization Review Programs

Such programs include prior authorization, concurrent review, discharge planning, and case management for high-cost patients (42). They are intended to discourage physicians from providing unnecessary or marginal services. However, some utilization review procedures may disallow interventions that physicians consider medically necessary and beneficial to patients (12,37).

Physicians commonly complain that they face inconvenience and hassles when they obtain prior authorization or appeal a denial of coverage (43). Physicians may believe that they are made to wait when they telephone, that they must speak with a series of bureaucrats, and that the amount of documentation requested is burdensome. Some physicians may decide that obtaining authorization, even for beneficial services, is not worth the hassle and time.

Practice Guidelines or Protocols

These specify how physicians should act in certain circumstances (19). They may limit inappropriate use of specialists or diagnostic tests, correct underuse of beneficial interventions, and reduce unjustified variations in practice. However, physicians may reject such guidelines as "cookbook medicine" or bureaucratic infringements on physicians' professional judgment.

Direct Limitations on Services

Some managed care systems restrict certain services. Most managed care plans have closed formularies that exclude certain expensive drugs and encourage the use of preferred drugs for which they have negotiated favorable prices.

Queuing

Queuing involves waiting for appointments. If appointments are scarce, visits for minor, self-limited problems will be reduced (43). Patients may decide that their problem is not serious enough to warrant attention. In many cases, the medical problem resolves before the date of the appointment. However, queuing may delay needed care for serious problems and reduce trust in the system.

Deselection

Some physicians fear that their contract with a managed care plan will not be renewed if they are identified as high utilizers of resources or appeal many utilization review decisions (44,45). Such concerns may lead physicians to provide fewer services, independently of any direct financial incentives to do so.

REFERENCES

1. Eddy DM. Connecting value and costs: whom do we ask, and what do we ask them? *JAMA* 1990;264:1737–1739.
2. Eddy DM. The individual versus society: is there a conflict? *JAMA* 1991;265:1146–1149.
3. Eddy DM. The individual versus society: resolving the conflict. *JAMA* 1991;265:2399–2406.
4. Boren SD. I had a tough day today, Hillary. *N Engl J Med* 1994;330:500–502.
5. Levit K, Cowan C, Braden B, et al. National health expenditures in 1997: more slow growth. *Health Aff (Millwood)* 1998;17:99–110.
6. Schwartz WB. The inevitable failure of current cost-containment strategies. Why they can provide only temporary relief. *JAMA* 1987;257:220–224.
7. Eddy DM. Health system reform: will controlling costs require rationing services? *JAMA* 1994;272:324–328.
8. Iglehart JK. The American health care system: managed care. *N Engl J Med* 1992;327:742–747.
9. Hillman AL. Financial incentives for physicians in HMOs: is there a conflict of interest? *N Engl J Med* 1987;317:1743–1748.
10. Rodwin MA. *Medicine, money, and morals: physicians' conflicts of interest.* New York: Oxford University Press, 1993:146.
11. Miller RH, Luft HS. Does managed care lead to better or worse quality of care? *Health Affairs* 1997;16:7–25.
12. Borowsky SJ, Davis MK, Goertz C, et al. Are all health plans created equal? The physician's view. *JAMA* 1997;278:917–921.
13. Blendon RJ, Brodie M, Benson JM, et al. Understanding the managed care backlash. *Health Affairs* 1998;17:80–94.
14. Kerr EA, Hays RD, Mittman BS. Primary care physicians' satisfaction with quality of care in California capitated medical groups. *JAMA* 1997;278:308–312.
15. Halm EA, Causino N, Blumenthal D. Is gatekeeping better than traditional care? *JAMA* 1997;278:1677–1681.
16. Kao AC, Green DC, Zaslavsky AM, et al. The relationship between method of physician payment and patient trust. *JAMA* 1998;280:1708–1714.
17. Levinsky NG. The doctor's master. *N Engl J Med* 1984;311:1573–1575.
18. Kassirer JP. Managing care—should we adopt a new ethic? *N Engl J Med* 1998;339:397–398.
19. Hillman AL. Managing the physician: rules versus incentives. *Health Aff (Millwood)* 1991;10:138–146.
20. Hall MA, Berenson RA. Ethical practice in managed care: a dose of realism. *Ann Intern Med* 1998;128:395–402.
21. Hillman AL. Health maintenance organizations, financial incentives, and physicians' judgments. *Ann Intern Med* 1990;112:891–893.

22. Latham SR. Regulation of managed care incentive payments to physicians. *Am J Law Med* 1996;22:399–432.
23. Orentlicher D. Paying physicians more to do less: financial incentives to limit care. *Univ Richmond Law Rev* 1996;30:155–197.
24. Pearson SD, Daniels N, Emanuel E. Ethical guidelines for physician compensation based on capitation. *N Engl J Med* 1998;339:689–693.
25. Grumbach K, Osmond D, Varanizan K, et al. Primary care physicians' experience of financial incentives in managed care systems. *N Engl J Med* 1998;339:1516–1521.
26. Ellrodt AG, Conner L, Riedinger M, et al. Measuring and improving physician compliance with clinical practice guidelines. *Ann Intern Med* 1995;122:277–282.
27. Miller TE. Managed care regulation: in the laboratory of the states. *JAMA* 1997;278:1102–1109.
28. Levinson DF. Toward full disclosure of referral restrictions and financial incentives by prepaid health plans. *N Engl J Med* 1987;317:1729–1731.
29. Gallagher TH, Alpers A, Lo B. HCFA's new regulations for financial incentives in Medicare and Medicaid managed care. *Am J Med* 1998;105:409–415.
30. Miller TE, Sage WM. Disclosing physician financial incentives. *JAMA* 1999;281:1424–1430.
31. Chassin MR, Hannan EL, et al. Benefits and hazards of reporting medical outcomes publicly. *N Engl J Med* 1996;334:394–398.
32. Ubel PA, Goold S. Recognizing bedside rationing: clear cases and tough calls. *Ann Intern Med* 1997;126:74–80.
33. Morreim EH. Gaming the system: dodging the rules, ruling the dodgers. *Arch Intern Med* 1991;151:443–447.
34. Povar G, Moreno J. Hippocrates and the health maintenance organization. *Ann Intern Med* 1988;109:419–424.
35. Sage WM. Physicians as advocates. *Houston Law J* 1999;35:1525–1630.
36. Wickline *v.* State of California, 228 Cal.Rptr. 661 (Cal. App. 1986).
37. Kaiser Family Foundation. Survey of physicians and nurses. www.kff.org. July, 1999.
38. Gallagher TH, Lo B, Chesney M, et al. How do managed care physicians respond to patients' requests for costly, unindicated tests? *J Gen Intern Med* 1997;12:663–668.
39. Bodenheimer T. Physicians and the changing medical marketplace. *N Engl J Med* 1999;340:584–588.
40. Bodenheimer T, Lo B, Casalino L. Primary care physicians should be coordinators, not gatekeepers. *JAMA* 1999;281:2045–2049.
41. Hillman AL, Pauly MV, Kerman K, et al. HMO managers' views on financial incentives and quality. *Health Aff (Millwood)* 1991;10:207–219.
42. Hoy EW, Curtis RE, Rice T. Change and growth in managed care. *Health Aff (Millwood)* 1991;10:18–36.
43. Grumet GW. Health care rationing through inconvenience: the third party's secret weapon. *N Engl J Med* 1989;321:607–611.
44. Blum JD. The evolution of physician credentialing into managed care selective contracting. *Am J Law Med* 1996;22:173–204.
45. Woolhandler S, Himmelstein DU. Extreme risk—the new corporate proposition for physicians. *N Engl J Med* 1995;333:1706–1708.

ANNOTATED BIBLIOGRAPHY

1. Kassirer JP. Managed care and the morality of the marketplace. *N Engl J Med* 1995;333:50–52.
   Eloquent plea that professional ethics is incompatible with a profit-oriented, entrepreneurial approach to medicine.
2. Pearson SD, Daniels N, Emanuel E. Ethical guidelines for physician compensation based on capitation. *N Engl J Med* 1998;339:689–693.
   Suggestions for a just system of incentives in managed care.
3. Hall MA, Berenson RA. Ethical practice in managed care: a dose of realism. *Ann Intern Med* 1998;128:395–402.
   Hall MA. *Making medical spending decisions.* New York: Oxford University Press, 1997.
   This article and book argue that financial incentives to physicians to limit care can be ethical and in fact are preferable to rules set by administrators.
4. Miller TE, Sage WM. Disclosing physician financial incentives. *JAMA* 1999;281:1424–1430.
   Analyzes rationale for disclosure of financial incentives to physicians.

35

Gifts from Drug Companies

Gifts from drug companies to physicians are ubiquitous, ranging from pens and mugs to meals at conferences. Although gifts and subsidies from drug companies may foster medical education and provide welcome perks to physicians and students, some gifts may impair the physician's judgment or create the impression of a conflict of interest. Consumer advocates and government officials are increasingly scrutinizing such gifts. This chapter presents the arguments for and against accepting gifts from drug companies or manufacturers of medical products and suggests guidelines for such gifts.

TYPES OF GIFTS

In 1997, drug companies spent over $6.3 billion on marketing events and drug representatives to visit physicians (1). This amount represents over $9000 per practicing physician in the United States. Gifts and subsidies from drug companies to physicians range from token to lavish.

Small Items

Individual physicians may receive items that bear the company or product name. These range from pens and message pads to more expensive items such as umbrellas, flashlights, and clocks. At one national meeting, 34% of gifts displayed and distributed by drug companies were of more than minimal value, including watches, tape recorders, and cameras (2). Drug companies may also distribute medical books and equipment such as reflex hammers.

Meals and Hospitality

Drug companies frequently provide lunch or refreshments at conferences in hospitals or medical schools. Conference organizers often solicit these subsidies in order to increase attendance. Companies also host dinners for physicians coupled with a talk. Drug companies may also offer tickets to sporting events.

Continuing Medical Education and Conferences

Drug companies may support hospital conferences by paying honoraria and travel expenses for speakers. In an era of financial constraints, such subsidies may enable hospitals or medical schools to invite nationally prominent experts. Drug companies also may subsidize continuing education courses and professional society meetings in exchange for setting up booths to display their products. In the past, some drug companies also offered physicians travel expenses or stipends to attend meetings.

In addition, drug companies organize their own educational meetings for physicians, which may be cosponsored by academic institutions. The companies typically have control over the program and provide travel, lodging, and entertainment expenses for physicians attending these meetings. Sometimes these meetings are held at resort locations that are more luxurious than sites of conferences by professional organizations (3).

REASONS FOR DRUG COMPANIES TO OFFER GIFTS

Enhance Product Recognition

As profit-making companies, drug companies strengthen recognition of their products through gifts bearing the drug's name. One commentator observed, "No drug company gives away its shareholders' money in an act of disinterested generosity" (4). One study showed that all-expenses-paid trips to vacation sites to attend symposia sponsored by a pharmaceutical company increased prescribing of two drugs two- and threefold (5). Almost all physicians who attended the symposia said beforehand that it would not influence their prescribing behavior. In another study, the vast majority of physicians reported that they paid little attention to drug advertisements and detail people (6). Respondents were then questioned about two commonly prescribed drugs that the scientific literature indicates are ineffective or only minimally effective. Between one-third and one-half of doctors regarded these drugs as effective (6). The study concluded that physicians were more influenced by commercial than by scientific sources of information about these drugs.

REASONS FOR ACCEPTING DRUG COMPANY GIFTS

Gifts Improve Transmission of Medical Knowledge

Through subsidies from drug companies, hospitals, medical schools, continuing education courses, and professional society meetings may be able to invite prominent speakers. Drug company subsidies may substantially reduce the cost of registration at professional meetings and courses, thereby allowing more physicians to attend. Even providing lunches for hospital conferences may improve educational programs by increasing attendance.

Gifts Do Not Impair Clinical Judgment

Many physicians consider it absurd to believe that small gifts from drug companies might compromise patient care decisions. Indeed, some physicians are insulted at the suggestion that accepting pens or note pads might impair their clinical judgment. They reject such allegations as moralistic overreactions.

Refusing Gifts Might Cause More Harm Than Benefit

Some argue that refusing all drug company gifts and subsidies would cause more overall harm than benefit. The price of drugs to consumers would not be lowered, because drug companies would probably reallocate the money to drug detailing or to advertising. In addition, medical education would suffer if drug company sponsorship of speakers and conferences ceased. In other words, patients might actually be harmed if physicians refused all gifts and subsidies from drug companies: they would pay the same amount for drugs, but their physicians would receive less education.

OBJECTIONS TO ACCEPTING DRUG COMPANY GIFTS

Table 35-1 summarizes objections to accepting gifts from drug companies.

Gifts Create the Expectation of Reciprocity

Gifts create relationships and obligations in the recipient, such as grateful conduct, social duties, and reciprocation (7). The problem is not that physicians would immediately change prescribing practices after receiving a free lunch. One writer has warned, "The sell is much more subtle. All the advertiser may expect is that, other things being equal, if you subsequently have to make a decision it is more likely to be in the favor of the advertiser" (8).

Gifts Impair Objectivity

Objectivity of presentations at conferences and continuing education courses may be compromised if the drug company selects speakers and topics, prepares slides for presentations, writes or edits talks, or trains the presenters (9). A speaker may selectively present or emphasize data favorable to one drug or class or drugs, rather than drawing from the overall body of available data (10). A balanced presentation would present all pertinent information, both favorable and unfavorable, about a drug.

When academic institutions sponsor continuing medical education programs, physicians expect the institution to select the speakers and topics in an independent manner, without drug company interference. Physicians attending conferences sponsored by academic institutions may not even know whether drug companies have determined the program and speakers. Because the bias introduced into programs supported by pharmaceutical companies is "almost never obvious" (9), it may have greater impact than clear-cut advertising by drug companies.

Gifts Increase the Cost of Health Care

Ultimately patients and their insurers pay for drug company gifts to physicians. Given the rising cost of drugs, it may be unseemly for physicians to receive gifts from drug companies. One physician criticized, "Am I supposed to believe that the members of a clinical department are so impoverished that they cannot buy their own pens or pizza and beer?" (8).

Gifts Demean the Profession

Depending on drug company subsidies to support continuing medical education programs demeans physicians (8). Physicians should consider how the public might react to evidence that physicians attend conferences only if lunch is provided or if the registration fee is subsidized.

TABLE 35-1. *Objections to accepting gifts from drug companies*

Gifts create the expectation of reciprocity.
Gifts impair objectivity.
Gifts increase the cost of health care.
Gifts demean the profession.
Gifts give the appearance of conflict of interest.

The public may infer that physicians do not consider it worthwhile to learn about medical progress and to keep up to date.

Gifts Give the Appearance of Conflict of Interest

Even if gifts from pharmaceutical companies do not actually influence a physician's therapeutic decisions, the appearance of bias and conflict of interest may be deleterious. After all, physicians are not choosing medications for their own use and paying the bills themselves; they are prescribing for their patients. Public trust in the medical profession might be compromised if patients worried that drug company gifts influence patient care decisions. Some patients might wonder about the objectivity of a physician who uses a pen or note pad bearing the name of a medication or drug company.

Outside of medicine, society has enacted strict rules regarding conflicts of interest that may undermine trust in public officials. Judges are expected to refuse gifts from individuals or companies who have a financial stake in their professional decisions. Government officials may not accept gifts of more than nominal value from persons or organizations who would be affected or gain financially from their decisions. By analogy, it may be inappropriate for physicians to accept drug company gifts that give even the appearance of a conflict of interest.

RECOMMENDED SOLUTIONS

Forbid Certain Practices

Certain types of gifts and support from drug companies are so likely to raise questions about bias and impropriety that they should be banned (9,11). For example, the American College of Physicians, the American Medical Association, the Accreditation Council for Continuing Medical Education, and the Pharmaceutical Manufacturers Association agree that it is unethical for physicians to accept direct payments to attend a meeting or lavish entertainment that has no clear educational or scientific justification. Course directors should retain complete control over the scientific program and choice of speakers when drug companies support continuing medical education programs sponsored by academic institutions. In addition, the company should not select the physicians who attend the program.

The Food and Drug Administration (FDA) proposed plans to regulate certain drug company involvements in medical education as promotional events rather than scientific exchange. To qualify as scientific exchange, programs must have independence, objectivity, balance, and scientific rigor (10). By "balance," the FDA means that a range of views must be presented, "leading to a free exchange of ideas rather than a preordained conclusion" (10). The FDA requires that drug companies have "neither express nor implied control over the scientific content of the program" (10). In particular, the FDA regards it as inappropriate for drug companies to "offer to suggest participants for a symposium, draft a journal article, or prepare slides for a presentation" (10).

Allow Certain Other Practices

Some types of gifts or support are generally considered acceptable. For example, at professional society meetings, drug companies often underwrite the printing of abstract books. In turn, they set up displays in an exhibition hall. Similarly, pens or note pads that bear the names of drug companies or their products are commonly regarded as acceptable.

Encourage Pooled Support by Drug Companies

Several drug companies might contribute support jointly for a professional meeting, continuing medical education course, or hospital conference series. Such pooled support, coupled with control over speakers and topics by the program directors, would be less likely to result in bias favoring one viewpoint or product compared with support from a single company. The drug company can then gain the general goodwill of the physicians without being suspected of trying to slant the educational material.

Disclose Gifts to the Public

Consumer advocates believe that the public needs to know about gifts from drug companies to physicians. Without such information, patients have no opportunity to make informed decisions regarding physician objectivity and integrity. It may be difficult to draw the line between what is acceptable and what is not. The Royal College of Physicians of London has suggested a helpful rule of thumb: "Would you be willing to have these arrangements generally known?" (12). This rule has been criticized because physicians might approve of gifts that the public would regard as improper. A more rigorous question—and one more to the point—would be, "What would your patients or the public think if they knew you had accepted these gifts?" In borderline cases, it would be judicious to err on the side of declining gifts.

In summary, gifts from drug companies may raise at least the appearance of conflicts of interest, increase the cost of health care, and impair objectivity. Physicians need to keep in mind that ultimately their primary concern should be the best interests of their patients, not their own personal convenience or well-being.

REFERENCES

1. Zuger A. Fever pitch: getting doctors to prescribe is big business. *New York Times*, January 11, 1998:A1.
2. Goldstein AO. Gifts to physicians from industry. *JAMA* 1991;266:61.
3. Goldfinger SE. A matter of influence. *N Engl J Med* 1987;316:1408–1409.
4. Rawlins MD. Doctors and the drug makers. *Lancet* 1984;2:276–278.
5. Orlowski JP, Wateska L. The effects of pharmaceutical firm enticements on physician prescribing patterns: there's no such thing as a free lunch. *Chest* 1992;102:270–273.
6. Avorn J, Chen M, Hartley R. Scientific versus commercial sources of influence on the prescribing behavior of physicians. *Am J Med* 1982;73:4–8.
7. Chren M, Landefeld S, Murray TH. Doctors, drug companies, and gifts. *JAMA* 1989;262:3448–3451.
8. Waud DR. Pharmaceutical promotions: a free lunch? *N Engl J Med* 1992;327:351–353.
9. American College of Physicians. Physicians and the pharmaceutical industry. *Ann Intern Med* 1990;112:624–626.
10. Kessler DA. Drug promotion and scientific exchange: the role of the physician investigator. *N Engl J Med* 1991;325:201–203.
11. Gifts to physicians from industry. *JAMA* 1991;265:501.
12. The relationship between physicians and the pharmaceutical industry: a report of the Royal College of Physicians. *J R Coll Physicians Lond* 1986;20:235–242.

ANNOTATED BIBLIOGRAPHY

1. American College of Physicians. Physicians and the pharmaceutical industry. *Ann Intern Med* 1990;112:624–626.
   Criticial analysis of drug company sponsorship of continuing medical education and medical conferences.
2. Chren M, Landefeld S, Murray TH. Doctors, drug companies, and gifts. *JAMA* 1989;262:3448–3451.
   Argues that gifts from drug companies create expectations of reciprocity that may compromise the physicians' responsibility to the interests of their patients.
3. Kessler DA. Drug promotion and scientific exchange: the role of the physician investigator. *N Engl J Med* 1991;325:201–203.
   Explains how the Food and Drug Administration plans to regulate as promotional activities drug company-sponsored activities that lack independence, objectivity, balance, and scientific rigor.
4. Waud DR. Pharmaceutical promotions: a free lunch? *N Engl J Med* 1992;327:351–353.
   Spirited article arguing that physicians should not accept any gifts from drug companies.

36

Disclosing Mistakes

Mistakes by physicians may cause serious harm or even death to patients. One study found that 1% of hospitalized patients were seriously injured by substandard care (1). Disclosure of mistakes to patients and colleagues is difficult for physicians, who may fear recriminations, loss of respect, and lawsuits. In one study, house officers who made serious mistakes told attending physicians only 54% of the time and told patients or families in only 24% of cases (2). In another survey, a third of physicians said they would not tell the family about a mistake that was fatal to the patient (3). The following case illustrates dilemmas posed by physicians' mistakes.

CASE 36.1. OVERDOSE OF INSULIN. *A patient with diabetes, hospitalized for congestive heart failure, is prescribed for by the intern and receives from the nurse double his usual dose of insulin. He develops hypoglycemia, seizures, and coma. Upon recovery, both the patient and his family ask physicians why the seizures occurred. The health care team wonders how to respond.*

The patient and family naturally want to know why his condition changed so dramatically. The physician is reluctant to tell the patient that a mistake occurred, fearing that the patient would get angry and perhaps sue. However, it is deceptive not to tell the patient of the mistake.

This chapter discusses the reasons for and against disclosing mistakes and suggests how physicians can respond to mistakes. In this chapter, "mistake" refers to acts or omissions for which the physician is responsible and that would have been judged wrong by knowledgeable peers at the time.

REASONS NOT TO DISCLOSE MISTAKES TO PATIENTS OR SURROGATES

Physicians commonly offer several reasons for not disclosing serious mistakes to patients or surrogates.

The Physician Is Not Really Responsible for the Mistake

Physicians understandably do not want to take the blame for someone else's mistake. Because many people are involved in the care of a patient, responsibility may be blurred. For example, the intern in Case 36.1 may believe that the resident or attending physician provided inadequate supervision. Alternatively, the physicians might claim that the nurse or pharmacist should have questioned the unusually high dosage. Perhaps the system is at fault, by requiring unreasonably long hours or causing results of laboratory tests to be delayed.

Determining the cause of a serious mistake is essential to assuring quality of care and preventing recurrences, but uncertainty over responsibility should not deter physicians from informing patients or surrogates about the mistake. Patients want to know that a mistake occurred and what the consequences will be. They are less concerned about which part of the health care system is to blame. Indeed, they may regard mutual recriminations among health care workers as attempts to shirk responsibility.

Disclosure Would Harm the Patient or Surrogate

Physicians may believe that if mistakes are disclosed, patients or surrogates might worry unnecessarily about other aspects of care. Such worry might cause stress or deter patients from seeking necessary care or accepting beneficial interventions in the future.

Disclosure Would Harm Health Care Professionals

Physicians may fear that patients or families may respond to disclosure of mistakes by becoming angry, bringing a lawsuit, or leaving the physician's practice. In a survey, 14% of patients said they would want to change physicians after a minor mistake, and 65% would change after a severe mistake such as the failure to follow up on a x-ray report showing a lung mass (4). The reluctance of physicians to acknowledge mistakes, however, creates a vicious circle. In one study, disclosure of mistakes did not increase malpractice claims (3a).

Disclosing a mistake may increase emotional distress for physicians. Accepting responsibility for a mistake may heighten feelings of remorse, guilt, and inadequacy (2). Colleagues and supervisors who are told of a mistake may be punitive rather than supportive (2).

Health care workers may be concerned that their reputations or careers will be damaged if they disclose a serious mistake. Their referrals, staff privileges, or license may be jeopardized. Trainees may also be concerned that supervisors who learn of a mistake will not recommend them for future positions.

REASONS TO DISCLOSE MISTAKES TO PATIENTS OR SURROGATES

There are several strong reasons to disclose mistakes to patients or their surrogates (Table 36-1).

Disclosure Respects Patients

In one survey, 98% of patients said that would want even minor errors disclosed to them (4). Unless the patient in Case 36.1 is told about the insulin overdose, he cannot understand this episode. He may well fear that the seizures and coma will recur or that he has a grave problem, such as a brain tumor. Fearing a recurrence, he may change jobs or cut back on activities such as driving or travel. According to the doctrine of informed consent, physicians have an affirmative duty to provide the patient or surrogate with pertinent information about the patient's condition and the options for care. This duty to disclose goes beyond merely responding honestly to questions.

TABLE 36-1. *Reasons to disclose mistakes to patients or surrogates*

Disclosure respects patients.
Disclosure benefits the patient.
Disclosure benefits the physician.
   Disclosure maintains the doctor's sense of integrity.
   Disclosure helps physicians to learn from the mistake.
Nondisclosure harms the physician.
   Nondisclosure damages the physician's reputation.
   Nondisclosure undermines public trust.

It may be helpful for physicians to imagine that the patient is a close relative. How would they feel if a dramatic change occurred in their relative's condition, and the health care team was not forthright about the cause of the change?

Disclosure Benefits the Patient

Disclosure of a mistake, by explaining the adverse event, may prevent anxiety about a recurrence. In addition, disclosure enables patients or surrogates to take steps to reverse the error or mitigate its harms. Patients might need additional treatment, close monitoring, or frequent visits to the physician. Patients or families are more likely to cooperate with such measures if they understand the reasons for them.

Disclosure might also allow patients to be compensated for serious harms. In Case 36.1, the patient required intensive care, a prolonged hospitalization, and a computed tomography (CT) scan following the mistake. It is unfair to require the patient to pay for the additional care, in addition to suffering physical harm. Furthermore, it seems inequitable if patients are not compensated for lost income or serious disability resulting from mistakes. Patients cannot negotiate such compensation unless they or their surrogates know that a mistake occurred.

Disclosure Benefits the Physician

Disclosure Helps to Maintain the Doctor's Sense of Integrity

When a serious mistake has been made, it seems callous and deceptive not to admit it. When a person harms another, the natural response is usually to say that one is sorry (5). Telling the patient or family about the mistake is a prerequisite to making amends and being forgiven.

Disclosure Helps Physicians to Learn From the Mistake

Disclosure requires physicians to accept responsibility for the mistake, rather than blaming others or "the system." Accepting such responsibility makes it more likely that the physician will make constructive changes in practice to prevent future errors (2).

Nondisclosure Harms the Physician

Nondisclosure Damages the Physician's Reputation

The patient or family will likely learn the cause of a dramatic complication, such as the seizures in Case 36.1, and will probably feel outraged and betrayed if they were not told promptly. Indeed, if they believe that a cover-up was attempted, the patient and family will probably be more angry than if the mistake was disclosed immediately. In a survey, patients said that would be more likely to sue after a mistake if the physician had not informed them of the mistake and they found out in some other way (4). Legal liability may be greater if the physician conceals negligent actions and the patient is harmed by reliance on such misrepresentation (5a).

Nondisclosure Undermines Public Trust

Nondisclosure may harm the profession as a whole, not just the individual physician. If the public perceives a pattern of nondisclosure, patients may believe that doctors are more concerned about protecting themselves than in doing what is best for patients. Such mistrust may affect all aspects of care, not just concerns about mistakes.

WHAT SHOULD PHYSICIANS SAY TO PATIENTS?

In Case 36.1, the physician clearly made a mistake, the patient suffered serious harm, and the mistake caused a poor outcome. Under these circumstances, the physician's responsibility to the patient should prevail over any self-interest in concealing the mistake. The physician should take the initiative in disclosing relevant information. First, when a definite mistake caused the patient serious harm, physicians should explicitly acknowledge that a mistake occurred and say that they are sorry (6). Second, the physician needs to explain the mistake and its consequences. Third, the physician should explain what can and will be done to mitigate the resulting harms.

Some risk managers may fear that disclosing mistakes encourages patients to sue. Some risk managers may recommend telling the patient and family in Case 36.1 only that the seizures were caused by low blood sugar. But the patient and family are likely to ask what caused his glucose to be low. The most appropriate ethical response by the risk manager in Case 36.1 would be to offer a fair out-of-court settlement. The patient should not be billed for additional care necessitated by the mistake (6).

SITUATION IN WHICH DISCLOSURE MAY NOT BE WARRANTED

In many cases, it is not clear that a mistake occurred, that the patient suffered harm, or that the mistake caused the harm. Under these circumstances, it would be reasonable not to disclose mistakes to the patient or family.

The Patient Suffered No Harm

Sometimes physicians make definite mistakes, but the patient suffers little or no harm.

CASE 36.2. INCORRECT PRESCRIPTION. *A physician prescribed a sulfonamide antibiotic to a patient with a history of allergy to those medications. The error was discovered by a nurse and the prescription changed after two doses. No adverse effects occurred.*

In Case 36.2, some physicians might argue that if the prognosis or future care of the patient is not altered, there is no point in telling the patient of the mistake. Such physicians might hesitate to burden patients with all the uncertainties and adjustments made in the course of care. In this view, patients would not benefit from knowing about "trivial" errors and might be harmed if they lost confidence in the physician and the hospital.

Even in this case, however, there are reasons to disclose the mistake. Disclosure is likely to strengthen the doctor–patient relationship because patients respect physicians for being honest. Disclosure might also promote patient well-being; as a result of this error, the diagnosis of drug allergy might be reconsidered. Furthermore, the patient himself may call attention to errors, for example, after noticing that the medication has been changed. If this occurs, the physician may find it difficult to explain the situation if she did not tell the patient of the mistake immediately.

The Mistake Did Not Cause the Poor Outcome

In other cases, the physician makes a mistake and the patient suffers a poor outcome, but the mistake did not cause the poor outcome.

CASE 36.3. FAILURE TO ADMINISTER APPROPRIATE TREATMENT. *A 52-year-old man had vomiting and ataxia, followed by stupor and coma. In the emergency department, he had a blood pressure of 200/105, which was not treated while a CT scan was obtained. He was found to have a cerebellar hemorrhage and died in the emergency department.*

In this case, standard care would be to lower blood pressure before obtaining the CT scan. However, once comatose, this patient's prognosis would be grim even if his blood pressure were reduced. The patient was so severely ill that he would almost certainly have died even if the mistake had not occurred.

In such situations, when telling the family about the patient's death, the physicians need not say that it resulted from a mistake. Physicians must recognize, however, that their belief that the mistake caused no harm to the patient may be biased or self-serving. Consultation with an experienced colleague may help the physician evaluate her actions realistically.

Even if a mistake is not mentioned, family members may ask physicians whether everything was done. This questions deserves both a literal and deeper response. On the literal level, it would be deceptive to say that everything was done when the physician knows that this was not the case. On another level, the survivors may be asking whether *they* should have acted differently or whether the patient suffered needlessly. The physician needs to acknowledge and respond to these concerns. For instance, the physician might say, "It's natural when someone dies suddenly to ask if anything more could have been done. We've been reviewing what we did, and families sometimes ask whether they could have done anything differently. In hindsight, we may all wish we had acted differently. However, in all likelihood he still would have died. . . . One thing that we can feel reassured about is that he didn't suffer."

No Mistake Occurred, Even Though the Patient Had a Poor Outcome

The patient may suffer a poor outcome after a procedure, although the physician did not make a mistake.

CASE 36.4. FORESEEABLE COMPLICATION OF AN INVASIVE PROCEDURE. *A 43-year-old man with interstitial lung disease undergoes a bronchoscopy and transbronchial biopsy. The procedure is performed skillfully. He suffers a pneumothorax that requires insertion of a chest tube for 2 days. He is informed of this risk prior to the procedure. The procedure is performed skillfully, with no apparent difficulties.*

In this case, the patient suffered a known complication. The patient agreed to the procedure and accepted the risks. Although the physician should express sadness that the complication occurred, there was no mistake.

DISCLOSING MISTAKES BY TRAINEES TO AN ATTENDING PHYSICIAN

In teaching hospitals, serious mistakes by trainees may not be reported to attending physicians (2).

Disclosure of Serious Mistakes by Trainees to Attending Physicians

It is understandable that students, house officers, and fellows may be reluctant to tell supervisors about mistakes. They may fear that grades, recommendations, or future positions may be jeopardized. Supervisors may also be judgmental and unsympathetic when told of mistakes.

Attending physicians, however, are ethically and legally responsible for patient care. They cannot perform this role adequately if significant information about the patient is withheld. Importantly, attending physicians may learn of such mistakes even if trainees do not disclose them. Most supervising physicians believe that failure to disclose mistakes is worse than making them in the first place (7). Although trainees are expected to make some errors, covering them up raises doubts about reliability, trustworthiness, and character.

Responses by Attending Physicians to Mistakes by Trainees

Once a trainee has a disclosed a mistake, the attending physician needs to respond on several levels.

Elicit and Acknowledge the Trainee's Emotional Distress

Appropriate emotional support needs to be provided. The supervisor can put the trainee's feelings in context: although it causes distress to admit a mistake, it is essential to do so if the trainee is to learn from the mistake (2). Understanding this link between emotional distress and learning may offer the resident some solace.

Review the Medical Issues and the Decisions

The supervisor can help the trainee learn from the mistake and make constructive changes in practice to prevent similar errors in the future. Such constructive changes might include seeking more advice, reading more about the problem, confirming clinical data personally, and paying more attention to detail (2).

Discussing mistakes can also help other trainees avoid similar errors. In addition, systematic problems that contributed to the mistake, such as inadequate backup or the lack of a computerized pharmacy system, can be identified and corrected.

Discuss Whether to Disclose the Mistake to the Patient or Surrogate

If disclosure is appropriate, the attending physician can inform the patient together with the trainee. Such joint discussions would provide trainees with emotional support and role modeling.

MISTAKES BY OTHER HEALTH CARE WORKERS

A physician may become aware of a definite mistake by another health care worker that seriously harmed a patient. For example, in Case 36.1, the overdose of insulin might have been made by a coworker on the primary team, another clinical service, or a different hospital. Even if the current physician did not make the mistake, the patient still needs to understand what happened and perhaps take action to mitigate the harms caused by the mistake. Thus, the current physician may question whether she should disclose the mistake to the patient.

Ethical Issues Regarding Mistakes by Other Health Care Workers

Ethically, the same standards should be applied to disclosing mistakes by other physicians as to disclosing one's own mistakes. If it would be appropriate for the patient to know that a mistake occurred, it should not matter that someone else was responsible. However, it is often more difficult to deal with mistakes by others.

There may be strong reasons for not disclosing the mistakes of other health care workers. The facts of the case may be unclear. Even if physicians review the medical record, they may not know what actually happened, particularly at another hospital. In addition, disclosure may conflict with the current physician's self-interest. The other person or institution may become irate or stop referring patients. Physicians in training who notice a serious mistake by a senior physician may fear retaliation (*see* Chapter 38). In addition, the patient or family may vent their anger on the current physician, who bears no responsibility for the mistake.

Responses to Mistakes by Other Health Care Workers

Faced with a clear and serious mistake by another health care worker, the current physician may take several approaches.

Wait for the Patient to Ask

As discussed previously, this strategy is ethically problematical because physicians have an affirmative obligation to disclose relevant information to patients, not only to answer patients' questions honestly.

Ask the Other Attending Physician to Disclose

Although this option may be easiest for the current physician, it may be problematical for the patient or family. The previous physician may choose not to tell the patient or may provide misleading information about the mistake.

Arrange a Joint Conference

A conference may be held with the current physician, the previous physician, and the patient or family. This approach allows the other physician to take the lead revealing the mistake, while ensuring that the discussion is appropriate. However, such a meeting may be impossible to arrange.

Tell the Patient

Although this approach leads to appropriate disclosure, it may undermine the relationships between the patient and the previous physician and between the two physicians. It is possible that the other doctor wanted to talk to the patient directly and would have carried out the discussion appropriately. If this approach is taken, it would be preferable to give the other physician the opportunity to talk to the patient first.

Ideally, the decision to acknowledge a mistake should be based on ethical guidelines, not expedience. Disclosure of mistakes is difficult. However, failure to disclose mistakes that cause serious harm undermines the credibility of physicians and compromises their integrity. Anticipating potential adverse consequences of disclosure allows physicians to cope with them. Ultimately the quality of medical care is enhanced if we are willing to admit our mistakes and learn from them.

REFERENCES

1. Brennan TA, Leape LL, Laird NM, et al. Incidence of adverse effects and negligence in hospitalized patients: results of the Harvard Malpractice Study I. *N Engl J Med* 1991;324:370–376.
2. Wu AW, Folkman S, McPhee SJ, et al. Do house officers learn from their mistakes? *JAMA* 1991;265:2089–2094.
3. Novack DH, Detering BJ, Arnold R, et al. Physicians' attitudes toward using deception to resolve difficult ethical problems. *JAMA* 1989;261:2980–2985.
3a. Kraman SS, Hamm G. Risk management: extreme honesty may be the best policy. *Ann Intern Med* 1999; 131:963–967.
4. Witman AB, Park DM, Hardin SB. How do patients want physicians to handle mistakes? A survey of internal medicine patients in an academic setting. *Arch Intern Med* 1996;156:2565–2569.
5. Hilficker D. Facing our mistakes. *N Engl J Med* 1984;310:118–122.
5a. Furrow BR, Johnson SH, Jost TS, Schwartz RL. Health law: cases, materials, problems, 3rd ed. St. Paul: West Publishing Co., 1997:385–388.

6. Wu AW, Cavanaugh TA, McPhee SJ, et al. To tell the truth: ethical and practical issues in disclosing medical mistakes to patients. *J Gen Intern Med* 1997;17:770–775.
7. Bosk CL. *Forgive and remember: managing medical failure.* Chicago: University of Chicago Press, 1979.

ANNOTATED BIBLIOGRAPHY

1. Hilficker D. Facing our mistakes. *N Engl J Med* 1984;310:118–122.
   Eloquent first-person account of a physician's reaction to serious mistakes and the need to acknowledge mistakes.
2. Wu AW, Folkman S, McPhee SJ, Lo B. Do house officers learn from their mistakes? *JAMA* 1991;265:2089–2094.
   House officers who accepted responsibility for serious mistakes were more likely to make constructive changes in practice but were also more likely to experience emotional distress. Attending physicians were told of serious mistakes only 54% of the time, and patients or families were told of the mistake in only 24% of cases.
3. Kohn L. Corrigan J, Donaldson M, eds. To err is human: building a safer health system. Washington, DC: National Academy Press, 2000.
   Recommends that a confidential system of reporting medical mistakes be established in order to prevent future mistakes.

37

Impaired Colleagues

Physicians who are impaired or incompetent may harm patients. Society relies on the medical profession to regulate itself (1), yet colleagues of impaired physicians are often reluctant to intervene, even in egregious cases. The following case illustrates common dilemmas regarding impaired colleagues.

CASE 37.1. DRINKING ALCOHOL WHILE ON CALL. *Dr. New, a young internist who has recently joined a group practice, is at a party. She overhears a senior colleague, Dr. Elder, answer a page. Dr. Elder has been drinking and has slurred speech. Over the phone he prescribes 1.25 mg of digoxin, an unusually large dose. From what she hears of the conversation, Dr. New suspects that she has previously covered for this patient, an elderly man with mild renal insufficiency, a recent hip fracture repair, and postoperative pneumonia.*

Dr. New is in a quandary. Although she suspects that a patient is at risk of a drug overdose, she cannot be sure. Should she intervene to protect the patient from this suspected mistake? If so, should she confront Dr. Elder directly or talk to the house officer or nursing supervisor covering the service? Even if she protects this patient, what about other patients Dr. Elder might harm? Dr. New wants to prevent harm to patients, but she is reluctant to jeopardize the career of an established physician as well as her own future.

This chapter discusses physicians' concerns about intervening with impaired colleagues, reasons to take action, and practical suggestions. Chapter 36, on mistakes, contains related materials. Mistakes by impaired or incompetent colleagues are more serious than other mistakes because they are more likely to be repeated.

CAUSES OF IMPAIRMENT AND INCOMPETENCE

Common causes of impairment include alcoholism, substance abuse, and psychiatric and medical illness, such as depression and Alzheimer's disease (2). Many impaired physicians can be treated effectively in programs that stress confidential rehabilitation rather than punishment (3). Physicians may also be incompetent because of inadequate knowledge and skills or careless behavior, for example, failing to round on patients.

REASONS FOR INTERVENING WITH IMPAIRED COLLEAGUES

Physicians have an ethical obligation to be competent, based on the ethical guidelines of refraining from causing harm and acting in their patients' best interests. There are also compelling ethical reasons for physicians to intervene with seriously impaired colleagues, even though the patients who may be harmed are not their own (Table 37-1).

TABLE 37-1. *Reasons for intervening with impaired colleagues*
Prevent harm to patients.
Carry out professional self-regulation.
Help the impaired colleague.

Prevent Harm to Patients

People have a duty to prevent serious harm to others when it can be done at minimal risk or inconvenience to themselves (4). Modern professional codes of ethics also require physicians to protect patients from impaired colleagues. The American College of Physicians Ethics Manual states, "It is the responsibility of every physician to protect the public from an impaired physician. . . . All steps must be taken to assure that no patient is harmed because of actions or decisions made by an impaired physician" (5). Colleagues of an impaired physician may be in a unique position to prevent harm to patients. Physician-peers have the expertise and the opportunity to evaluate the quality of care rendered by colleagues (1).

In other occupations, workers whose impairment may endanger the public are aggressively identified. For example, airline pilots and train engineers are required to submit to drug testing before hiring, after accidents, and on a random basis (6). A commercial pilot who is suspected of drinking while on duty may be removed from the cockpit.

Critics charge that in comparison impaired physicians are treated laxly. It seems inconsistent to forbid pilots to drink while on duty but to allow physicians to drink while on call.

Carry Out Professional Self-Regulation

Society grants the medical profession considerable autonomy to regulate itself through selecting applicants for medical school and residency, defining standards of education and practice, certifying physicians, and disciplining members. The rationale for such professional control is that laypeople do not have the expertise to determine whether physicians are impaired or incompetent. In return for such autonomy, society expects the profession to screen out practitioners who might endanger patients. Public trust in the medical profession will be undermined if people believe that physicians are covering up for impaired or incompetent colleagues. In addition, society might take away the power to regulate impaired or incompetent physicians.

Help the Impaired Colleague

Impaired physicians may harm themselves and their families as well as their patients; they may have serious automobile accidents, violent episodes, or lapses in judgment. Furthermore, impaired physicians may destroy their livelihood and their families' economic security. Intervening with impaired colleagues may help them to avert such destructive outcomes.

CONCERNS ABOUT INTERVENING WITH IMPAIRED COLLEAGUES

Strong evidence that physicians are reluctant to intervene with impaired colleagues comes from state licensing boards. Compared with the estimated prevalence of impairment, state boards receive few reports about impaired physicians (7). There may be several reasons for such reluctance.

Uncertainty That Patients Are at Serious Risk

Physicians may be uncertain that colleagues suspected of impairment are actually placing patients at risk. In Case 37.1, although Dr. New has good reason to suspect that Dr. Elder may have harmed a patient, she cannot be certain. She does not know the complete story. Perhaps the patient needed a high dose because he had uncontrolled atrial fibrillation or intestinal malabsorption.

Reluctance to Criticize Colleagues

Physicians rely on the skills, knowledge, and judgment of colleagues, and it would be difficult to practice medicine without such reliance. Physicians may hesitate to admit that a colleague is impaired because it is uncomfortable to mistrust their colleagues.

Physicians may also be reluctant to delve into matters that are often considered private, such as alcohol consumption. Dr. New might be reluctant to act on the basis of a personal telephone conversation that she accidentally overheard.

Doctors are understandably reluctant to undermine a colleague's reputation and livelihood. On a subconscious level, physicians may identify with impaired colleagues. If they question a colleague's competence, might other physicians in turn criticize them harshly after a minor mistake?

Retaliation Against Whistleblowers

Whistleblowers often face personal retaliation, despite their good intentions. If Dr. New confronts Dr. Elder, he may get angry or tell her to mind her own business. If she tells other people, colleagues might label her a snitch or a tattletale. Dr. Elder may accuse her of trying to ruin his reputation or trying to build up her own practice. He might even retaliate by criticizing her work and discouraging other physicians from referring patients to her. Legal retaliation might also be a concern. Dr. Elder might sue her for defamation of character or lost income. Even the threat of a lawsuit, its concomitant cost, and adverse publicity might deter Dr. New from pursuing the matter. Dr. New's natural concern about her own career may conflict with her desire to prevent harm to vulnerable patients.

LEGAL ISSUES REGARDING IMPAIRED COLLEAGUES

Many states have adopted laws concerning reporting of impaired or incompetent colleagues (1,8).

Reporting Laws

The specific provisions of reporting laws vary from state to state. In Massachusetts physicians must report to the state licensing board colleagues whom they suspect are practicing medicine while impaired. Other states permit such reporting but do not require it. Most states grant legal immunity from civil suits to physicians who report colleagues in good faith.

Diversion Programs

Many states have set up voluntary programs to treat and rehabilitate impaired physicians (3). The goal is to allow rehabilitated physicians to continue to practice or to return to work. Physicians entering such programs may be granted confidentiality and immunity from disciplinary actions. In some states, while physicians participate in the program, their medical licenses may be suspended or put on probation. In many states, the licensing board has asked local medical societies to conduct these programs, so that rehabilitation programs are clearly differentiated from punishment. Several states have reported success at rehabilitating impaired physicians in such programs (2).

The Health Care Quality Improvement Act

In 1986 Congress passed legislation regarding reporting of incompetent physicians (9). This law requires hospitals and state licensing agencies to report to a federal agency most disciplinary actions related to professional incompetence or misconduct. In addition, insurance companies must report malpractice payments above $10,000. These reports are entered into the National Practitioner Data Bank. To prevent incompetent or impaired physicians from simply resigning from one hospital staff, relocating, and continuing to practice elsewhere, hospitals are required to obtain information from the National Practitioner Data Bank when physicians apply for hospital privileges and periodically thereafter.

The law also confers legal immunity on individuals and hospitals who report impaired colleagues in good faith. Specifically, immunity is given to individuals who provide "information to a professional review body regarding the competence or professional conduct of a physician." In addition, peer review bodies and individuals who work with or assist them are granted legal immunity. Note, however, that these provisions may not protect Dr. New in Case 37.1 if she attempts to deal with Dr. Elder outside the formal peer review process.

DEALING WITH IMPAIRED COLLEAGUES

Physicians might deal with an impaired colleague in several ways (Table 37-2).

Protect Patients From Immediate Harm

If Dr. New believes that the patient may be seriously harmed by Dr. Elder's order, she should take immediate action. She might say to Dr. Elder, "I'm sorry to intrude, but I thought I heard you say 1.25 mg of digoxin. I'm afraid the nurses might have heard the wrong dose as well." If the matter is not resolved satisfactorily, Dr. New could call the hospital and ask the nursing supervisor at the hospital to look into the case. Dr. New should also intervene if Dr. Elder is apparently drunk on call, even if she had no direct evidence that he had made a questionable medical decision. If Dr. Elder does not agree to have a colleague take calls for him, it would be prudent to notify another senior physician or the chief of the department and arrange for someone else to take calls, at least until Dr. Elder regains sobriety.

TABLE 37-2. *Dealing with impaired colleagues*

Protect patients from immediate harm.
Determine whether further action is needed.
Talk with the colleague directly.
Report the problem to responsible officials.

Determine Whether Further Action Is Needed

After preventing immediate harm to patients, Dr. New needs to assess whether additional actions are needed. Gathering more information about the impaired colleague can usually be done discreetly.

Because whistleblowing is emotionally difficult and personally risky, physicians might take steps to prevent harm to patients, without reporting the impaired or incompetent colleague to appropriate officials or confronting him directly. Many physicians would not refer patients to such a colleague but would otherwise let the matter drop. Other physicians cover up for impaired colleagues rather than confront them. For example, a physician may review the colleague's work and correct his errors. Such oversight helps to protect patients. Although well-intentioned, such actions are ineffective in the long run. To try to monitor all the clinical activities of an impaired or incompetent colleague is impractical and also counterproductive, because it allows him to deny the impairment.

Talk With the Colleague Directly

In many situations, a physician will want to talk with an impaired colleague directly, particularly if the colleague is a friend. Although such conversations are uncomfortable, they can be quite effective. The matter can be resolved if the impaired colleague agrees to seek help, for example, by enrolling a rehabilitation program. Alternatively, physicians impaired by physical illness may decide to retire or to restrict the scope of their practice.

Report the Problem to Responsible Officials

Dr. New does not need to solve the problem of an impaired colleague by herself. She needs only to decide whether there is sufficient suspicion of impairment to warrant further investigation. In Case 37.1, Dr. New directly observed a situation of potential harm to a patient. She can discharge her ethical obligations by reporting impaired colleagues to officials, who can investigate and take appropriate action. Such officials include the chief of service, the chief of staff of the hospital, or, if a trainee is involved, the director of a training program or student clerkships. These individuals are responsible for ensuring the quality of patient care and the competence of medical staff. Furthermore, most health care organizations have employee assistance programs to help impaired workers (3). Because Dr. New has just joined the practice, she may feel more comfortable asking the chief of service to pursue the matter than talking to Dr. Elder directly. In cases of egregious impairment or incompetence, notifying the state licensing board directly might also be advisable. The circumstances of the case often determine how physicians prefer to respond to an impaired or incompetent colleague. In one survey, most house officers said they were willing to confront a fellow house officer who was impaired by alcohol but preferred to tell the chief resident or the chief of medicine about an attending physician who was similarly impaired. However, house officers were less comfortable confronting a fellow house officer who was incompetent rather than impaired and preferred to refer such matters to a more senior physician (10).

In summary, there are understandable practical reasons why physicians hesitate to intervene with impaired colleagues. However, there are cogent ethical reasons for physicians to take action to prevent impaired colleagues from harming patients. Pragmatically, there are ways to do so that are safe for whistleblowers.

REFERENCES

1. Report 39. *Reporting impaired, incompetent or unethical colleagues.* Report of the Council on Ethical and Judicial Affairs of the American Medical Assocation. Chicago: American Medical Assocation, 1992.
2. Aach RD, Girard DE, Humphrey H, et al. Alcohol and other substance abuse and impairment among physician in residency training. *Ann Intern Med* 1992;116:245–254.
3. O'Connor PG, Spickard A Jr. Physician impairment by substance abuse. *Med Clin North Am* 1997;81:1037–1052.
4. Beauchamp TL, Childress JF. *Principles of biomedical ethics,* 3rd ed. New York: Oxford University Press, 1989:120–193.
5. American College of Physicians. *American College of Physicians ethics manual. Ann Intern Med* 1992;117: 947–960.
6. Modell JG, Mountz JM. Drinking and flying—the problem of alcohol use by pilots. *N Engl J Med* 1990;323: 455–461.
7. Feinstein RJ. The ethics of professional regulation. *N Engl J Med* 1985;312:801–804.
8. Walzer RS. Impaired physicians: an overview and update of the legal issues. *J Legal Med* 1990;11:131–198.
9. Health Care Quality Improvement Act, 42 U.S.C.A. §§11101–11151 (1990).
10. Reuben DB, Noble S. House officer responses to impaired physicians. *JAMA* 1990;263:958–960.

ANNOTATED BIBLIOGRAPHY

1. Report 39. *Reporting impaired, incompetent or unethical colleagues.* Report of the Council on Ethical and Judicial Affairs of the American Medical Association. Chicago: American Medical Association, 1992.
   Discusses ethical and practical issues regarding impaired physicians.
2. Ethics case study: the dilemma of dealing with an impaired colleague. *ACP Observer* 1991;11:10–11.
   Stresses the goals of protecting patients while helping the impaired colleague.
3. Aach RD, Girard DE, Humphrey H, et al. Alcohol and other substance abuse and impairment among physicians in residency training. *Ann Intern Med* 1992;116:245–254.
   Discusses how to help house officers suffering from substance abuse and other causes of impairment.

38

Ethical Dilemmas Facing Students and House Staff

In their training, most clinicians have entered a patient's room to perform a procedure knowing that someone else could do it far more skillfully.

CASE 38.1. PERFORMING AN INVASIVE PROCEDURE. *Obviously tired after a 5-hour wait in the emergency room, a woman with an asthma exacerbation is finally admitted to the floor. "Oh no, not another needlestick!" she groans, as a medical student approaches to draw arterial blood gases. The medical student gulps inwardly, aware that his previous attempts at drawing blood gases have been unsuccessful or required multiple punctures.*

The self-interest of trainees in learning may conflict with the best interests of their patients. Learning clinical skills and taking responsibility may present inconvenience, discomfort, or even risk to patients. Ethical conflicts also arise when trainees observe unethical or substandard care by other physicians. Both trainees and patients benefit when these issues are discussed openly, rather than hidden from view. Ideally, the welfare of the patient should be paramount.

LEARNING ON PATIENTS

In their training, medical students may worry that they are taking unfair advantage of patients but hesitate to voice their concerns to their supervisors (1). They fear that their reputation or career may suffer if others believe they are reluctant to accept responsibility.

Introducing Trainees to Patients

CASE 38.2. INTRODUCING STUDENTS AS PHYSICIANS. *The attending physician introduces a medical student beginning a third-year clerkship to the patient as "Doctor." When the student raises concerns about this, the attending physician insists that students have to get over their "hangups" about taking responsibility. According to the attending physician, patients who seek care at a teaching hospital know that students will be taking care of them. If they did not agree, they would not come to a teaching hospital.*

Introducing students as physicians is not uncommon (2). On name tags, 27% of medical schools do not identify students as medical students, student doctors, or student physicians (3). There are several reasons why trainees are not introduced as such (4). First, trainees may fear that if their status is disclosed, patients will not trust them to provide care. Second, some physicians argue that patients who come to a teaching hospital have given "implied consent" for trainees to care for them. Third, other physicians contend that introducing trainees will cause unwarranted worry to patients.

There are compelling reasons to introduce students truthfully. Patient trust cannot be built on misrepresentation. A patient who is misled about a health care provider's role may feel betrayed if he discovers the trainee's true status. The legal doctrine of informed consent requires physicians to disclose pertinent information to the patient (*see* Chapter 3). The identity of trainees who will be providing care may be highly relevant to patient decisions. State laws and accreditation requirements may also require that trainees disclose their educational status to patients (4). The argument that patients who seek care at teaching hospitals have given implied consent to be "teaching material" is untenable. The concept of "implied consent" applies only to emergency situations in which delaying treatment to obtain consent would seriously harm the patient.

Protecting patients from unnecessary worry is also an unconvincing reason to withhold information. Most patients agree that trainees enhance the quality of their care and want to contribute to a trainee's education (5,6). If physicians are concerned that patients will worry inappropriately, they should provide more information about teaching hospitals, not less. Trainees are accessible around the clock, have more time to answer questions, and are closely supervised. Overall, primary teaching hospitals have a lower rate of adverse patient events due to negligence than nonteaching hospitals (7).

Some trainees resort to unfamiliar titles, such as "clinical clerk." Such a term is the literal truth and avoids the consequences of explicitly calling oneself a student. However, the term "clinical clerk" is unacceptable because it is incomprehensible to patients and intended to mislead. "Student physician" is commonly used and emphasizes the special medical training that the student has received.

Learning Basic Clinical Skills

To learn to take a history, perform a physical examination, draw blood, and start intravenous lines, medical students to practice on patients. Although patients are not subjected to any serious medical risks, they may be inconvenienced, lose privacy, or experience some discomfort. Out of respect for patients, the attending physician or resident should ask permission beforehand. When asked, almost all patients agree to have students listen to a heart murmur or perform a history and physical examination. Although it is reasonable to ask patients to spend an hour with a student, it is inappropriate to ask them to spend 3 hours for an exhaustive student examination, to miss their meals, or to lose sleep.

Learning Invasive Procedures

Invasive procedures performed by trainees may raise ethical concerns. In Case 38.1, medical students need practice in order to learn how to perform arterial punctures skillfully. When trainees learn invasive procedures such as lumbar puncture or insertion of central lines, their first patients may experience increased discomfort or even risk. The trainee's self-interest in learning and long-term goal of benefiting future patients may therefore conflict with the short-term goal of providing the best care to current patients.

Trainees frequently do not discuss their participation in invasive procedures with patients (2). One reason for avoiding the issue is the fear that patients will request more experienced physicians (8). Such requests would be understandable. Physicians might consider whether they would be willing to have a trainee perform the procedure on a close relative, or would request a more experienced physician.

In the spirit of informed consent, patients need to understand who will be performing invasive procedures and what additional risk, if any, can be attributed to trainees. Such information may be highly pertinent to the patient's decision to undergo a procedure at that institution. For surgical procedures, almost all patients want the attending surgeon to tell them what the resident will do during the operation (5). In one study, all obstetrical patients believed that student participation should be requested rather than assigned (9). In another study, patients considered it very important to know that a medical student is going to make the incision, hold retractors, perform rectal or pelvic examinations under anesthesia, suture incisions, or intubate them (8). Furthermore, patients consider such disclosure more important than medical students do (8).

The attending physician should take responsibility for telling patients about the participation of students and residents in their care and introduce the trainees (5). Patient concerns about unskilled trainees are best resolved by providing more information, not less. When informed and given a choice, most patients allow trainees to do procedures. In one study, 80% of patients said they would want to know the experience of the person performing a lumbar puncture (10). However, 52% of patients would allow a closely supervised medical student to attempt a first lumbar puncture on them, and 66% would allow a resident to do so. Patients prefer that discussions of student participation be carried out before elective surgery and with the student not present (5,9). Patient requests to have a more experienced physician perform the procedure should be honored if possible.

Trainees should carry out procedures only under adequate supervision, except in dire emergencies. Without supervision, the patient may be placed at unnecessary risk, and the trainee will not have an optimal learning experience. The hospital has a responsibility to provide such supervision, and the trainee also has a responsibility to ensure it before starting the procedure. The senior physician should take over if the trainee encounters problems during the procedure.

Learning on Unconscious or Dead Patients

Trainees may face further dilemmas when they are asked to learn on unconscious or newly dead patients without explicit consent to do so. For example, an attending physician may tell the medical student and intern that they should perform pelvic examinations on a patient under general anesthesia. He says that such examinations are excellent learning experiences because it is easier to palpate the ovaries when the patient is anesthetized. However, pelvic examinations performed under anesthesia without explicit permission violate patient privacy and autonomy (*see* Chapter 41).

Similar ethical dilemmas arise regarding learning invasive procedures on newly dead patients without the consent of the next of kin. For instance, after a patient on their service dies, the resident may tell the intern and student to practice intubation and insertion of a central venous catheter. "The patient is dead; you can't hurt her, but you might hurt a live patient if you don't practice." Such practice increases skill and thereby benefits future patients (11). However, invasive procedures might disfigure the body and outrage family members. Dead patients are not "teaching material." They deserve to be treated with respect.

Some physicians suggest that practicing invasive procedures be permitted unless relatives specifically object. However, unless family members are informed that such a practice occurs, they may not know to raise objections (11). A better policy would be to obtain consent from survivors for practicing invasive procedures on newly dead patients (12). When consent is sought in a candid and compassionate manner, most family members give permission (13,14). Permission from survivors also helps trainees to resolve their own ambivalence or anguish about learning on patients and to appreciate how their training depends on the altruism of other people (13).

TAKING TOO MUCH CLINICAL RESPONSIBILITY

Trainees sometimes assume too much decision-making responsibility, without adequate supervision (1). For instance, a resident on a busy service may tell a subintern to sign his name on the physicians' order sheet, saying "You're clearly a good student, and you can page me if you have a real question." However, it is unrealistic to expect the student to distinguish routine orders from serious management decisions. Errors in judgment or dosage can occur even in "routine" orders. Furthermore, the resident is giving the student a mixed message: call me for serious problems, but if you're a good student you won't bother me. Discouraging trainees' questions also reduces opportunities for learning. Students who insist on adequate supervision implicitly criticize the resident and may experience retaliation in grades and evaluations. They may be labeled as "not a team player," insecure, or reluctant to assume responsibility.

The training system may place the student in an untenable situation by exerting pressure to take too much responsibility or failing to set clear expectations or provide adequate supervision. The institution should set clear expectations for supervision of trainees and establish a mechanism for students as well as residents to ask for help. A satisfactory resolution may require systemwide changes. The attending physician might get more directly involved in patient care and supervision, freeing up the resident. The team might transfer some patients to another team or be assigned an additional house officer.

Trainees are ultimately accountable for taking too much responsibility and potentially harming patients. Ethically, trainees should know their own limitations and not exceed them.

UNETHICAL BEHAVIOR OR SUBSTANDARD CARE BY OTHER PHYSICIANS

Trainees may be involved in cases in which senior physicians appear to violate ethical guidelines (15).

CASE 38.3. FAILURE TO OBTAIN INFORMED CONSENT FOR STERILIZATION. *An attending obstetrician performs a tubal ligation on a 32-year-old Latina woman on Medicaid who has just delivered her sixth child by cesarean section. According to the chart, the patient refused sterilization at her last prenatal visit. The resident who delivered the baby and served as the translator for the patient is outraged. The delivery room nurse confirms that no informed consent was obtained, but cautions, "Don't ruin your career over this."*

Some disagreements reflect reasonable differences of clinical judgment or misunderstanding by the trainee. In Case 38.3, however, the attending physician is clearly violating the ethical guideline of respecting patient autonomy as well as laws on informed consent. The resident felt outraged at the event, frustrated at being powerless, guilty that she did not intervene, and ashamed that she had become an accomplice in an unethical deed. She believed that the attending physician's action was both sexist and racist.

Trainees who are involved in a patient's case may also observe grossly substandard care by senior physicians, as when they fail to round on patients, write progress notes, or answer pages. In cases of clearly inadequate care, the trainee has an ethical obligation to protect patients and to not mislead them. In addition, there is an ethical obligation to try to prevent harm to future patients if a pattern of impairment exists (*see* Chapter 37). However, there are also strong countervailing pragmatic considerations, as we discuss next.

Risks to Whistleblowers

Fear of retaliation is a legitimate practical concern for trainees (16). The obstetrics resident in Case 38.3 did not want to risk a bad recommendation for the rotation or unfavorable treatment during the rest of her training. As in all walks of life, whistleblowers may suffer harm even if their accusations prove to be valid. Ideally, the well-being of the patient should take priority over the self-interest of the trainee. Individual trainees need to decide how much personal risk as a whistleblower they are willing to accept, relative to the harm they might prevent.

Suggestions for Trainees

Involve Other Physicians

Often trainees feel that they have to resolve these troubling situations by themselves. However, they can discuss the situation with trusted colleagues and senior physicians. This serves several purposes. Trainees can verify that they have observed unethical misconduct or markedly substandard care, not merely a reasonable difference of clinical judgment. Such reality testing is often crucial for their peace of mind and sense of integrity. In addition, other people might provide emotional support, give advice, and intervene constructively. The chief resident, clerkship or residency director, and chief of service have an obligation to address issues of unethical or incompetent behavior (16). Furthermore, every hospital should have procedures, such as quality assurance programs or a patient ombudsperson, for investigating such cases (16).

Decide What to Tell the Patient

In addition to informing appropriate senior physicians, the trainee needs to consider what to tell patients, if anything. There are strong reasons why patients should have truthful information about events that will affect their future medical care and life plans. The sterilized woman in Case 38.3 cannot make informed decisions about reproduction and contraception if she does not know that a tubal ligation was performed.

Trainees do not need to inform the patient personally of what happened, if they inform some responsible person, such as the chief of service. In some circumstances, however, trainees should personally inform the patient. If the patient asks the trainee directly what happened, a misleading answer would be inappropriate. Furthermore, when no one else informs the patient, trainees may mislead the patient by keeping silent.

Protect Your Own Interests

If the harm to patients is serious, the ethical ideal is for trainees to fulfill their obligations to patients, even at some risk to their careers. However, trainees should also minimize risks to themselves. Measures such as writing an angry note in the chart or directly accusing the attending of being unethical are likely to inflame the situation. Involving more senior physicians can reduce the risk of reprisals. Trainees who are unwilling to be identified as the accuser can still discuss the episode with the quality assurance committee or chief of staff. In this way, if other people are willing to come forward, there will be corroborating evidence. In addition, trainees should keep records of how they raised their concerns.

In summary, medical students, house officers, and fellows face unique clinical dilemmas. The interests of trainees in learning clinical medicine and invasive procedures may conflict with the interests of patients. In addition, the ethical guideline of preventing harm to patients may conflict with their career advancement or the reputation of the institution. The ethical ideal is for all trainees to act in the best interests of the patient, even at some personal risk or disadvantage.

REFERENCES

1. Christakis DA, Feudtner C. Ethics in a short white coat: the ethical dilemmas that medical students confront. *Acad Med* 1993;68:249–254.
2. Cohen DL, McCullough LB, Kessel RWI, et al. A national survey concerning the ethical aspects of informed consent and the role of medical students. *J Med Educ* 1988;63:821–829.
3. Silver-Isenstadt A, Ubel PA. Medical student name tags: identification or obfuscation. *J Gen Intern Med* 1997;12:669–671.
4. Marracino RK, Orr RD. Entitling the student doctor: defining the student's role in patient care. *J Gen Intern Med* 1998;13:266–270.
5. Kim N, Lo B, Gates EA. Disclosing the role of residents and medical students in hysterectomy: what do patients want? *Acad Med* 1998;73:339–341.
6. Magrane D, Jannon J, Miller CT. Obstetric patients who select and those who refuse medical students' participation in their care. *Acad Med* 1994;69:1004–1006.
7. Brennan TA, Hebert L, Laird NM, et al. Hospital characteristics associated with adverse events and substandard care. *JAMA* 1991;265:3265–3269.
8. Silver-Isenstadt A, Ubel PA. Erosion in medical students' attitudes about telling patients they are students. *J Gen Intern Med* 1999;14:481–487.
9. Magrane D, Jannon J, Miller CT. Student doctors and women in labor: attitudes and expectations. *Obstet Gynecol* 1996;88:298–302.
10. Williams CT, Fost N. Ethical considerations surrounding first-time procedures: a study and analysis of patient attitudes toward spinal taps by students. *Kennedy Inst Ethics J* 1992;3:217–233.
11. Orlowski JP, Kanoti GA, Mehlman MJ. The ethics of using newly dead patients for teaching and practicing intubation techniques. *N Engl J Med* 1988;319:439–441.
12. Goldblatt AD. Don't ask, don't tell: practicing minimally invasive resuscitation techniques on the newly dead. *Ann Emerg Med* 1995;25:86–90.
13. Benfield DG, Flaksman RJ, Lin TH, et al. Teaching intubation skills using newly deceased infants. *JAMA* 1991;265:2360–2363.
14. McNamara RM, Monti S, Kelly JJ. Requesting consent for an invasive procedure in newly deceased adults. *JAMA* 1995;273:310–312.
15. Satterwhite WM, Satterwhite RC, Enarson CE. Medical students' perceptions of unethical conduct at one medical school. *Acad Med* 1998;73:529–531.
16. Council on Ethical and Judicial Affairs of the American Medical Association. Disputes between medical supervisors and trainees. *JAMA* 1994;272:1861–1865.

ANNOTATED BIBLIOGRAPHY

1. Marracino RK, Orr RD. Entitling the student doctor: defining the student's role in patient care. *J Gen Intern Med* 1998;13:266–270.
   Analyzes why medical students often are not introduced to patients as medical students.
2. Goldblatt AD. Don't ask, don't tell: practicing minimally invasive resuscitation techniques on the newly dead. *Ann Emerg Med* 1995;25:86–90.
   Cogently argues that permission should be sought from next of kin before practicing invasive procedures on patients who have just died.

SECTION VI

Ethical Issues in Clinical Specialties

39

Ethical Issues in Pediatrics

Ethical issues in pediatrics are difficult because young children cannot understand what is best for them or make informed decisions about their own care. In addition, children are dependent on their parents or guardians. The immaturity and vulnerability of children require that decisions be made differently in pediatrics than in adult medicine.

HOW ARE ETHICAL ISSUES IN PEDIATRICS DIFFERENT?

Young Children Cannot Make Informed Decisions

Children cannot weigh risks and benefits, compare alternatives, or appreciate the long-term consequences of decisions. Autonomy, a basic ethical guideline in adult medicine, is not pertinent to decisions for young children. Children's preferences, choices, and actions should not be given the same respect as the decisions of informed, competent adults. Children's objections to beneficial interventions do not have the same ethical force as informed refusals by adults.

Because children are immature, an adult must make decisions for them. Parents are presumed to be the appropriate decision-makers (1). Parents are given considerable discretion in how they wish to raise their children. However, parental power is not absolute and is limited by the welfare the child.

The Best Interests of the Child Must Be Protected

Decisions for children should be guided by their best interests. In the United States, children are considered to have an open future. It is in a child's best interests to have the opportunity to grow, develop, and fulfill their potential as individuals. Although children are molded by parental values, when they reach maturity, they can make their own choices about their lives.

Because children cannot look after their own welfare, they must be protected from the consequences of unwise decisions, either by themselves or others. It is tragic if a child dies or suffers serious, permanent physical harm because simple, effective medical treatment was not provided. Hence children need protection if their parents or guardians make decisions about their medical care that are contrary to their best interests.

Physicians Should Be Advocates for Children

Doctors are in a unique position to identify situations in which the health and well-being of the child are jeopardized by parental decisions or the child's actions. Pediatricians are given special responsibilities to protect such a child, because if they do not intervene, the child may suffer serious, long-lasting harm.

Physicians Should Respect the Child's Potential to Become an Autonomous Adult

Although young children are not autonomous, their potential automony in the future deserves respect. Pediatricians need to provide children with information about their condition and the opportunity to participate in decisions about their care, to the extent this is developmentally appropriate (1). As children grow, their involvement in their own care should increase. Physicians need to respect adolescents' growing ability to make informed decisions, while realizing that most adolescents are dependent on their parents emotionally and financially.

WHAT STANDARDS SHOULD BE USED IN MAKING DECISIONS FOR CHILDREN?

Because children cannot make informed decisions, beneficience, or the best interests of the child, replaces autonomy as the primary ethical guideline in pediatrics.

The Best Interests of the Child

The "best interests" of the child are often vague and difficult to interpret. People may disagree over which factors comprise a child's best interests, which outcomes and risks are acceptable, and how to balance the benefits of intervention with the concomitant burdens. Promoting some of the child's interests may set back other interests of the child.

A child's best interests include both the duration and quality of life. For example, in deciding about chemotherapy for a child with cancer, parents naturally consider not only the projected survival but also the likely side effects of treatment and the expected level of functioning. However, while quality of life judgments seem unavoidable, they may be ethically problematical. Concerns are particularly strong when the quality of one child's life is compared with that of other children. It is difficult to predict the future quality of life of a child. Healthy people tend to underestimate the quality of life of persons with chronic illness. Some people believe that Down syndrome is a fate worse than death, when in fact such children can experience happiness and are prized by their parents. Despite these shortcomings, the concept of "best interests" is important because it emphasizes that children deserve respect as individuals separate from their parents, with their own interests and rights.

The Preferences of the Child

To the extent that children have the capacity to make informed decisions about their medical care, their choices should be respected. Chapter 10 discusses how to determine whether a patient has the capacity to make medical decisions. Even when children are not capable of giving informed consent, their assent to interventions is still ethically important.

It is disturbing to force interventions on children who are actively resisting them. A child's objections are not necessarily decisive; for instance, a child who objects to shots should still receive immunizations. However, forced therapy becomes more ethically problematical if children are older, the effectiveness of the intervention is less clear, or the side effects are more common, more serious, or longer lasting. The pediatrician should listen to and respond to the child's reasons for dissenting from treatment. If interventions are carried out over the child's objections, it is appropriate for the pediatrician to offer an apology to the child (2).

The Interests of Parents and Family Members

Although the best interests of the child are of primary concern, parents and other family members have interests that must be respected. What is best for an individual child must be balanced against what is best for the family as a whole or for other members of the family. Parents cannot be expected to devote all their energy and resources to one child, even though they should be expected to make some sacrifices. Pediatricians should help provide parents with emotional and social support, so that they are not overwhelmed by the burdens of care.

WHO SHOULD MAKE MEDICAL DECISIONS FOR CHILDREN?

The Presumption of Parental Decision-Making

Parents are presumed to be the appropriate decision-makers for children. Generally love motivates parents to do what is best for the child. In most cases, parents concur with pediatricians' recommendations, for example, agreeing to antibiotics for otitis media, bronchodilators for asthma, and surgery for appendicitis. In addition, parents have long-term relationships with and obligations to their children. U.S. culture prizes parental responsibility, the integrity of the family, and strong parent–child relationships. Parents or guardians have considerable latitude in raising children. Within limits set by society, parents have great discretion to inculcate their values in children and to make choices about rearing their children. For example, children must attend school, but parents may choose public school, a private school, a religious-based school, or home schooling. Similarly, parents are asked to give permission for medical care for the child. Pediatricians speak of parental permission rather than consent in order to distinguish what people may decide for themselves from what they may decide for others. Although informed adults have a right to refuse any medical intervention, parents do not have absolute power to refuse care for their children (1,2).

Exceptions to Parental Decision-Making

In some cases, the presumption of parental decision-making may be invalid. Some parents may be estranged from their children or unwilling to be involved in their care. Other parents lack the capacity to make informed decisions because of alcohol or substance abuse, developmental disability, or immaturity. Strictly speaking, parents should make decisions for children unless a court has appointed someone else as guardian. The courts, however, may be too slow for medical decisions to be made in a timely manner. In practice, physicians often make informal arrangements for another relative to make decisions when parents are absent or incapable of making decisions.

Emergencies

In emergencies, when a parent or guardian is not available, and delay in treatment would jeopardize the child's life or health, the physician should provide appropriate treatment without parental permission (3,4). The rationale is that it would violate the child's best interests to delay emergency treatment until approval is obtained.

Disagreements Between Parents and Pediatricians

Pediatricians are understandably distressed when parents make medical decisions that are not in the child's best interests or when a child's care at home is suboptimal. Physicians can help families deliberate by eliciting their concerns and questions, pointing out overlooked considerations, and recommending what they believe is best for the child. They need to try to persuade parents to accept effective interventions that have few side effects. In addition, physicians, together with social workers and nurses, can mobilize emotional support and social resources to help the parents provide better care.

Overriding parents through the legal system should be a last resort (5). Lifestyles that physicians may find objectionable, such as alcohol abuse or an untidy home, do not in themselves constitute neglect. Even if a child with asthma or diabetes is not receiving medications regularly, disrupting the parent–child bond causes emotional distress for the child. Foster placement or institutionalization may be worse for the child than care from well-meaning parents trying to cope with difficult circumstances.

In some situations, however, physicians need to oppose parental actions or decisions. Physicians and other health care workers must report to child protective services agencies about cases of suspected child abuse or neglect. The privacy of the parents and children is overridden in order to protect vulnerable children from the possibility of serious harm. To be justified in reporting a case, physicians do not need definitive proof of abuse and neglect, only sufficient information to warrant a fuller investigation. In evaluating possible child abuse, pediatricians should treat parents with respect, keeping in mind that most parents are trying their best to deal with a difficult situation. Intervention may enable parents to obtain enough assistance and support to prevent further abuse. In extreme cases, however, the child may be removed from parental custody by protective service agencies.

Another situation in which physicians should override parental decisions is when parents cannot be persuaded to accept life-saving therapy that has few side effects. For instance, if parents refuse antibiotics for bacterial meningitis in a previously healthy child, physicians should apply for an emergency court order to authorize treatment.

The Adolescent Patient

As children mature, they develop the capacity to make informed decisions about their health care (6). By statute, adolescents over 18 years of age can give informed consent or refusal for medical care without parental involvement. The law may also allow younger minors to make their own decisions about health care (3,7,8). Since statutes vary from state to state, pediatricians need to be familiar with the laws in their jurisdiction.

Mature Minors

"Mature minors" are capable of giving informed consent. Ethically speaking, mature minors should be allowed to consent to or refuse medical treatment, just like adults. Pediatricians need to evaluate an adolescent's capacity to give informed consent and to help him obtain appropriate support from parents or other adults. Physicians need to assess the adolescent's understanding of the proposed intervention, the alternatives, the risks and benefits of each, and the likely consequences. Generally adolescents over 14 or 15 years of age can be shown to have such decision-making capacity, whereas younger children often have difficulty entertaining different alternatives, appreciating the consequences of decisions, and appraising their future realistically (6). In most cases, mature minors benefit from discussing medical decisions with their parents, and physicians should encourage such discussions.

Emancipated Minors

Adolescents who are living apart from parents and managing their own finances, are married, have children, or have served in the armed forces are termed "emancipated" minors. Most states regard them as *de facto* adults, capable of consenting to their own medical care. Some states require a judicial hearing and declaration of emancipation.

Treatment of Specified Conditions

Most states allow minors to assent to treatment without parental permission for sensitive conditions, such as sexually transmitted diseases, contraception, pregnancy, substance abuse, and psychiatric illness (9). The rationale is not that adolescents who make such decisions are making informed decisions. Indeed, these conditions may impair judgment or result from unwise choices. The justification is that requiring parental permission would deter many adolescents from seeking treatment for important public health problems (10).

Parental Requests for Treatment

Parents may request that the physician test an adolescent for illicit drug use or pregnancy, without telling the child (11). While such requests are generally motivated by concern, surreptitious testing is unacceptable because it violates the adolescent's emerging autonomy, undermines trust in the physician, and compromises future care.

THE RELATIONSHIP OF THE PEDIATRICIAN TO THE CHILD AND PARENTS

Disclosure of information to children, confidentiality, and truth-telling may raise ethical dilemmas. These actions are important because they show respect for the child, lead to beneficial consequences, and foster trust in the medical profession.

Disclosure of Information to Children

To obtain assent from children, pediatricians need to provide them with pertinent information in terms they can understand. Pediatricians need to ask children if they want information and if so to provide it in terms the child can comprehend. Children who do not want information or cannot understand medical details may still want to know what will be done to them.

Some parents do not want their children to know about serious diagnoses, such as cancer or human immunodeficiency virus (HIV) infection (12,13). Pediatricians should elicit the parents' concerns and fears. Parents may believe that the child will not be able to handle bad news or that peers will reject the child. Physicians can explain how children may have better coping, fewer psychosocial problems, and enhanced adherence to treatment if they understand their diagnosis and the proposed therapy (13). Parental requests for secrecy are particularly difficult when adolescents are capable of making health care decisions. Generally, physicians can persuade parents to allow disclosure of information to the child, provide developmentally appropriate information, and help the child cope with the news.

Physicians should never promise parents that the child will not learn the diagnosis. Other members of the health care team may disclose it. In addition, pediatricians should provide forthright answers when children ask directly about their diagnosis. Deception would compromise the physician's integrity and patients' trust in the medical system.

Confidentiality

As Chapter 5 discusses, confidentiality is not absolute. For example, it may be broken when disclosure has been authorized by parents or adolescents or when child abuse occurs. Pediatrics presents several unique issues involving confidentiality.

Disclosure to Schools

Pediatricians may need to disclose health information to schools. Whenever information is disclosed, physicians should disclose only information that is truly needed. For example, a school needs only to know that the child's absence was medically indicated, not the diagnosis. Pediatricians may also need to arrange for the child to receive medications at school. It is useful for pediatricians to discuss how parents, the child, and school personnel may respond to inquiries about the child's health in ways that maintain confidentiality.

Adolescents' Requests for Confidentiality

Adolescents may wish to keep certain information confidential from their parents. For instance, they may not want parents to know that they are receiving care for certain psychiatric conditions, sexually transmitted diseases, pregnancy, or substance abuse (9,14). Assurances of confidentiality increase the willingness of adolescents to disclose sensitive information to physicians and to seek health care (15). State laws generally protect confidentiality in such situations (9). Doctors should routinely offer adolescents an opportunity to talk privately, apart from their parents.

Pediatricians generally should encourage adolescents to discuss medical decisions with their parents, who usually provide useful support and advice situations (9). In many situations, it will be impossible to keep the parents from learning about the child's condition, because of the practicalities of obtaining treatment, the nature of the condition, or insurance arrangements. Doctors can offer to help adolescents disclose information to their parents. In some situations, however, disclosure may be counterproductive or dangerous, as when domestic violence is likely. In such situations, it might be best for the child to confide in a trusted adult relative.

Pediatricians should routinely discuss confidentiality with adolescent patients (9). Assuring adolescents of confidentiality encourages them to assume responsibility for their health and health care (15). Many physicians provide absolute rather than conditional assurances of confidentiality (16), and unconditional assurances increase adolescents' willingness to return for future care (16). However, most adolescents themselves believe that confidentiality should be overridden when the patient plans to commit suicide or is a victim of physical or sexual abuse (10). Furthermore, as Chapter 5 discusses, overriding confidentiality is ethically appropriate and legally mandated in such situations. Hence physicians should explain that confidentiality is not absolute but that exceptions are made only in limited situations (9).

Parental notification for abortion is particularly controversial, as Chapter 41 discusses (17). A number of states require minors who seek abortions to either have parental permission or obtain a judicial waiver.

REFUSAL OF MEDICAL INTERVENTIONS

The physician's response to refusal of treatment will depend on the clinical circumstances, the benefits and burdens of treatment, and in some cases on the wishes of the child (18).

Refusal of Interventions of Limited Effectiveness or Great Burdens

Parents may refuse interventions that have limited effectiveness, impose significant side effects, require chronic treatment, or are controversial. In such situations, the parents' informed refusals should be decisive. Refusal of life-sustaining interventions may be ethically appropriate even if the patient's life expectancy may be shortened. If physicians believe that the intervention is in the child's best interests, they can attempt to persuade the parents.

Refusal of Effective Interventions With Few Side Effects

Parents sometimes refuse treatments for life-threatening conditions even though these treatments are highly effective in restoring the child to previous health, are short-term, and have few side effects (19). For example, Jehovah's Witnesses commonly refuse blood transfusions for children who suffer acute trauma. Similarly, Christian Scientist parents often refuse antibiotics even for curable life-threatening infections such as bacterial meningitis. Physicians who are unable to persuade parents to accept such interventions should seek a court order to administer the treatment (20). A court order is important because it signifies that society believes that the parent's refusal is unacceptable. As one court declared, while "parents may be free to become martyrs themselves," they are not free to "make martyrs of their children" (21).

In some situations, physicians defer to parental refusals of effective, safe interventions because the child would be harmed by conflict between the parents and the medical system. For instance, some parents object to immunizations because of religious objections, concerns about side effects, or opposition to modern medicine. Immunizations are required for entrance into school, although many states allow parents to refuse based on religious or other objections. Even when no exceptions are permitted, requirements for immunization may not be enforced. If the number of unimmunized children is small and herd immunity exists, it may not seem worth alienating the parents. However, if an epidemic does break out, the risk to unimmunized children increases, and public health officials rapidly enforce requirements for immunization.

Refusal of Effective Therapy With Significant Side Effects

The most difficult decisions involve interventions that are highly effective in serious illness but also highly burdensome, such as bone marrow transplantation in acute lymphocytic leukemia or combination chemotherapy in testicular carcinoma. In this situation, the preferences of the child may be important. If an older child or adolescent makes an informed decision to undergo such treatment, physicians should support that decision.

If parents continue to refuse therapy after repeated attempts at persuasion, some physicians seek court orders to compel treatment. In doing so, physicians need to take into account the harm to long-term parental cooperation with the child's care. At the very least, physicians need to listen to the parent's objections, show respect for their opinions, and respect the ongoing responsibility parents have for other aspects of the child's life.

Child's Refusal of Interventions

In some cases, children may refuse effective treatments. The physician's response should depend on the seriousness of the clinical situation, the effectiveness of treatment, the side effects, the reasons for refusal, the parents' preferences regarding treatment, and the burdens of insisting on treatment. It is difficult to force adolescents to take ongoing therapies, such as insulin shots for diabetes or inhalers for asthma. The most constructive approach is to try to understand the patient's reasons for refusal, to address them, and to provide psychosocial support. In several recent cases, adolescents have run away from home rather than accept cancer chemotherapy that has significant side effects (22). Because it is physically difficult as well as morally troubling to force such treatment on adolescents, these refusals have been accepted, particularly when the parents have supported the child's refusal.

HANDICAPPED INFANTS

The federal Child Abuse Amendments of 1984 and subsequent regulations, commonly called "Baby Doe Regulations," apply to decisions to withhold medical treatment from disabled infants less than 1 year old. Their intent is to ensure such interventions as surgery for duodenal atresia or tracheal-esophageal fistula in infants with Down syndrome. They limit the circumstances in which interventions may be withheld. Under these regulations, treatment other than "appropriate nutrition, hydration, or medication" need not be provided if (a) the infant is irreversibly comatose; (b) treatment would merely prolong dying; (c) treatment would not be effective in ameliorating or correcting all life-threatening conditions; (d) treatment would be futile in terms of survival; or (e) treatment would be virtually futile and would be inhumane. Decisions to withhold medically indicated treatment may not be based on "subjective opinions" about the child's future quality of life. In addition, hospitals are encouraged to establish ethics committees, called infant care review committees, to advise physicians in difficult cases.

The Baby Doe Regulations have been sharply criticized (23). Many terms, such as "appropriate" and "futile," are subject to conflicting interpretations. Parents are not included in decision-making, despite their customary role as surrogates. Commentators point out that the regulations often are not literally followed nor strictly enforced. Physicians should appreciate that these laws and regulations do not require physicians to provide treatment that in their judgment is inappropriate.

REFERENCES

1. American Academy of Pediatrics Committee on Bioethics. Informed consent, parental permission, and assent in pediatric practice. *Pediatrics* 1995;95:314–317.
2. Bartholome WG. A new understanding of consent in pediatric practice: consent, parental permission, and child assent. *Pediatr Ann* 1989;18:262–265.
3. Holder AR. Disclosure and consent problems in pediatrics. *Law Med Health Care* 1988;16:219–228.
4. American Academy of Pediatrics Committee on Pediatric Emergency Medicine. Consent for medical services for children and adolescents. *Pediatrics* 1993;92:290–291.
5. American Academy of Pediatrics Committee on Bioethics. Guidelines on foregoing life-sustaining medical treatment. *Pediatrics* 1994;93:532–536.
6. Weithorn LA, Campbell SB. The competency of children and adolescents to make informed treatment decisions. *Child Dev* 1982;53:1589–1599.
7. Holder AR. Minors' rights to consent to medical care. *JAMA* 1987;257:3400–3402.
8. Sigman GS, O'Connor C. Exploration for physicians of the mature minor doctrine. *J Pediatr* 1991;119:520–525.
9. Society for Adolescent Medicine. Confidential health care for adolescents: position paper of the Society for Adolescent Medicine. *J Adolesc Health* 1997;21:408–415.
10. Cheng TL, Savageau JA, Sattler AL, et al. Confidentiality in health care. A survey of knowledge, perceptions, and attitudes among high school students. *JAMA* 1993;269:1404–1407.
11. American Academy of Pediatrics Committee on Adolescence. Screening for drugs of abuse in children and adolescents. *Pediatrics* 1989;84:396–397.
12. Sigman GS, Kraut J, LaPuma J. Disclosure of a diagnosis to children and adolesents when parents object. *Am J Dis Child* 1993;147:764–768.
13. American Academy of Pediatrics Committee on Pediatric AIDS. Disclosure of illness status to children and adolescents with HIV infection. *Pediatrics* 1999;103:164–166.
14. Council on Scientific Affairs of the American Medical Association. Confidential health services for adolescents. *JAMA* 1993;269:1420–1424.
15. Ford CA, Millstein SG, Halpern-Feisher BL, et al. Influence of physician confidentiality assurances on adolescents' willingness to disclose information and seek future health care. *JAMA* 1997;278:1029–1034.
16. Ford CA, Millstein SG. Delivery of confidentiality assurances to adolescents by primary care physicians. *Arch Pediatr Adolesc Med* 1997;151:505–509.
17. American Academy of Pediatrics Committee on Adolescence. The adolescent's right to confidential care when considering abortion. *Pediatrics* 1996;97:746–751.
18. Fleischman AR, Nolan K, Dubler NN, et al. Caring for gravely ill children. *Pediatrics* 1994;94:433–439.
19. Asser SM, Swan R. Child fatalities from religion-motived medical neglect. *Pediatrics* 1998;101:625–629.
20. Wadlington W. Medical decision making for and by children: tensions between parent, state, and child. *Univ Illinois Law Rev* 1994;1994:311–336.
21. Prince *v*. Massachusetts, 321 U.S. 158 (1944).
22. Traugott I, Alpers A. In their hands: adolescents' refusal of treatment. *Arch Pediatr Adolesc Med* 1997;151:922–927.
23. Kopelman LM, Irons TG, Kopelman AE. Neonatologists judge the "Baby Doe" regulations. *N Engl J Med* 1988;318:677–683.

ANNOTATED BIBLIOGRAPHY

1. American Academy of Pediatrics Committee on Bioethics. Informed consent, parental permission, and assent in pediatric practice. *Pediatrics* 1995;95:314–317.
   Lucid discussion of distinctions between assent by children, permission from parents for care, and informed consent by adults.
2. Society for Adolescent Medicine. Confidential health care for adolescents: position paper of the Society for Adolescent Medicine. *J Adolesc Health* 1997;21:408–415.
   Thoughtful and current review, with practical suggestions on handling dilemmas regarding confidentiality.
3. Fleischman AR, Nolan K, Dubler NN, et al. Caring for gravely ill children. *Pediatrics* 1994;94:433–439.
   Discussion of end-of-life decision making in pediatrics.
4. Traugott I, Alpers A. In their own hands: adolescents' refusal of life-sustaining treatment. *Arch Pediatr Adolesc Med* 1997;151:922–927.
   Dilemmas that occur when adolescents are old enough to run away rather than accept life-sustaining interventions.

40

Ethical Issues in Surgery

Surgery differs from other specialties in ways that have significant ethical implications. First, surgeons intentionally cause short-term injury to the patient in order to achieve longer term therapeutic goals. Although all medical interventions involve risk, surgical side effects are certain, not merely possible. Because of the surgical wound and anesthesia, patients experience pain, need to heal, and have a scar. Second, in the operating room, patients turn over control of their bodies to the surgical team. Events in the operating room are out of view of the patient and family. Third, operations are not standardized in the sense that drug therapies have standard dosages. Individual surgeons vary in their choice of incision, use of electrocautery and stapling, and selection of suture material or implanted devices. In an individual patient, the operative approach may need to be modified because of anatomic variation.

HOW ARE ETHICAL ISSUES IN SURGERY DIFFERENT?

As a result of these clinical features, some ethical considerations are particularly important for surgeons.

First, acting for the welfare of the patient takes on added importance because patients are completely dependent on the surgical team during operations. Patients cannot look out for their best interests during surgery.

Second, informed consent for surgery is especially important because surgery is a major bodily invasion. Decisions to undergo operative risks will depend on the patient's personal values and assessment of quality of life. Some operations, such as mastectomy, colostomy, or amputation, dramatically alter patients' body image, sense of self, and daily functioning. However, informed consent may be more difficult because surgeons often have no prior relationship with the patient. Furthermore, surgeons must discuss before the operation such intraoperative decisions such as how the operation might be modified because of intraoperative findings. In other specialties, physicians can come back to the patient or surrogate to discuss changes in care necessitated by the response to the initial plan.

Third, individual surgeons are held responsible for the outcomes of surgery. Deaths in the operating room or after surgery raise the question of whether the surgeon made a mistake in judgment or technique. Postoperative deaths need to be reported to the coroner. In surgical morbidity and mortality conferences, surgeons must justify why they operated and how the case was managed (1). Increasingly, surgeon-specific clinical outcomes are tracked and made available to the public or insurers. Moreover, surgeons feel more personally responsible for outcomes, because of their "hands-on" involvement in care, than do other physicians.

Fourth, technical competency is essential for surgeons because poor manual skills may harm patients. Even after completion of formal training, surgeons need to learn new techniques, such as laparoscopic procedures. Learning procedural skills differs from learning cognitive skills. More senior physicians can supervise medical decision-making by trainees so that the risk of mistakes is greatly reduced. However, with procedural skills, the trainee has manual control of the procedure and can make a mistake before the supervising surgeon can intervene.

DISCLOSURE OF INFORMATION DURING THE INFORMED CONSENT PROCESS

To make informed decisions about surgery, patients need pertinent information about the operation, the benefits and risks, the likely consequences, and the alternatives.

Disclosure of Alternative Approaches

Evidence-based medicine has demonstrated that for many conditions no alternative is clearly superior. For benign prostatic hypertrophy (BPH) or localized breast cancers, several approaches have similar outcomes. In BPH, transuretheral resection of the prostate, medical treatment, and watchful waiting are all acceptable approaches. For breast cancer, lumpectomy followed by radiation offers survival rates similar to more extensive surgery but has different anatomical and psychological consequences. Legally, a number of states require that women with breast cancer be informed of breast-conserving treatments (2). The patient's preferences regarding surgery and side effects will be decisive. Hence the surgeon should discuss all standard options with the patient, even if the doctor personally believes that one is superior. However, surgeons do not need to discuss alternative or unconventional therapies whose effectiveness has not been demonstrated or that have not been adopted by a respected subset of physicians.

Disclosure of Provider-Specific Outcomes

For major operations, patients who are risk adverse may want to select a hospital or surgeon with excellent outcomes. Such patients naturally want to know which providers have the best outcomes for the operation. Outcomes published in the literature may not represent everyday clinical practice and may mask considerable variation among providers. To enhance informed patient decisions, surgeons should inform patients of the complication rates in their practice or their institution (3,4).

Computerized databases allow the mortality rates for common operations, such as coronary artery bypass and graft, to be calculated on the level of individual hospitals and surgeons. Such information may be highly pertinent to patients who are choosing a surgeon or hospital. Surgeons commonly raise several objections to public disclosure of such outcomes data. Risk adjustment for case mix and severity of illness may be inadequate. Hence hospitals and surgeons with sicker, more complicated patients may appear to have worse outcomes than they actually do. Data may also be misleading because of random variation in relatively small samples and changes in personnel or organization since statistics were collected. New York State and Pennsylvania publish surgeon-specific outcomes for coronary bypass surgery, which are risk-adjusted for several variables (5,6). Surgeons and hospitals have an opportunity to examine the data before they are released, so that any errors can be corrected. Although current methodologies are imperfect, the antidote is for surgeons to provide more explanation, not to withhold information that patients would regard as important.

Disclosure of the Experience of the Surgeon

Generally, more experienced surgeons have better outcomes (4). Thus the surgeon's experience with the operation is information that reasonable patients would consider relevant when selecting a hospital or surgeon. In teaching hospitals, residents and students usually play a role in the surgery. In one study, over 90% of women undergoing hysterectomy wanted the attending surgeon to tell them that a resident would participate in the operation as well as what the resident would do (7). The patients wanted faculty physicians to take the lead in disclosing such information. Almost all patients also wanted to meet the resident before the operation.

Patients should be informed of the roles of trainees during surgery and how they will be supervised (4). Patients consider it very important to know that a medical student is going to make the incision, hold retractors, perform rectal or pelvic examinations under anesthesia, suture incisions, or intubate them (8). Furthermore, patients consider disclosure of such procedures more important than do medical students, and preclinical students place significantly more importance on such disclosure than do clinical students (8). Even though anesthetized patients suffer no discomfort as a result of students performing procedures in the operating room and would not know of such actions, they want to be notified and give permission. The faculty surgeon might say: "Dr. X is a senior level resident in our training program and will be performing portions of your operation; I will be assisting and supervising Dr. X throughout (9)."

Similar issues of disclosure arise when experienced surgeons learn new techniques, such as laparoscopic surgery (4). Initially, complication rates are higher with laparoscopic surgery than with open techniques, and operating times are longer. With more experience by the surgeon, complication rates become comparable to those of open procedures. For patients, it is important to know the experience of a surgeon with a new technique, particularly if the outcomes would be significantly better with a more experienced surgeon.

Surgeons may fear that if patients are told that they are inexperienced with a technique or are still in training, patients will not trust them to do the operation. Supervised experience promotes mastery of surgical techniques and will benefit future patients. However, generally patients respond favorably to having trainees participate in operations. Most patients believe that residents are adequately supervised and can respond quickly if complications develop, although patients also realize that inexperience in residents may lead to substandard care (7).

Changes in the Operation Due to Unanticipated Findings

A surgeon may encounter unexpected findings that require a substantially different operation than was discussed during the informed consent process. For example, suppose that during a cholecystectomy, the surgeon finds a gastric mass that is suspicious for carcinoma. Should the surgeon biopsy the mass, and if so, should the surgeon resect the tumor if the biopsy shows carcinoma? The surgeon may believe that an opportunity to cure gastric carcinoma may be missed if biopsy and resection are not done. Furthermore, a second operation would subject the patient to additional risk. On the other hand, the patient may be shocked to find that the surgeon performed a more extensive operation than discussed, even if the surgeon did so in order to benefit him.

How can the surgeon resolve this dilemma between acting for the good of the patient and respecting his autonomy? Some surgeons seek blanket consent to change the operation if unexpected findings occur. However, this contingency is so rare that it is not efficient to discuss it with all patients preoperatively. A sound approach is to contact the next of kin in the waiting area. If the family agrees with the surgeon's recommendations, the patient's best interests and autonomy are both served. It would also be acceptable to carry out the biopsy if the family cannot be immediately located, with plans to resect the mass only if consent from a family member can be obtained in time.

Such cases of incidental findings need to be distinguished from cases in which the operation needs to be changed because of a complication. For instance, a surgeon may nick the spleen, and a splenectomy may be required to control the bleeding. In this instance, the surgeon should proceed with splenectomy and explain to the patient after the operation that a splenectomy was done because of the intraoperative complication.

MAY A SURGEON DECLINE TO OPERATE?

In some cases, a surgeon may determine that an operation is not indicated because the risks of surgery greatly outweigh the possible benefits (10). What should the surgeon do if the patient or referring physician insists on surgery? Different reasons for not operating need to be distinguished. Some reasons are patient centered. The surgeon may believe that an operation will not benefit the patient. For instance, a patient with chronic abdominal pain may believe that the pain is due to gallbladder disease and seek a cholecystectomy (10). However, if there is no objective evidence of gallstones, the surgeon may conclude that the patient's symptoms are not caused by gallstones and that therefore cholecystectomy will not benefit the patient. A cholecystectomy in this situation would be futile in a strict sense (*see* Chapter 9).

In other situations, the surgeon may judge that although the operation might benefit the patient, the risks are prohibitive, as the following case illustrates.

CASE 40.1. DECISION TO NOT OPERATE IN A VERY HIGH-RISK PATIENT. *A 64-year-old man admitted for a myocardial infarction continues to have chest pain, ischemic changes on his cardiogram, and congestive heart failure. He is found to have multiple diffuse coronary lesions that cannot be revascularized. He also develops a urinary tract infection from a Foley catheter. Despite antibiotics, he subsequently develops pyelonephritis, intrarenal abscesses, and septic shock. The patient becomes confused and unable to participate in decisions. The referring physician and family urge an operation to drain the abscesses, because they believe that without it the patient will certainly die. Percutaneous drainage guided by computed tomography is not feasible. The family appreciates that the surgery is risky, but they believe it offers the patient the only chance of survival. However, the surgeon believes that the patient's coronary disease is so unstable that he is extremely unlikely to survive an abdominal operation.*

Traditionally, surgeons are permitted great discretion not to perform interventions that they believe are not in the patient's best interests. In this situation, the surgery cannot be considered futile in a strict sense because there is a small possibility that the patient would benefit from it. Indeed, the prospect of success exceeds the 1% threshold that some writers have suggested for "futility" (*see* Chapter 9). Often surgeons justify a refusal to operate by the shorthand declaration, "This patient is not a surgical candidate." Such surgical decisions are rarely challenged and discussed, whereas unilateral decisions by internists to withhold medical interventions are controversial and extensively debated.

Is there an acceptable ethical basis for this distinction between surgeons and internists? Surgeons are considered more responsible for the harmful consequences of operations than are internists for the harmful effects of drugs they prescribe. In both situations the physician is responsible for the recommendation to carry out an intervention or not. However, making a surgical incision causes much more certain and direct harm to the patient than writing a prescription. Even though the patient or surrogate consents to the operation, the surgeon still has the responsibility to justify to peers the decision to operate. Furthermore, because surgery requires manual manipulations, it is undesirable to require surgeons to perform operations they deem inadvisable. An operation by an unwilling surgeon may place the patient at additional risk because of lapses of concentration or lack of confidence.

It is important to delineate the scope of the surgeon's refusal to operate because of unacceptable risks. The key questions are what risk is prohibitive and who determines this level. Patients have different thresholds for risk, and some may accept unfavorable odds of success and severe short-term harms. Surgeons need to take into account the patient's values and assessment of risk. They should decline to operate only if the risks are dramatically greater than the likely benefits, not just slightly increased. Surgeons need to guard against overstating the risks of the operation because consciously or unconsciously they believe that the operation seriously compromises their own interests, as opposed to the best interests of the patient. Furthermore, surgeons must be careful to base decisions on medical outcomes, not their personal judgments that the patient's quality of life is unacceptably poor.

Other reasons for not operating may be surgeon centered. The surgeon may believe that the risk of contracting human immunodeficiency virus (HIV) infection or hepatitis C during an operation is unacceptable in view of the limited benefits to the patient. For example, an orthopedic surgeon may believe that a total hip replacement on a patient with the acquired immunodeficiency syndrome presents an unacceptable risk of occupational HIV infection because bone fragments may penetrate gloves, even double gloves. In other cases, a surgeon may be reluctant to take on complex, high-risk cases that may worsen their complication rates or length of hospital stays. In turn, poor outcomes may make it more difficult to secure referral contracts from managed care organizations. Yet another factor may be reimbursement (10). A surgeon may believe that she has accepted more than her fair share of charity cases and cannot afford to take on additional uncompensated cases. In these situations, the self-interest of the surgeon must be acknowledged as a natural and legitimate concern. However, they must be put into perspective and addressed directly. Chapter 43 discusses the risk of occupational HIV infection in detail. Ultimately, the ethical ideal is for physicians to place the best interests of the patient ahead of their own self-interest.

In some cases, patients decline an operation recommended by a surgeon, have surgery by someone else, and after they experience an unsatisfactory outcome return to the first surgeon to request that she fix the complications (11). Such patients may believe that only the first surgeon can set things right. In making a decision whether to operate, the surgeon needs to be aware of her feelings, which may include anger, resentment, and pride. Such feelings may stand in the way of objective judgment. The surgeon has no obligation to operate in such a situation, because the patient broke off the doctor-patient relationship. In many cases, it will be desirable to refer the patient to a colleague who can start the doctor–patient relationship with a fresh slate. The surgeon has the option of reestablishing that relationship or not. In contrast, the surgeon would be responsible for addressing the complications of an operation that she had performed.

REQUESTS TO CARRY OUT SURGERY IN WAYS THAT INCREASE RISK

Patients may consent to an operation but refuse specific interventions or techniques. Such restrictions may make their operation riskier and more complicated. These decisions need to be distinguished from patient refusals of the operation itself.

CASE 40.2. EMERGENCY SURGERY ON A JEHOVAH'S WITNESS. *A 74-year-old Jehovah's Witness is admitted after a motor vehicle accident with a ruptured spleen, a hematocrit of 18%, hypotension, chest pain, and ischemic changes on electrocardiogram. He refuses blood transfusions but agrees to surgery, understanding that he might die without transfusions. The surgeon declares, "I accept his right to refuse transfusions, but he can't make me operate with one hand tied behind my back."*

In this case, the patient has a clear indication for laparotomy and splenectomy. In this patient's religion, surviving the accident is less important than avoiding the taint of transfusions, which would result in everlasting damnation (*see* Chapter 11). Generally Jehovah's Witnesses have operative outcomes that are similar to patients who receive transfusions. However, severe anemia places this patient at greater risk for myocardial infarction and renal failure. The hospital course will be more complicated without transfusion support, and the length of stay and overall cost will probably be greater. In the managed care era, such outcomes may adversely affect contracts or referrals.

Some surgeons may be angry because of the need for additional time and effort and the reduced margin for error. Many surgeons intuitively make a distinction between respecting the patient's refusal of transfusions and following the patient's request to have the surgery under restrictive conditions. Philosophers state this more formally, distinguishing negative and positive rights. Negative rights are claims to be left alone; they protect patients from unwanted interventions on their bodies. Positive rights require others to act in certain ways. Negative rights are generally considered stronger than positive rights. Thus it makes sense to grant patients a strong right to refuse unwanted interventions, but much weaker claims to specify how surgeons carry out their work.

Faced with requests to carry out operations with specific restrictions, surgeons in most cases have a legal right to decline to operate and to transfer care of the patient to another surgeon. However, this right may be suspended in emergency cases when there is no suitable replacement. In many cases a more fruitful approach is to consider how the surgery might be managed to minimize additional risks. Use of cell savers, hemodilution, and administration of erythropoeitin may reduce perioperative risk to more acceptable levels. Moreover, surgeons should keep in mind the ethical ideal that the patient's best interests are paramount. If the surgery is medically necessary, a skilled and experienced surgical team offers the patient the best chance at a favorable outcome.

In Case 40.2, the Jehovah's Witness raised his refusal of transfusion without the physician having to broach the topic. In other situations, the patient expresses objections to certain aspects of the proposed operation only because the physician brings up the issues.

CASE 40.3. PATIENT REFUSAL OF EMERGENCY COLOSTOMY (12). *A 74-year-old man is admitted to the hospital with an acute abdomen. A KUB reveals free air under the diaphragm. The surgeon believes that the patient has perforated a peptic ulcer or a carcinoma of the colon. The surgeon explains that if the perforation is in the colon, she will perform a colostomy, which may not need to be permanent. The patient adamantly refuses a colostomy. "A friend had one and had one complication after another. He was so ashamed of that bag. I'd rather be dead than go through that humiliation." There is no time for the patient to talk to people who have adapted well to a colostomy. Technically, an end-to-end anastamosis is possible, but it has a much higher risk of complications.*

The surgeon consults a colleague about the case. He says, "In an emergency, I never discuss the details of the surgery. All the patient needs to know is that he needs an operation to save his life and that the risks of surgery are small compared with the alternatives. Too much information can be dangerous, because there is no time to correct misunderstandings. All this discussion about a colostomy is probably moot. Chances are, he'll have a perforated ulcer. Even if he perforated his colon, you may be able to take the colostomy down later. I wouldn't do an end-to-end anastamosis. How would you justify it at a morbidity and mortality conference if he got a complication?

In Case 40.3, the ethical dilemma is the patient may be making an irreversible decision that he would greatly regret later. The surgeon believes that the patient's refusal is based on an unrealistic appraisal of a colostomy. Because it is an emergency, the patient cannot talk to other people who have adapted to a colostomy. In elective situations, most patients can be persuaded to accept a colostomy. A surgeon dedicated to acting in the patient's best interests would want to do the less risky operation, knowing that most patients adapt to a colostomy. From this perspective, it would also be unfortunate if the patient refused surgery because he feared an outcome that might not happen or might not be permanent. The colleague's concern about the morbidity and mortality conference is not just a desire to avoid personal criticism; the professional standard of care is based on what a reasonable patient would find beneficial and what a reasonable surgeon would do under the circumstances.

On the other hand, a surgeon dedicated to patient autonomy will respect the patient's refusal of colostomy, even if that decision may not be truly informed. From this viewpoint, it would be tragic if the patient had to live with what she considers a mutilation of her body and had no prior discussion or opportunity to object. A patient's preferences about therapy depend not only on the likelihood of survival and postoperative complications, but also on the nature of the surgery and the quality of life afterwards (13,14). A patient might consider a colostomy is so unacceptable that he would literally rather die than have the operation.

The surgeon in Case 1 has several options. One option is to refuse to operate unless the patient agrees to a colostomy if needed. However, this option may leave the patient worse off than having an end-to-end anastamosis. Also, if the on-call surgeon declines to operate, it may be difficult to find a colleague to take over the case in a timely manner.

A better approach is to try to persuade the patient to accept the colostomy. Often this can be done despite severe time constraints. The surgeon can ask the patient to talk his decision over with his family, friends, primary care physician, or the chaplain, and the surgeon could explain to them why a colostomy is preferable. In addition, the surgeon may be able to persuade the patient by paradoxically giving him control. "If you decide that you won't accept the colostomy after talking to your family and your primary care doctor, I'll agree to do the surgery in the other, riskier way. I won't force you to have an operation you don't want. But before you decide, I'd like to understand better what about the colostomy troubles you. I'd also like you to understand why I think the colostomy is the best operation for you." If persuasion fails, it is ethically appropriate for the surgeon to agree to do an end-to-end anastamosis. In this situation, both the patient and the surgeon would need to accept the higher risk of complications with this technique.

In trying to persuade patients, some surgeons may be tempted to misrepresent what they will do in the operating room. For example, they may say they will try to do an end-to-end anastamosis if possible but reserve the right to do a colostomy if necessary. However, the surgeon actually may plan to do a colostomy except in the highly unlikely possibility that she believes the end-to-end anastamosis would carry no additional risk. For reasons discussed in Chapter 6, such misrepresentation is problematical and undermines both patient trust and the physician's integrity.

In summary, the unique clinical circumstances of surgery impose special ethical obligations on surgeons regarding informed consent, decisions not to operate, and patient requests to carry out the operation in certain ways.

REFERENCES

1. Bosk CL. *Forgive and remember: managing medical failure.* Chicago: University of Chicago Press, 1979.
2. Nattinger AB, Hoffman RG, Shapiro R, et al. The effect of legislative requirements on the use of breast-conserving surgery. *N Engl J Med* 1996;335:1035–1040.

3. Arnold RM, Shaw BW, Purtillo R. Acute high-risk patients: the case of transplantation. In: McCullough LB, Jones JW, Brody BA, eds. *Surgical ethics*. New York: Oxford University Press, 1998:97–115.
4. Gates EA. New surgical procedures: can our patients benefit while we learn? *Am J Obstet Gynecol* 1997;176: 1293–1298.
5. Schneider EC, Epstein AM. Use of public performance reports: a survey of patients undergoing cardiac surgery. *JAMA* 1998;279:1638–1642.
6. Chassin MR, Hannan EL, DeBuono BA. Benefits and hazards of reporting medical outcomes publicly. *N Engl J Med* 1996;334:394–398.
7. Kim N, Lo B, Gates EA. Disclosing the role of residents and medical students in hysterectomy: what do patients want? *Acad Med* 1998;73:339–341.
8. Silver-Isenstadt A, Ubel PA. Erosion in medical students' attitudes about telling patients they are students. *J Gen Intern Med* 1999;14:481–487.
9. McCullough LB, Jones JW, Brody BA. Informed consent: autonomous decision-making of the surgical patient. In: McCullough LB, Jones JW, Brody BA, eds. *Surgical ethics*. New York: Oxford University Press, 1998:15–37.
10. Sugarman J, Harland R. Acute yet non-emergent patients. In: McCullough LB, Jones JW, Brody BA, eds. *Surgical ethics*. New York: Oxford University Press, 1998:116–132.
11. Case from David Bradford, M.D.
12. Case from Kimberly Kirkwood, M.D.
13. McNeil BJ, Weichselbaum R, Pauker SG. Speech and survival: tradeoffs between quality and quantity of life in laryngeal cancer. *N Engl J Med* 1981;305:982–987.
14. McNeil BJ, Weichselbaum R, Pauker SG. Fallacy of the five-year survival in lung cancer. *N Engl J Med* 1978;299:307–401.

ANNOTATED BIBLIOGRAPHY

1. McCullough LB, Jones JW, Brody BA, eds. *Surgical ethics*. New York: Oxford University Press, 1998.
   Monograph covering ethical issues in various surgical contexts. Chapters are jointly written by a surgeon and an ethicist.
2. Gates EA. New surgical procedures: can our patients benefit while we learn? *Am J Obstet Gynecol* 1997;176: 1293–1298.
   Argues that surgeons should disclose their own experience and outcomes during the informed consent process.

41

Ethical Issues
in Obstetrics and Gynecology

Ethical dilemmas in obstetrics and gynecology are particularly difficult because the care of pregnant women and the care of the fetus are inextricably linked. Furthermore, decisions about reproduction and sexuality rest on values that are intensely private and may be socially contested.

HOW ARE ETHICAL ISSUES
IN OBSTETRICS AND GYNECOLOGY DIFFERENT?

Reproductive Health is Highly Personal, but Third Parties Seek to Influence It

Decisions in obstetrics and gynecology involve highly intimate and personal topics, such as sexuality, reproduction, and childbearing. Many women want control over their reproductive decisions and have strong preferences regarding family planning and childbirth. At the same time, public leaders and religious groups may hold strong views regarding children, family, and the appropriate role of women. These third parties may seek to shape women's decisions regarding reproductive health. In the past, some women were sterilized over their objections and without procedural safeguards (1,2). Currently, debates over abortion in the United States are passionate and highly politicized.

Feminist critics assert that society and physicians exercise control over women through policies regarding reproductive health care and that domination and exploitation are common. Some women also believe that the doctors and society have transformed the experience of pregnancy and childbirth into an overly technological and professionalized procedure.

Reproductive Health Involves Philosophical Quandaries That Science Cannot Resolve

Decisions about conception, pregnancy, and childbirth inevitably raise philosophical or religious questions that science can neither validate nor refute.

- Is the fetus a person, with moral and legal rights?
- When does personhood begin: at conception, viability, birth, or some other point?
- Does the pregnant woman have an ethical right of reproductive liberty that encompasses a right to abortion?

Theologians, philosophers, public leaders, and the public have debated these conundrums without reaching agreement or common ground. Consensus is unlikely to emerge, and public policies need to be developed despite deep disagreements.

New Reproductive Technologies Raise Unprecedented Dilemmas

Assisted reproductive technologies raise complex dilemmas because pregnancy can occur in unprecedented ways. With in vitro fertilization (IVF) and gamete donation, different individuals can fill the roles of genetic, gestational, and childrearing parents. Dramatic dilemmas have arisen regarding the disposition of frozen embryos after a couple has separated, IVF with donated oocytes for postmenopausal women, and "surrogate motherhood," in which the gestational mother has no genetic link with the fetus and will not raise the child after birth. Such dilemmas force people to reconsider fundamental, often unspoken beliefs regarding parental responsibility and roles.

The Obstetrician Has Two Patients, the Pregnant Woman and the Fetus

Fetal movements and fetal heartbeat can be visualized with ultrasound and other imaging techniques. Doctors can diagnose many conditions in utero, such as congenital abnormalities or fetal distress. Furthermore, physicians can treat the fetus through interventions on the mother. Fetal treatments include prenatal vitamins, tocolytic agents in premature labor, corticosteroids in prematurity, and fetal blood transfusion for Rh isoimmunization. In light of this ability to diagnose and treat fetal disorders, it seems reasonable to consider the fetus a patient, as well as the pregnant woman, when the pregnant woman intends to carry the fetus to term and presents for prenatal care (3).

Everyone hopes that children will be born healthy. It is tragic when a child is born with a preventable illness or congenital anomaly. The pregnant woman has some moral responsibility to reduce harms and provide benefit to the child who will later be born (4). Physicians have a responsibility to represent the interests of such future children, who cannot represent themselves. These moral responsibilities are based on the desire to prevent harms to children who will be born; they do not depend on the belief that the fetus is a person with rights (4).

Interventions directed to the fetus are also interventions on the pregnant woman. They may cause side effects in the mother or have important consequences for other aspects of her life. In premature labor, terbutaline causes tremor and anxiety in the pregnant woman. Long-term bed rest for premature labor may prevent the pregnant woman from caring for her other children or working at a job that supports her family. Most pregnant women accept side effects, inconvenience, and disruption of their life for the sake of the child who will be born. However, it is unreasonable to expect a pregnant woman to adopt every intervention that might benefit the fetus, regardless of the degree of benefit, risks, or impact on her life. Responsibilities to a fetus who will become a child have limits; logically they should not exceed responsibilities that parents have to living children (5). Parents have no obligation to provide all potentially beneficial interventions to children after birth or to minimize all harms to their children.

INFORMED CONSENT IN OBSTECTRICS AND GYNECOLOGY

Although informed consent is important in all medical specialties, several situations in obstetrics and gynecology raise particular ethical issues regarding consent.

Provision of Information Regarding Family Planning and Abortion

Some physicians have strong moral and religious objections to these interventions (6). They believe it would violate their conscience not only to write a prescription for birth control or perform an abortion, but also to discuss these options with patients. Physicians are not obligated to carry out actions that would violate their fundamental moral beliefs or their conscience. Physicians are free to withdraw from the care of a patient as a last resort if a mutually acceptable plan cannot be negotiated. However, it is problematical if physicians provide care without informing patients of options that are medically acceptable (7). In other clinical settings, physicians have an affirmative duty to disclose all medically appropriate options with the patient, even if they would not personally recommend them (*see* Chapter 3). Thus respecting the physician's conscience may conflict with respecting the patient's autonomy.

How can this dilemma be resolved? At a minimum, physicians should tell patients that there are options for care they will not discuss for religious or moral reasons, but that other physicians are willing to discuss. For the sake of continuity of care, physicians should inform patients at the onset of their moral objections to abortion or family planning. It is ethically problematical for physicians to use their role to impose their moral or religious views on patients.

Similar dilemmas arise when a health care organization, such as a Catholic hospital, does not provide family planning or abortion services (8). While there are strong reasons to respect an institutional policy based on religious beliefs, it is also important to inform women who present for care or schedule appointments that certain options will not be provided at that institution. Another question is whether such organizations can forbid individual physicians to provide information to patients about family planning or abortion, write prescriptions, or refer patients to other organizations for such services (8). Individual physicians should have the scope to discuss and recommend interventions that in their judgment are medically appropriate. To restrict such communication on the basis of an organization's policies or religious mission is to impose its views on both patients and health care providers. It is simplistic to believe that all physicians who work for an institution share the moral beliefs that animate the institutional policy, particularly as many health care organizations merge.

Reproductive Health for Adolescents

Girls under 18 years of age, who often are sexually active, may seek care for contraception, sexually transmitted diseases, or pregnancy. Many people believe that allowing minors to obtain such care without parental consent undermines family values and encourages promiscuity and irresponsibility. In most states, however, adolescents may seek reproductive health care without parental consent. The rationale is that it is preferable for adolescents to have access to such care, rather than forego care because they are reluctant or unable to obtain parental approval. Often adolescents have exaggerated fears that their parents will not understand or will reject them. In most cases, it is in the adolescent's best interest to involve parents in their care, and physicians should encourage them to do so. However, in some cases, adolescents may have compelling reasons for not involving parents, for example, in cases of domestic violence or incest.

Routine Prenatal Testing

During pregnancy, women commonly have screening tests for rubella, Rh type, diabetes, syphilis, and gonorrhea. Like many ambulatory tests, the woman usually assents to routine therapy, rather than giving full informed consent. By assent, we mean the woman agrees with the recommendation of her physician but does not discuss the risks and benefits of each test, and its alternatives. By routine therapy, we mean standard interventions that are provided unless the patient actively objects. Another way to describe routine testing is that women have the right to opt of out testing but do not need to give affirmative consent. Most states require mandatory prenatal testing for syphilis (9). The ethical justification for routine and mandatory prenatal screening tests is prevention of harm to children who will be born, the failure of completely voluntary testing to achieve the desired level of testing, and the belief that the infringement of the woman's autonomy is acceptably small.

Prenatal HIV Testing

Until recently, prenatal human immunodeficiency virus (HIV) testing has been treated differently from other prenatal screening tests. Written informed consent and pretest counseling have been required for HIV testing. Such procedures were required because HIV testing may result in significant psychosocial risks, such as stigma and discrimination. Early in the epidemic there was no intervention that could prevent vertical transmission of HIV infection. However, single-agent antiretroviral therapy reduces the incidence of perinatal HIV infection from 25% to 8.3% (10), and combination antiretroviral therapy is likely to reduce transmission to virtually zero. Although perinatal HIV infection has declined dramatically, many pregnant women are still not tested for HIV under voluntary testing policies. Requirements for pretest counseling and written consent are viewed as barriers to testing (11).

To maximize perinatal HIV prevention, various policies have been adopted to increase prenatal HIV testing (11). Several states require clinicians to offer voluntary prenatal HIV testing. A few states require pregnant women to sign an acknowledgment that they were offered HIV testing. In effect, pregnant women in these states need to sign a form to refuse HIV testing. Opponents object that this approach discriminates against pregnant women and that such signatures may be used against them, for example, in child custody hearings. Four states allow routine prenatal HIV testing without specific consent, unless the mother objects. In Texas, women must be told that the test will be done unless they object. Universal routine prenatal testing has been recommended (11,12) and is likely to become more widely adopted.

Although mandatory prenatal testing has been proposed (13), no state has adopted it. Mandatory testing is a much more serious violation of the woman's autonomy than routine testing. Furthermore, mandatory testing may polarize the doctor–patient relationship and make women less willing to accept long-term antiretroviral therapy.

Obstetrical Emergencies

Some obstetrical decisions need to be made in crisis situations. An uncomplicated pregnancy at term may unexpectedly and rapidly become an emergency if severe fetal distress develops or if the umbilical cord is wrapped around the fetus' neck. Decisions to perform a cesarean section may need to be made within minutes in order to prevent severe, irreversible harm to a child. As with any emergency situation, the consent process may be truncated if delaying care to obtain consent would cause serious harm and if most patients would agree to the intervention if given an opportunity to consent. The process of informed consent during labor also may be more difficult because fatigue, pain, medications, and emotional factors may compromise the pregnant woman's ability to make informed decisions. Almost all pregnant women agree to recommended nonelective cesarean sections (14). In an emergency, a cesarean section may be performed on the basis of the assent by the pregnant woman, rather than informed consent. That is, the patient agrees to the doctor's recommendations, without being informed of all the risks and benefits of the procedure.

Sterilization

Sterilization without a woman's consent is a grave violation of her autonomy. In the early 1900's, nonvoluntary eugenic sterilization was carried out in the United States on women who had mental retardation, resided in psychiatric institutions, and were prisoners (1,15). African-American women were disproportionately subjected to nonvoluntary sterilization. In reaction to these abuses, many states have enacted procedural requirements, such as waiting periods, to ensure that sterilization decisions are voluntary and informed (1,15).

Sterilization is commonly considered for severely mentally disabled individuals. Caretakers may be convinced that the woman cannot care for a child. Today, a court hearing generally is required in order to sterilize a woman who is not capable of giving informed consent (1,15).

ABORTION

Debates over abortion in the United States are contentious. Pro-life advocates contend that the fetus is a person with a right to live and that abortion is intentional killing of a person, a form of murder. Pro-choice advocates claim that women have a right to control their bodies and their reproductive choices and often contend that a fetus becomes a person only after birth. Disagreements on abortion are associated with different views on the role of women and the meaning of women's lives (15). While pro-life activists tend to view motherhood as the "most important and satisfying role" for a woman, pro-choice activists tend to believe that motherhood is "only one of several roles, a burden when defined as the only role" for a woman (16). Debates have become increasingly polarized, and adherents of one view are unlikely to be persuaded to change their minds (3,5).

The Supreme Court has made several important rulings on abortion. In Planned Parenthood *v.* Casey, the Supreme Court affirmed the core of the 1973 Roe *v.* Wade decision, which protected a woman's right to choose to abort her fetus. In Casey, the court held that states may ban abortion after fetal viability, as long as exceptions were made to protect the health or life of the woman, and as long as the restriction's "purpose or effect [was not] to place substantial obstacles in the path of a woman seeking an abortion before the fetus attains viability" (17). A number of states require parental notification if minors seek an abortion; these states must have a procedure for adolescents to seek judicial authorization for the procedure instead of parental notification. Because state laws on abortion vary, physicians must understand the laws in their state.

In caring for patients, physicians have responsibilities that should transcend their own personal views. As in any clinical situation, physicians need to respond to the patient's emotional needs, educate the patient about alternatives for care, and help ensure that difficult decisions are made after due deliberation. Physicians may offer recommendations, but they need to distinguish what they would do for themselves from what they judge to be best in view of the patient's individual situation and values.

Some requests for abortion are particularly problematical. For example, a pregnant woman may seek an abortion on the basis of the sex of her fetus, even though there is no sex-linked genetic disease. The woman may come from a culture where male children are more prized or may desire a son or daughter after having all children of the opposite sex. Parents commonly have a preference regarding the sex of the child. However, it is not morally justified for a physician to perform an abortion on a healthy fetus solely because of its sex (18). There is little ethical justification for treating females and males differently in this situation. If the physician cannot persuade the woman to withdraw her request, the doctor is justified in withdrawing from the case.

MATERNAL/FETAL CONFLICT

Most pregnant women agree with their physician's recommendations. However, in some cases women may reject recommendations despite continued attempts at persuasion.

Patient Requests for Interventions Whose Risks Outweigh the Benefits

Pregnant women may request interventions whose balance of benefits to risks physicians consider unfavorable. For example, young pregnant women at low risk for genetic abnormalities may request amniocentesis or chorionic villus sampling. Such women may desire information about the fetus and reassurance that the pregnancy is progressing normally, even though there is little likelihood of a serious abnormality. In the case of chorionic villus sampling or amniocentesis, risks to the fetus need to be taken into account. If the risk for serious congenital abnormalities is very low, it may be less than the risk of complications such as miscarriage.

How should the physician respond to such requests? The physician can check that the mother understands the benefits and risks of the procedure and the availability of other tests for congenital abnormalities, such as alpha fetoprotein screening. In addition, the physician can help the woman deliberate about the decision and make a recommendation. Ultimately, however, the woman's choice should be decisive.

Care of Pregnant Women With Other Medical Problems

When pregnant women have serious medical problems, such as cancer, depression, or seizures, physicians are understandably concerned that treatments for those conditions may have adverse effects on the developing fetus. However, such concern for the fetus must not lead physicians to withhold effective therapies inappropriately from the woman. First, physicians need accurate information about the effects of therapies on the fetus. Often physicians overestimate the risks to the fetus. Second, in such conditions as tuberculosis or epilepsy, aggressive treatment for the pregnant woman promotes the physical health of the child who will be born (19). Furthermore, it will be in the best interests of the child for the mother to be healthy. Finally, the pregnant woman should make informed decisions about the care of her medical problems. She should decide what risks to the fetus are acceptable in view of the overall benefits of the intervention. It is inappropriate for physicians to withhold effective interventions from the mother or to insist that the pregnant woman obtain an abortion as a condition of treatment.

Substance and Alcohol Abuse During Pregnancy

Some state laws hold mothers responsible for harms to a fetus. Women have been criminally prosecuted and incarcerated for drug or alcohol use during pregnancy. In several states, doctors are required to report drug-using pregnant women to state authorities (1,2). The South Carolina Supreme Court held in 1997 that women who neglect, abuse, and thus endanger their fetus can be prosecuted under current child abuse statutes (20). Critics object that these policies undermine trust in physicians, may deter women from seeking prenatal care or being candid, discriminate against women of color, and cause more harm than benefit in the long run (21). A more constructive approach is to focus on substance abuse treatment, rather than punishment (22,23).

Forced Cesarean Section Deliveries

If a pregnant woman cannot be persuaded to accept a cesarean section that the physician believes is required, some doctors seek court authorization for the operation. Recent court rulings hold that a competent pregnant woman may refuse a cesarean section, even if the welfare of a viable fetus is at stake (21,24–26). These rulings articulate why forced cesarean sections are ethically untenable. Courts note that competent adults may refuse treatment, that cesarean sections are a significant bodily invasion, and that the medical need for the procedure is often overstated. In many cases in which court orders were sought for cesarean section, the woman delivered vaginally without complications (21,27). Additional objections are that forced cesarean sections compromise women's trust in physicians and discriminate against women who do not speak English and women of color.

ASSISTED REPRODUCTIVE TECHNOLOGIES

Physicians may doubt whether a woman seeking infertility treatment would be a good parent. Because physicians take an active and essential role in assisted reproductive technologies, they feel a moral responsibility for the well-being of the child who may be born (18). Many physicians would hesitate to provide infertility treatments to women with drug addiction, serious developmental delay, or severe psychiatric illness. Some physicians may be reluctant to assist single, unmarried, or lesbian women.

Concern for the well-being of children who will be born is laudable. Physicians should help women and couples seeking assisted reproductive technologies appreciate the difficulties of infertility treatments and childrearing. The physician may also make recommendations based on the patient's situation, needs, and goals. However, physicians should distinguish concerns that are based on clinical evidence from their personal views of parenthood and family. Some characteristics, such as marital status, have little power to predict whether an individual would be a good parent (18). Many married couples fail as parents, while many individuals who are single or have nontraditional relationships succeed. At the other extreme, it would be irresponsible for physicians to provide assisted reproductive technologies to women who are incapable of giving informed consent or to women who have abused their children.

Some women over 40 years of age seek infertility treatment (18). Many such women are committed to raising a child, have strong social support, and have carefully considered their decision. It seems arbitrary to exclude them from assisted reproductive technologies solely on the basis of age. Because having a child is such a private decision, attempts by physicians to impose their views of who is worthy of being a parent are problematical.

STUDENT PARTICIPATION IN GYNECOLOGICAL AND OBSTETRICAL CARE

Pelvic examinations done under anesthesia offer opportunities for students to master this difficult skill. Because a woman's muscles are relaxed under anesthesia, a more thorough examination is possible. Senior physicians sometimes ask students to perform pelvic examinations on an anesthetized patient in the operating room without her consent. Some individuals believe that explicit consent is not needed because, by agreeing to the surgery, the patient implicitly consents to examinations by medical students. This conception of "implied consent" is incorrect. Implied consent refers to emergency care when patients are not capable of giving consent and no surrogate is available (*see* Chapter 3). Agreeing to surgery is not tantamount to consenting to a pelvic exam by an unknown medical student who is not participating in her ongoing care. Women want to be informed about the extent of a student's involvement in their care. In one study, all the women surveyed believed that students should ask specific permission to perform a pelvic examination on an anesthetized patient (28). Although patient consent to participation by trainees in their care is always important (*see* Chapter 38), it is particularly important for pelvic examinations because of patient modesty and privacy.

REFERENCES

1. Dubler NN, White A. Fertility control: legal and regulatory issues. In: Reich WT, ed. *Encyclopedia of bioethics.* revised ed. New York: Simon & Shuster Macmillan, 1995:839–847.

2. Brown GF, Moskowitz EH. Moral and policy issues in long-acting contraception. *Annu Rev Public Health* 1997;18:379–400.
3. McCullough LB, Chervenak FA. *Ethics in obstetrics and gynecology.* New York: Oxford University Press, 1994.
4. Steinbock B. Maternal-fetal relationship: ethical issues. In: Reich WT, ed. *Encyclopedia of bioethics.* revised ed. New York: Simon & Shuster Macmillan, 1995:1408–1413.
5. Murray TH. *The worth of a child.* Berkeley: University of California Press, 1996:96–114, 142–166.
6. Thorp JM, Wells SR, Bowes WA, et al. Integrity, abortion, and the pro-life perinatologist. *Hastings Center Rep* 1995;25:27–28.
7. Blustein J, Fleishman AR. Integrity, abortion, and the prolife perinatologist. *Hastings Center Rep* 1995;25:22–26.
8. Gallagher J. Religious freedom, reproductive health care, and hospital mergers. *J Am Med Womens Assoc* 1997;52:65–68.
9. Acuff KI. Prenatal and newborn screening: state legislative approaches and current practice standards. In: Faden RR, Geller G, Powers M, eds. *AIDS, women and the next generation.* New York: Oxford University Press, 1991:121–165.
10. Connor E, Sperling R, Gelber R, et al. Reduction of maternal-infant transmission of human immunodeficiency virus type 1 with zidovudine treatment. *N Engl J Med* 1994;331:1173–1180.
11. Stoto MA, Almario DA, McCormick MC, eds. *Reducing the odds: preventing perinatal transmission of HIV in the United States.* Washington, DC: National Academy Press, 1999.
12. American Academy of Pediatrics and American College of Obstetricians and Gynecologists. Human immunodeficiency virus screening. *Pediatrics* 1999;104:128.
13. Segal AI. Physician attitudes toward human immunodeficiency virus testing in pregnancy. *Am J Obstet Gynecol* 1996;174:1750–1755.
14. Lescale KB, Inglis SR, Eddleman KA, et al. Conflicts between physicians and patients in non-elective cesarean delivery: incidence and adequacy of informed consent. *Am J Perinatal* 1996;13:171–176.
15. American Academy of Pediatrics Committee on Bioethics. Sterilization of minors with developmental disabilities. *Pediatrics* 1999;104:337–340.
16. Luker K. *Abortion and the politics of motherhood.* Berkeley: University of California Press, 1984.
17. Planned Parenthood of Southeastern Pennsylvania *v.* Casey, 112 US 674 (1992).
18. The New York State Task Force on Life and the Law. *Assisted reproductive technologies.* New York: The New York State Task Force on Life and the Law, 1998:165–169, 177–213.
19. Eller DP, Patterson CA, Webb GW. Maternal and fetal implications of anticonvulsant therapy during pregnancy. *Obstet Gynecol Clin* 1997;24:523–534.
20. Whitner *v.* State, 492 S.W.2d 777 (S.C. 1977).
21. Johnsen DE. Maternal-fetal relationship: legal and regulatory issues. In: Reich WT, ed. *Encyclopedia of bioethics,* revised ed. New York: Simon & Shuster Macmillan, 1995:1413–1418.
22. Chavkin W. Mandatory treatment for drug use during pregnancy. *JAMA* 1991;266:1556–1561.
23. Board of Trustees AMA. Legal interventions during pregnancy: court-ordered medical treatments and legal penalties for potentially harmful behavior by pregnant women. *JAMA* 1990;264:2663–2670.
24. Curran WJ. Court-ordered cesarean sections receive judicial defeat. *N Engl J Med* 1990;323:489–492.
25. Levy JK. Jehovah's Witnesses, pregnancy, and blood transfusions: a paradigm for the autonomy of all pregnant women. *J Law Med Ethics* 1999;27:171–189.
26. Goldblatt AD. Commentary: no more jurisdiction over Jehovah. *J Law Med & Ethics* 1999;27:190–193.
27. Nelson LJ, Milliken N. Compelled medical treatment of pregnant women: life, liberty and law in conflict. *JAMA* 1988;259:1060–1066.
28. Bibby J, Boyd N, Redman C, et al. Consent for vaginal examination by students on anaesthetised patients (letter). *Lancet* 1988;2:1150.

ANNOTATED BIBLIOGRAPHY

1. The New York State Task Force on Life and the Law. *Assisted reproductive technologies.* New York: The New York State Task Force on Life and the Law, 1998.
Comprehensive, balanced discussion of ethical and legal issues regarding assisted reproductive technologies.
2. Stoto MA, Almario DA, McCormick MC, eds. *Reducing the odds: preventing perinatal transmission of HIV in the United States.* Washington, DC: National Academy Press, 1999.
Consensus recommendations for universal routine prenatal HIV testing.
3. McCullough LB, Chervenak FA. *Ethics in obstetrics and gynecology.* New York: Oxford University Press, 1994.
Monograph on ethical issues in obstetrics and gynecology, with philosophical orientation.

42

Ethical Issues in Psychiatry

Some patients with severe psychiatric illness are not autonomous because they are not capable of making informed decisions about health care or controlling their behavior. Effective treatment of the psychiatric illness may restore their decision-making capacity. Rather than respecting their choices, physicians need to protect such patients against the consequences of their uninformed decisions and actions.

HOW ARE ETHICAL ISSUES IN PSYCHIATRY DIFFERENT?

Severe Impairment Caused By Serious Psychiatric Illness

Patients with severe psychiatric illness may be unable to make informed decisions, to care for themselves, to distinguish right from wrong, or to control their aggressive impulses. When dominated by their illness, patients may not be the same persons, with the same values, preferences, and judgment they have when their illness is treated. Patients with severe psychiatric illness may have little insight into the nature of their illness and its impact on their thinking and have an impaired ability to judge the benefits of treatment. Such patients may not be considered morally or legally responsible for their actions.

The Opportunity to Restore the Patient's Decision-Making Capacity

Physicians are in a unique position to identify such patients, to protect them from harm, and to prevent harm to unsuspecting third parties. Society therefore has given physicians the role of intervening in such cases, both to protect third parties from harm and to help such patients obtain treatment that may restore their ability to control their thoughts and behaviors. Intervention is particularly justified because successful treatment of psychiatric illness treats the underlying cause of the patients' impaired decision-making capacity and restores their authentic character. Thus, a short-term infringement on the patient's freedom, such as involuntary hospitalization, may restore the long-term autonomy of the patient.

Risk of Abuses

Involuntary psychiatric interventions, such as hospitalization against the patient's wishes, is a serious deprivation of liberty. In the past, many psychiatric patients were subjected involuntarily to extreme measures, such as lengthy confinement in inhumane institutions and psychosurgery. Today the public is unwilling to allow physicians—no matter how well-intentioned—unlimited discretion to hospitalize psychiatric patients against their will. Regulations and procedures for involuntary commitment have been established. Physicians need to ensure that involuntary confinement is instituted only when it is truly appropriate.

Importance of Confidentiality

Confidentiality is particularly important with psychiatric conditions. In therapy, patients reveal their innermost emotions, fears, and fantasies. Confidentiality respects the highly personal nature of such information and encourages patients to seek care for mental illness and to be candid with physicians. In addition, confidentiality protects patients from stigma and discrimination, which patients with psychiatric illness may face even if their disease is in remission.

INVOLUNTARY PSYCHIATRIC COMMITMENT

Involuntary commitment is a dramatic exception to the ethical guideline of respecting the liberty of persons. Ordinarily people cannot be detained against their will merely because they have threatened to take their own lives or to harm others. The American criminal justice system generally does not permit preventive detention on the basis of threats or plans to harm another person. Because it infringes on freedom so profoundly, involuntary psychiatric commitment must be carefully justified.

Rationale for Involuntary Commitment

Severe psychiatric illness may render patients incapable of making informed decisions. Driven by their mental illness, patients may not be able to control actions that harm themselves or others. Intervention is warranted to prevent serious, irrevocable harm. Furthermore, involuntary commitment may promote their long-term autonomy after their mental illness is treated or goes into remission. Thus depriving mentally incapacitated patients of their liberty for a short time may allow them to regain the capacity to make informed decisions (1). After their depression, bipolar disorder, or schizophrenia is treated, most patients no longer choose to kill themselves or harm others.

Standards for Involuntary Commitment

Criteria for involuntary commitment differ among states, but typically require that patients be, as a result of mental illness:

• Dangerous to themselves, for example, suicidal, or
• Unable to care for themselves, for example, unable to provide food, clothing, and shelter, or
• Dangerous to others, for example, through a threat, attempt, or an overt act of harm.

In addition, patients in several states may be involuntarily committed if a severe deterioration in their condition is likely without treatment and they cannot give consent to treatment. Under such laws, the underlying rationale for commitment is the patient's need for treatment, rather than danger to self or others (1).

Procedures for Involuntary Commitment

Because involuntary commitment procedures vary across the states, physicians need to be familiar with the law in their state. The following provisions are typical. Initially, patients may be held against their will on an emergency basis for brief periods (typically a few days). During an emergency, patients can also be treated against their will to prevent serious physical injury to themselves or others or, in some states, to prevent irreversible deterioration in their condition. A judicial hearing must be held to determine whether the patient may be confined for a longer period.

Legal hearings are time consuming, and many physicians believe that they are an unwarranted intrusion of the legal system into medical practice. However, many laypeople have a sharply different perspective. Because involuntary psychiatric hospitalization is a serious deprivation of liberty and has been abused in the past, the public demands rigorous safeguards.

Physicians may threaten to initiate commitment proceedings, unless the patient "voluntarily" consents to hospitalization. This practice is coercive and ethically suspect (1). Voluntary hospitalization helps physicians by reducing paperwork and eliminating the need for a judicial hearing. However, patients may not realize that by agreeing to voluntary hospitalization, they are waiving their right to a judicial hearing to determine whether commitment is appropriate. An alternative strategy has been suggested as showing more respect to patients (1). Psychiatrists should first tell patients that plans for involuntary hospitalization will be instituted and explain their right to a judicial hearing. After patients understand the commitment procedures, they may be offered the opportunity to sign into the hospital voluntarily.

SUICIDAL PATIENTS

When patients attempt or threaten suicide, physicians have an ethical obligation to intervene. It is essential for physicians to understand the rationale for suicide intervention and to be able to assess the seriousness of suicide threats.

Rationale for Suicide Intervention

The ethical justification for suicide intervention is preventing serious, irreversible harm to persons with impaired decision-making capacity. Patients who are suicidal are almost always impaired by severe depression or other mental illness (2). Their actions therefore are not competent, informed choices, but rather are the product of their mental illness. Interventions to prevent suicide provide time to treat the underlying mental illness or let it enter a remission. Empirical studies demonstrate the effectiveness of suicide prevention. If persons are prevented from committing suicide, only about 10% to 20% subsequently kill themselves (2).

Even strong proponents of patient autonomy recognize the need to intervene to prevent nonautonomous persons from seriously harming themselves (3). Furthermore, short-term interventions to determine whether a person is acting in an autonomous manner or suffers from severe psychiatric impairment is justified if the patient might take his or her life if left alone. This situation can be readily distinguished from the ethically problematical situation of restricting the liberty of autonomous persons in order to prevent them from harming themselves.

Interventions to prevent suicide include arranging for voluntary psychiatric treatment, mobilizing assistance from family and friends, removing the means of suicide, getting patients to promise to call for help before they take their lives, and, as a last resort, imposing involuntary commitment. To varying degrees, these interventions restrict patient liberty. Infringements should be the minimum needed to protect the patient from harm. In some cases, it may be unclear whether patients who are threatening suicide are making an autonomous decision or not. It is ethically prudent to intervene temporarily to ascertain if the threat is serious and if the patient's decision-making capacity is impaired. If involuntary commitment is deemed necessary, it should be continued only as long as necessary to protect the patient.

Physicians need to appreciate that they do not have the power to prevent all patients from committing suicide. After discharge, patients who are determined to kill themselves can find the means and opportunity to do so. In addition, some patients with terminal illness, whose decision-making capacity is unimpaired, may make a deliberate and firm decision to end their lives. The ethics of so-called "rational suicide," particularly physician-assisted suicide, is hotly debated (*see* Chapter 19).

When is a Patient Suicidal?

Many individuals make suicidal gestures that, although representing a "cry for help," may not warrant involuntary commitment. Such persons may be successfully treated through less restrictive measures, such as outpatient care or voluntary hospitalization. Hence physicians must determine which patients truly need involuntary hospitalization.

When patients are severely depressed or mention suicide, physicians should ask specific questions to determine the likelihood of a serious suicide attempt. Fears that raising the topic of suicide will suggest it to depressed patients or will encourage persons to kill themselves are unfounded and deter physicians from gathering crucial information and initiating effective treatment. Many depressed patients feel relieved to discuss suicide with a caring and nonjudgmental physician.

Certain characteristics identify persons who are more likely to attempt suicide or to succeed in killing themselves (1,4).

- Patients who have the intent to commit suicide, a specific plan for doing so, and the means to carry out the plan. Access to lethal and violent means of suicide indicates particularly high risk. Similarly, it is more serious when the proposed method of the suicide attempt makes rescue unlikely, as when patients have arranged to be alone for an extended period.
- Persons who have made preparations, such as giving away possessions or saying good-bye.
- Persons who view their situation as hopeless or have ideas of reuniting with a deceased person.
- Persons who are so excruciatingly depressed or agitated that it is difficult for the physician to interview them.

Mitigating the Adverse Consequences of Involuntary Hospitalization

When suicidal patients are involuntarily hospitalized, they may feel betrayed. Patients may view the physicians who committed them as adversaries who can no longer be trusted. Such feelings may make psychiatric therapy difficult. Physicians should try to minimize the confrontational aspects of the situation and stress shared therapeutic goals. An experienced psychiatrist has suggested saying: "It would be a shame if you killed yourself while your depression clouded your judgment. Let's get you undepressed; then, if you still want to kill yourself, I know I can't stop you" (1). Such a statement demonstrates concern, suggests that therapy may effectively lead to remission of the mental illness, and reassures patients that ultimately they are in control.

PATIENTS WHO ARE DANGEROUS TO OTHERS

Patients with serious psychiatric illness may tell physicians about plans to kill or injure third parties, actual attempts, or overt acts of harm. The physician may be in a unique position to prevent serious harm to the threatened person. Psychiatric patients who cannot control their violent impulses may not be deterred by social norms and criminal sanctions. In this situation, the landmark Tarasoff case established that confidentiality should be overridden in order to prevent serious harm to third parties (5).

The Tarasoff Case and the Duty to Prevent Harm

A university student, Prosenjit Poddar, confided to his psychologist that he was planning to kill a woman, readily identifiable as Tatiana Tarasoff, who had rejected him romantically. The therapist and his superiors at the student health service decided that Poddar should be committed involuntarily and asked the campus police to detain him. The police did so but released him because he appeared rational. The director of psychiatry ordered therapy notes and correspondence with the police destroyed and ordered no action to place Poddar under involuntary detention. Subsequently Poddar went to Tarasoff's home and stabbed her to death. Her parents sued the Regents of the state university, the employers of the therapists, and the police for failing to detain a dangerous patient and to warn the victim or others of her danger. The California Supreme Court rejected the first claim because of governmental immunity. On the second claim, the court ruled that a therapist who determines, or should have determined, that the patient presents "a serious danger of violence to another" has a "duty to exercise reasonable care to protect others against dangers emanating from the patient's illness" (5). Thus, the court declared a duty to protect potential victims, not just warn them. The court rejected several arguments raised by the defendants, namely, that they had owed no duty of care to Tarasoff, that predictions of violence by psychiatric patients are inherently inaccurate, and that confidentiality is essential to psychotherapy. The court ruled that the special relationship between a patient and his doctor or psychotherapist supports "affirmative duties for the benefit of third persons." In this case, fallibility of predications of violence was not an issue because the therapists had determined that Poddar was dangerous. Furthermore, the confidentiality of psychotherapy communication must be balanced against the need to avert danger to others. "The protective privilege ends where the public peril begins" (5).

Therapists feared that the decision would undermine the doctor–patient relationship. They predicted that patients would be deterred from seeking mental health services and disclosing their violent thoughts, that warning potential victims would be ineffective, and that issuing a warning would effectively end therapy with a patient (6). However, empirical studies have shown that these anticipated effects have not occurred to a significant degree (6).

Most states require therapists to protect identifiable persons threatened with serious violence by psychiatric patients (6). Generally the duty is limited to identifiable patients and actual threats. In most states, therapists can meet this legal duty by warning the potential victim or the police or hospitalizing the patient (6).

Steps to Prevent Harm

The duty to prevent harm to potential victims of psychiatric patients requires several steps (7). First, the physician needs to evaluate the threat of violence. As with asking about suicide, physicians need to appreciate that asking about violence does not give patients the idea of harming others or encourage them to do so. Asking, "Do you ever think about harming someone else?" may help to elicit intentions and plans to seriously hurt others (8). Because past violence is a strong predictor of future violence, the physician should ask if the patient has ever caused death or serious injury to another person (1).

Predictions of violence by physicians may be quite inaccurate. In one study, 53% of patients whom clinicians predicted would be violent in fact committed violent acts over the subsequent

6 months; in comparison, 36% of patients whose psychiatrists had no concerns about violence committed violent acts (9). Violence was more serious in those patients whom psychiatrists had predicted would be violent. For women, however, the accuracy of predictions of violence was no greater than that expected by chance alone. Within the limits of clinical judgment, doctors need to do the best job they can to evaluate their patients' potential for violence. The standard of care is what a reasonable physician would do under the circumstances.

After determining that the threat of violence is severe and probable, the physician must decide how to respond. Warning the threatened victim is specifically required by law in many states. Other actions might also protect the victim, such as notifying the police, changing the patient's medications, increasing the frequency of therapy sessions, having the patient give up weapons, attempting to hospitalize the patient voluntarily, or committing the patient involuntarily (10).

Physicians should notify patients before they override confidentiality and explain why they are obliged to do so (10). Physicians should discuss with patients threats against third parties as part of therapy (8). Such discussions may help maintain a therapeutic relationship. Patients may give permission for the physician to warn the threatened person (1). Many patients are ambivalent about violence and may welcome help in finding other ways to express their emotions or deal with interpersonal conflicts. In addition, when beginning therapy with patients who have a history of violence, physicians might discuss the situations in which confidentiality may be overridden (1).

REFUSAL OF PSYCHIATRIC TREATMENT

Patients who are involuntarily committed to psychiatric institutions may still be deemed competent to refuse psychiatric treatment (1). Because competency is determined with regard to specific tasks, it is possible that a patient who is not competent to refuse commitment may still be competent to refuse medications. Confining patients but not treating them with effective medications has been criticized as "rotting with their rights on" (11). To critics, it is cruel and pointless to withhold from severely impaired patients the very treatments that are likely to restore their autonomy. In this view, short-term involuntary treatment, which may improve the underlying psychiatric illness, is a lesser infringement on the patient's freedom than prolonged involuntary hospitalization without treatment.

Nonetheless, many states have made it more difficult to administer treatments to involuntarily committed psychiatric patients. The rationale is that the goal of involuntary hospitalization—prevention of harm to self or others—can sometimes be accomplished by confinement without treatment. In addition, patients and the public may view the risks and benefits of psychiatric therapies differently than physicians. Many psychiatric patients want to discontinue medications because of the side effects. Patients may also reject drugs that are altering their brain and personality. Furthermore, past abuses have led the public to mistrust physicians' unilateral judgments that treatment is beneficial and necessary.

The ethical guideline of preventing harm is generally regarded as having more moral force than the guideline of doing good (*see* Chapter 4). Thus the obligation to prevent harms to nonautonomous psychiatric patients or to third parties is stronger than the duty to help psychiatric patients recover from their illness. First, forced administration of medications to unwilling patients is intrusive and inhumane. Second, it may be impractical in the long run. Even if psychiatric medications were forcibly administered to inpatients, patients can (and often do) discontinue therapies after discharge. Third, beneficence could become an open-ended burden. Physicians could expend great effort in trying to help severely disturbed patients who do not want treatment, without any significant improvement.

Several states have procedures to deal with such refusals of treatment by involuntarily hospitalized psychiatric patients. These states require a court hearing if a psychiatric patient who has been involuntarily committed refuses treatment (1). The court determines whether the patient is competent to make an informed decision to refuse treatment. If so, the refusal must be honored. If the patient is not competent, the court decides whether the treatment will be provided.

The patient's capacity to make informed decisions therefore is crucial to whether their refusal of therapy will be respected. Chapter 10 discusses decision-making capacity. Assessing the decision-making capacity of psychiatric patients may be particularly difficult (12). People with major depression may underestimate the benefits of treatment and overestimate the risks (13). They may be convinced that the treatment will fail or that they will experience a serious side effect of therapy. Depressed patients may also believe that they deserve to suffer and that treatment may interfere with such suffering. Similarly, manic patients may believe that nothing is wrong with them and therefore reject treatment as unbeneficial. Both depressed and manic patients can give seemingly logical reasons for their decisions, yet their underlying premises about medical care are false, and they assess the benefits and risks of treatment inaccurately. Thus, they are unable to make informed decisions about their care.

Empirical studies have described refusals of antipsychotic medications. In one study, only 7% of inpatients refused antipsychotic medication for longer than 24 hours (14). Patients refused because of psychotic or idiosyncratic thought processes in 30% of cases, side effects of medications in 35%, denial of mental illness in 21%, and alleged ineffectiveness of medications in 12%. Cases were resolved in several ways. In 50% of cases, the patient eventually took medication voluntarily. Typically the nursing staff, psychiatrists, or family persuaded the patient. In 23% of cases, antipsychotic drugs were either discontinued by the psychiatrist, or the patient was discharged without medication. In other words, the physician probably did not consider these medications essential. Finally, in 18% of cases, the psychiatrists obtained a court order for involuntary administration of the medication. In all cases that went to court, the judge authorized involuntary treatment.

REFUSAL OF MEDICAL TREATMENT BY PSYCHIATRIC PATIENTS

Patients with serious psychiatric illness may refuse recommended therapy for concurrent medical problems. As with other patients who refuse interventions, physicians should ask whether the patient has intact decision-making capacity. A psychiatric diagnosis *per se* does not imply that a patient lacks the capacity to make an informed decision about treatment. A competent patient's refusal should be respected if attempts at persuasion are unsuccessful. If the patient lacks decision-making capacity, then decisions should be based on advance directives or made by surrogates (*see* Chapters 12 and 13). Decisions may be especially perplexing when psychiatric patients who lack decision-making capacity actively resist treatment that is clearly in their best interests. Forced treatment may be difficult to carry out if the patient actively protests or resists. It may also be counter-productive because issues of control and independence may be problems that the patient needs to resolve. Overriding the patient's refusal may make it more difficult for him to take responsibility and control over other aspects of his life. Finally, the possibility of forced treatment is illusory. In a structured inpatient setting, the staff may be able to ensure that the patient is taking the medicine through cajoling, negotiation, and threats. For example, health care workers may threaten to withhold visiting privileges, outings, or cigarettes. The crucial issue, however, is whether the patient will continue to take medicines after discharge. This may be more likely if the patient believes that taking the medication is best for him.

In conclusion, when psychiatric patients are suicidal, unable to care for themselves, or dangerous to others, physicians have ethical as well as legal obligations to prevent harm. This obligation may override the ethical guidelines of respecting patient autonomy and maintaining confidentiality. In fulfilling this duty, physicians also need to use their clinical skills and judgment to encourage effective treatment for the underlying psychiatric disorders.

REFERENCES

1. Appelbaum PS, Gutheil TG. *Clinical handbook of psychiatry and the law*, 2nd ed. Baltimore: Williams & Wilkins, 1991.
2. Miller RD. Need-for-treatment criteria for involuntary civil commitment: impact in practice. *Am J Psychiatry* 1992;149:1380–1384.
3. Beauchamp TL, Childress JF. *Principles of biomedical ethics*, 4th ed. New York: Oxford University Press, 1994:271–287.
4. Blumenthal SJ. Suicide: a guide to risk factors, assessment, and treatment of suicidal patients. *Med Clin North Am* 1988;72:937–971.
5. Tarasoff v. Regents of the University of California, 551 P2d 334 (Cal 1976).
6. Appelbaum PS. Almost a revolution: mental health law and the limits of change. New York: Oxford University Press, 1994:71–113.
7. Appelbaum PS, Zonana H, Bonnie R, Roth LH. Statutory approaches to limiting psychiatrists' liability for their patients' violent acts. *Am J Psychiatry* 1989;146:821–828.
8. Simon RI. Clinical approaches to the duty to warn and protect endangered third parties. Clinical psychiatry and the law. Washington, DC: American Psychiatric Press, Inc., 1987:307–336.
9. Lidz C, Mulvey EP, Gardner W. The accuracy of predictions of violence to others. *JAMA* 1993;269:1007–1011.
10. Appelbaum PS. Tarasoff and the clinician: problems in fulfilling the duty to protect. *Am J Psychiatry* 1985;142:425–429.
11. Appelbaum PS, Gutheil TG. "Rotting with their rights on": constitutional theory and clinical reality in drug refusal by psychiatric patients. *Bull Am Acad Psychiatry Law* 1979;7:306–315.
12. Gutheil TG, Bursztajn HJ, Brodsky A, Alexander V. Affective disorders, competence, and decision making. Decision making in psychiatry and the law, 2nd ed. Baltimore: Williams & Wilkins, 1991:153–170.
13. Grisso T, Appelbaum P. Assessing competence to consent to treatment: a guide for physicians and other health professionals. New York: Oxford University Press, 1998:49–51.
14. Hoge SK, Appelbaum PS, Lawlor T. A prospective multicenter study of patients' refusal of antipsychotic medication. *Arch Gen Psychiatry* 1990;47:949–956.

ANNOTATED BIBLIOGRAPHY

1. Appelbaum PS, Gutheil TG. *Clinical handbook of psychiatry and the law*, 2nd ed. Baltimore: Williams & Wilkins, 1991.
   Excellent book on ethical and legal issues regarding psychiatric patients. Contains practical clinical advice on managing patients with severe psychiatric disorders.
2. Appelbaum PS. *Almost a revolution: mental health law and the limits of change*. New York: Oxford University Press, 1994.
   Lucid discussion of the ethical and policy issues regarding involuntary commitment and treatment.

SECTION VII

Current Controversies

43

Transmission of HIV Infection in Health Care Settings

In 1990, Kimberly Bergalis, a 23-year-old woman who contracted human immunodeficiency virus (HIV) infection during dental care, dramatized public alarm concerning HIV-infected health care workers. Ms. Bergalis asserted that she should have been told about the dentist's HIV infection: "I'm not asking that we be able to live in a risk free world. I want people to be able to choose their risks. I didn't have a choice to walk out of the office and seek another dentist" (1). She harshly criticized public health officials. "Whom do I blame?. . . Anyone who knew . . . [the dentist] was infected and had full-blown AIDS and stood by not doing a damn thing about it. You are all just as guilty as he was" (2).

This chapter discusses the transmission of HIV infection in medical settings. The most common situation is exposure of health care workers to patients' blood. Transmission of HIV infection in the opposite direction, from health care workers to patients, is much less common, but it evokes strong emotional reactions. In analyzing these difficult issues, this chapter emphasizes how protecting persons from HIV infection must be balanced against preventing discrimination against persons infected with HIV.

TRANSMISSION FROM PATIENTS TO HEALTH CARE WORKERS

CASE 43.1. NEEDLESTICK EXPOSURE OF HEALTH CARE WORKER TO A PATIENT'S BLOOD. *An intern starting an intravenous line jabs his thumb with a needle that is contaminated with the patient's blood. The patient has no risk factors for HIV. After the physician explains the risk of occupational HIV infection, the patient refuses to be tested. "I already told you I don't have any risk factors. If my company finds out that I got an AIDS test, they are going to wonder why. I could lose my health insurance. Also I don't want people at work thinking I use drugs or am gay." Upset by the patient's refusal, the physician considers drawing an extra tube of blood the next morning and obtaining an HIV antibody test without the patient's consent.*

If the patient is seropositive, the physician has a 0.3% risk of contracting HIV after a percutaneous exposure (3). Postexposure prophylaxis with antiretroviral therapy is recommended in Case 43.1 if the source is seropositive and is not needed if the patient is seronegative (3). The injured physician in Case 43.1 therefore believes that the patient is unreasonably withholding vital information, which would clarify his prognosis and need for prophylaxis. Moreover, if the physician develops HIV infection or hepatitis, documentation that the patient was an infected source may be needed for a disability claim.

The physician's desire to test the patient surreptitiously, while understandable given his anxiety, is legally and ethically problematic. Generally HIV testing without written consent from the patient is illegal, although some states permit HIV antibody testing in situations like Case 43.1 without the patient's consent (4). Ethically speaking, HIV testing over the patient's objections violates the patient's autonomy and privacy.

All too often, the situation in Case 43.1 becomes polarized and confrontational. The patient asserts a right to refuse HIV testing, while the physician claims a countervailing right to know the patient's HIV status. A better approach is anonymous testing of the patient who is the source of blood. The results could be placed in the physician's occupational medicine file, not in the patient's medical record. The name of the source patient need not be disclosed. This approach maintains the confidentiality of the patient, while allowing the physician to know whether he is at risk.

TRANSMISSION FROM HEALTH CARE WORKERS TO PATIENTS

The Risk of Transmitting HIV from Health Care Workers to Patients

Estimates of Risk

In medical settings, HIV can be transmitted from health care workers to patients only during invasive procedures in which a seropositive health care worker's blood might "contact the patient's body cavity, subcutaneous tissues, and/or mucous membranes" (5). The Centers for Disease Control and Prevention (CDC) distinguishes exposure-prone invasive procedures from other clinical activities. Exposure-prone invasive procedures present a "recognized risk of percutaneous injury to the health care worker and—if such an injury occurs—the health care worker's blood is likely to contact the patient's body cavity, subcutaneous tissues, and/or mucous membranes" (5). Such procedures include digital palpation of a needle tip in a body cavity or the simultaneous presence of the health care worker's finger and a sharp object "in a poorly visualized or highly confined anatomical site" (5). Infected health care workers who adhere to universal precautions and who do not perform invasive procedures "pose no risk for transmitting HIV or HBV [hepatitis B] to patients" (5).

Two clusters of transmission from an HIV-infected health care worker to patients have been documented. A Florida dentist transmitted HIV to five patients, including Ms. Bergalis (6). Also an HIV-infected orthopedic surgeon was reported to transmit infection to a patient who underwent two lengthy operations (7). In other investigations, no cases of HIV transmission were identified in detailed studies of 22,759 patients of 53 HIV-infected health care workers who performed invasive procedures (8). Thus large-scale epidemiological studies have documented that the overall risk of transmission from HIV-infected health care workers to patients during invasive procedures is very low. Highly active antiretroviral therapy and the adoption of new equipment and operative techniques probably reduce the risk even further (9).

Public Perception of Risk

The magnitude of a risk is only one factor in people's perception of risks (10). Familiar and voluntary risks are generally more acceptable than unfamiliar, involuntary, and uncertain risks, even if the latter are far less likely (11–13). For example, people usually fear the risk of death in an automobile accident far less than the risk of death in a nuclear accident, even though the latter is much less likely. The risk of nosocomial HIV infection seems especially ominous. HIV infection is fatal and can be transmitted to loved ones. Like Ms. Bergalis, patients may feel betrayed if a physician or dentist places them at any risk beyond that caused by their illness or treatment. Patients could completely avoid the risk by seeking care from a seronegative physician.

Public Health Dilemmas

There are several public health dilemmas regarding transmission of HIV from seropositive health care workers who perform invasive procedures.

- Should health care workers who perform invasive procedures be tested for HIV?
- Should HIV-infected health care workers who perform invasive procedures inform patients that they are seropositive?
- Should the practice of such health care workers be restricted?

Reasons for Restrictions on HIV-Infected Health Care Workers

There are several reasons to restrict the clinical activities of certain HIV-infected health care workers (10). The ethical guideline of nonmaleficence requires physicians to avoid harming their patients. Physicians also have a fiduciary duty to act in the best interests of their patients, even at some harm to their own interests. The guideline of respect for patients requires physicians to obtain informed consent for procedures. Physicians generally must disclose to patients information that a reasonable person would find material to the decision at hand. A very small risk may need to be disclosed if it is serious or if patients would find it material to the decision at hand (14). Most patients would want to know that their surgeon is infected with HIV (15).

Reasons Against Stringent Restrictions on HIV-Infected Health Care Workers

There also are strong arguments against restricting the clinical activities of HIV-infected health care workers (10,16). Attempts to achieve absolute patient safety would compromise other important ethical guidelines. Health care workers have a right to privacy and freedom from discrimination. The guidelines of beneficence and justice also require that the resources devoted to reducing the risk of nosocomial infection be proportionate to the expected benefits.

The Risk to Patients Is Very Small

Numerous epidemiological studies have shown that the risk that an HIV-infected health care worker will transmit the infection to a patient is very low (8). The risk has probably been further reduced by highly active antiretroviral therapies and by infection control measures such as double gloving and modifications in operating technique (9). The Society for Healthcare Epidemiology of America, the professional organization of infection control officers, has recommended that no restrictions be placed on otherwise qualified seropositive health care workers, because the risk of transmitting HIV to patients is so small (9).

HIV-Infected Health Care Workers Would Suffer Discrimination

Under the Americans with Disabilities Act, employees with infectious diseases may be restricted in their jobs only if they pose a significant risk to others, not simply a conceivable or identifiable risk. As noted, epidemiological studies indicate that the risk of transmission of HIV from an infected health care worker to a patient is very low. Arguably, this is not a "significant" risk.

HIV-infected health care workers suffer considerable job discrimination, even those who followed infection control guidelines, were not impaired, and in many cases did not even perform invasive procedures at work (17,18). If mandatory HIV testing of health care workers who perform invasive procedures is enacted, there would be a risk of breaches of confidentiality and employment discrimination.

Restricting All HIV-Infected Health Care Workers Would Have Undesirable Consequences

Trying to eliminate the risk of nosocomial HIV infection would be very costly (4), would deter health care workers from caring for HIV-infected patients, and would make it more difficult for public hospitals, which care for large numbers of HIV-infected patients, to recruit nurses, house staff, and staff physicians (19). These undesirable consequences would make all citizens worse off in the long run (16). For example, many public hospitals are also regional trauma centers and base stations for paramedics (10).

Approaches to Policy Dilemmas

In 1991, the CDC issued guidelines for HIV-infected health care workers. Are these guidelines still appropriate today? The CDC recommended that "health care workers who perform exposure-prone invasive procedures should know their HIV antibody status" (5). However, it rejected mandatory HIV testing of such health care workers as not cost-effective. In 1999, the case for mandatory testing is even weaker in light of new information about the very low risk of transmission and about discrimination against HIV-positive health care workers.

The CDC also recommended that an expert review panel decide on a case-by-case basis which invasive procedures a seropositive health care worker may or may not perform and when patients must be told that a health care worker is infected. Such panels would consider "the skill and technique of the individual infected health care worker and the health care worker's physical condition, as well as the specific invasive procedure being performed" (20).

Congress required states to adopt the CDC recommendations or their equivalent in order to receive federal Medicaid and Medicare funds (21). However, states vary considerably in whether they require seropositive health care workers to be reported to the health department or licensing board, whether they restrict the practice of HIV-infected health care workers, and whether they use expert panels to determine the need for such restrictions (22).

Expert advisory panels have generally allowed the infected health care worker to continue to practice, except when poor infection control is documented. Expert panels are trying to specify invasive procedures that the HIV-infected health care worker may safely perform, without having to notify his patients in advance that he is seropositive (22). Generally exposure-prone invasive procedures can be eliminated from the health care worker's practice or modified to reduce risk to acceptable levels. These expert advisory panels give great attention to maintaining the health care worker's confidentiality.

Responding to Patients' Questions About the Physician's HIV Status

Health care workers can expect patients to ask them about nosocomial HIV infection and specifically whether they are infected. According to the CDC guidelines, health care workers have no ethical duty to disclose their HIV antibody status if they present no significant risk to their patients. Physicians should consider how to respond to patients' questions (10). There is nothing to gain and much to lose by responding in a defensive, brusque, or confrontational manner, or by calling patient concern "unfounded hysteria" (23). Physicians need to listen to patients' concerns and acknowledge their fears.

Only after responding to patients' emotions should physicians try to put the risk of nosocomial HIV infection in perspective. Researchers of risk perception offer several cautions. Perceptions of risk will not be changed merely by reassuring patients that a risk is low or by comparing it with other risks (11–13). Comparisons that appear to trivialize a risk are counter-productive. People reject the suggestion that because they accept risks of greater magnitude, they should also accept the risk in question (24).

Exposure of Patients to a Health Care Worker's Blood

CASE 43.2. PATIENT EXPOSED TO BLOOD OF HEALTH CARE WORKER. *During pelvic surgery, a gynecologist nicks his finger with a suture needle, which then recontacts the patient. The gynecologist has never been tested for HIV antibodies, but has no risk factors. The gynecologist wonders what, if anything, he should say to the patient.*

Patient exposure is most common when the health care worker injures himself with a suture needle or sharp instrument, which then recontacts the patient. In one study, such an exposure occurred in 2% of surgical operations (25).

In Case 43.2, the physician may believe that the risk to the patient is vanishingly small and fear losing his livelihood if the patient's test results are positive for HIV antibodies. However, the patient needs to know that an exposure occurred in order to make informed decisions about postexposure prophylaxis for HIV and hepatitis B and to take precautions about spreading possible infection. Informing patients of actual exposure is recommended by professional organizations (9). It may be preferable for someone other than the seropositive physician to talk to the patient, for example, an infection control or HIV specialist. The discussion need not divulge the name of the infected physician, only the fact of exposure to a health care worker's blood and the possible consequences.

Impairment in HIV-Infected Health Care Workers

Seropositive health care workers may not observe infection control precautions or may be physically or mentally impaired. In these situations, their physicians face a dilemma because maintaining confidentiality conflicts with protecting the seropositive health care worker's unsuspecting patients.

CASE 43.3. SEROPOSITIVE HEALTH CARE WORKER WHO MAY POSE RISK TO PATIENTS. *An internist is caring for an HIV-infected gynecologist. The gynecologist reveals that he does not follow infection control precautions strictly, continuing to work even if he has cuts or dermatitis. Because he takes highly active antiretroviral therapy, which reduces the level of HIV antigen in the blood, he does not believe that he is contagious. The gynecologist has a mild neuropathy, most likely caused by HIV infection or antiretroviral therapy. Unable to convince the gynecologist to change his practice, the internist wonders whether she should take any further steps to protect the gynecologist's patients, such as talking to the chief of the medical staff.*

A reasonable balance needs to be set between the interests of seropositive health care workers and the interests of patients. If seropositive health care workers observe infection control precautions, have no physical or mental impairment, and eliminate exposure-prone invasive procedures, their rights prevail over the extremely small risk to patients. However, if precautions are violated or impairment is present, the risk to patients is increased and warrants restrictions on practice. In Case 43.3, silence by the internist would place patients at risk, undermine public trust in the profession, and fuel demands that HIV-infected health care workers refrain from all patient care. Public health regulations should clarify that seropositive health care workers that perform exposure-prone invasive procedures need to be reported to state officials if they are impaired or do not follow infection control guidelines.

In conclusion, the HIV epidemic polarizes society. Those who view themselves as potential unsuspecting victims seek to reduce their risk by testing others and restricting those who are seropositive. However, there is increasingly strong evidence that the risk of transmission during invasive procedures from seropositive health care workers to patients is very low. Policies to protect patients from harm must also respect the privacy of infected health care workers and protect them from unwarranted discrimination.

REFERENCES

1. Barringer F. AIDS from a healer, scorn from others. *New York Times*, February 9, 1991:A1.
2. Golden T. Dental patient torn by AIDS calls for laws. *New York Times*, June 22, 1991:A5.
3. CDC. Public health service guidelines for management of health care worker exposures to HIV and recommendations for postexposure prophylaxis. *MMWR* 1998:47(RR-7):1–33.
4. National Commission on AIDS. *Preventing HIV transmission in health care settings*. Washington, DC: National Commission on AIDS, 1992.
5. CDC. Recommendations for preventing transmission of human immunodeficiency virus and hepatitis B virus to patients during exposure-prone invasive procedures. *MMWR* 1991;40:1–9.
6. Ou CY, Ciesielski CA, Myers G, et al. Molecular epidemiology of HIV transmission in a dental practice. *Science* 1992;256:1165–1171.
7. Institut de Veille Sanitaire. Transmission du VIH à une patiente par un chiruigien infecte. www.rnsp-sante.fr/publications/sida2/chirugien. January 21, 1998.
8. Robert LM, Chamberland ME, Cleveland JL, et al. Investigations of patients of health care workers infected with HIV. The Centers for Disease Control and Prevention database. *Ann Intern Med* 1995;122:653–657.
9. AIDS/TB Committee of the Society for Healthcare Epidemiology of America. Management of healthcare workers infected with hepatitis B virus, hepatitis C virus, human immunodeficiency virus, or other bloodborne pathogens. *Infect Control Hosp Epidemiology* 1997;18:349–363.
10. Lo B, Steinbrook R. Health care workers infected with the human immunodeficiency virus: the next steps. *JAMA* 1992;267:1000–1005.
11. National Research Council. *Improving risk communication*. Washington, DC: National Academy Press, 1989.
12. Nelkin D. Communicating technological risk: the social construction of risk perception. *Annu Rev Public Health* 1989;10:95–113.
13. Slovic P. Perception of risk. *Science* 1987;236:280–285.
14. Appelbaum PS, Lidz CW, Meisel A. *Informed consent: legal theory and clinical practice*. New York: Oxford University Press, 1987.
15. Gerbert B, Maguire BT, Hulley SB, et al. Physicians and the acquired immunodeficiency syndrome. *JAMA* 1989;262:1969–1972.
16. Daniels N. HIV-infected professionals, patient rights, and the "switching dilemma." *JAMA* 1992;267:1368–1371.
17. Gostin L. The HIV-infected health care professional: public policy, discrimination, and patient safety. *Law Med Health Care* 1990;18:303–310.
18. Elovitz ME. Why the debate on restricting health care workers with HIV should end: a response to Professor Closen. *NY Law School Rev* 1996;41:141–149.
19. Barnes M, Rango NA, Burke GR, et al. The HIV-infected health care professional: employment policies and public health. *Law Med Health Care* 1990;18:311–330.
20. CDC. Revised recommendations for preventing transmission of human immunodeficiency virus and hepatitis B virus to patients during exposure-prone invasive procedures. *MMWR* 1991;40:1–9.
21. Treasury, Postal and General Government Appropriations Act of 1992 (effective October 28, 1991).
22. Danila R, Chelstrom L, O'Boyle C. Management of the health care worker with a bloodborne pathogen—1998. Presentation at expert panel meeting, Centers for Disease Control and Prevention, 1998.
23. American College of Surgeons. The surgeon and HIV infection—a statement.
24. National Research Council. *Improving risk communication*. Washington, DC: National Academy Press, 1989: 96–100.
25. Bell DM, Shapiro CN, Culver DH, et al. Risk of hepatitis B and human immunodeficiency virus transmission to a patient from an infected surgeon due to percutaneous injury during an invasive procedure: estimates based on a model. *Infect Agents Dis* 1992;1:263–269.

ANNOTATED BIBLIOGRAPHY

1. Lo B, Steinbrook R. Health care workers infected with the human immunodeficiency virus: the next steps. *JAMA* 1992;267:1000–1005.
   This article discusses ethical and policy issues regarding transmission of HIV from infected health care workers to patients and describes the 1991 CDC guidelines.
2. AIDS/TB Committee of the Society for Healthcare Epidemiology of America. Management of healthcare workers infected with hepatitis B virus, hepatitis C virus, human immunodeficiency virus, or other bloodborne pathogens. *Infect Control Hosp Epidemiol* 1997;18:349–363.
   Summary of current knowledge about transmission of bloodborne infections from health care workers to patients, together with policy recommendations.
3. Centers for Disease Control and Prevention. www.cdc.gov/nchstp/hiv_aids
   Website gives latest epidemiological information, together with CDC recommendations.

44

Ethical Issues
in Organ Transplantation

Kidney, heart, and liver transplantation may allow patients with end-stage disease to return to active lives, yet the need for organ transplantation far exceeds the supply of donated organs. In 1998, over 21,000 Americans received a solid organ transplant (1). Over 60,000 persons were on the waiting list for organ transplants at the end of 1998, a fourfold increase over 1988 (1). Each year over 4000 patients die while waiting for a transplant (1). This chapter discusses ethical dilemmas regarding the donation of organs, the selection of recipients, and the cost of transplantation.

DONATION OF ORGANS

Ethical Concerns about Donation

In organ donation, interventions are performed on one patient in order to benefit another person. The ethical guideline of nonmaleficence is violated if donation harms donors or hastens their death. The goal of care for donors should be their well-being. This focus not only protects donors but also maintains public trust that physicians never compromise the care of one patient in order to benefit another. This potential conflict of interest between the donor and transplant recipient can be addressed in several ways. First, there must be informed consent from a living donor or permission from an appropriate surrogate of a cadaveric donor. Second, the risks to donors must be circumscribed. Persons may not serve as living donors if they have medical conditions that significantly increase operative risk or, in the case of kidney donation, might impair renal function in the future. Third, the determination of death in cadaveric donors must be accurate. Unpaired organs may not be removed from patients who are not dead. Fourth, physicians must avoid even the perception of conflicts of interest. Decisions about the care of the potential donor must be separate from decisions about procurement and transplantation. The physician for the potential donor may not be part of the transplantation team.

The Current System for Donation

The United States has a voluntary system for organ donation, based on the ethical guidelines of respecting patient autonomy and fostering altruism. The Uniform Anatomical Gift Act allows persons to donate their organs for transplantation. Persons may complete an organ donor card giving permission to use their organs for transplantation after their death. Usually this card is attached to the driver's license. Only 13% to 28% of Americans have signed donor cards (2). One reason for such low rates is fear that patients who have consented to organ donation will receive suboptimal care (2). Although the donor card can be legally binding, in practice permission for organ donation is sought from the next of kin after the donor's death (3). Only about one-half of relatives of patients with brain death give permission for organ donation (2). Many families do not understand the concept of brain death, and some perceive the organ procurement process as insensitive (2). In some cultures, donating organs would be unthinkable (4,5). For instance, some Asian or Latino families may believe that bodies or spirits can suffer after death if organs are removed.

Because the supply of donated organs does not meet the need for transplantation, several policies recently have been adopted (2).

Required Request Laws

About one-fourth of families of eligible donors are not offered the opportunity to donate organs (1). Hospitals are now required to refer eligible families to local Organ Procurement Organizations (OPOs) and to ensure that they are given an opportunity to donate organs (6). The rationale is that more families would volunteer to donate organs if they were offered the opportunity to do so. However, such laws have had little impact on donations.

Routine Notification Laws

Hospitals now must also notify their local OPO of all deaths. The OPO can then contact eligible families to offer them the opportunity to donate (1).

Greater Use of Live Donors

"Emotionally related donors," including spouses, friends, and relatives by marriage, have donated kidneys and portions of livers and lungs (7). With kidney transplantation, outcomes are as good as parental donors and better than cadaveric donors (8). Sacrifices for the benefit of another person are generally considered morally good and commendable (9), yet misgivings persist about performing an operation on a healthy person for the benefit of another person (10). In addition, consent may be problematical because relatives may feel that they cannot refuse to donate (9).

Broadening the Criteria for Acceptable Cadaver Donors

Liberalized criteria allow kidney donors to be older and have diabetes and hypertension. By 1996, donors over age 50 years comprised over one-fourth of cadaver donors (2). However, expanding the donor pool lowers graft and recipient survival (2).

Harvesting Organs from Non-Heart-Beating Cadaver Donors

Such donors are declared dead by cardiorespiratory criteria. In contrast, most cadaver donors are declared dead by brain criteria and have beating hearts. With non-heart-beating cadaver donors, organs may be damaged during the time between declaration of death and retrieval of the organs. Two approaches to this problem have been carried out in a small number of cases (2,11,12).

In one approach, donors are patients on whom life-sustaining interventions will be withdrawn. They are transported to the operating room, where life support is withdrawn, death declared using cardiorespiratory criteria, and organs promptly retrieved. This approach has been criticized for several reasons (2,11–13). First, the definition of death may be manipulated. The cardiopulmonary criterion for death is irreversible cessation of circulatory and respiratory functions (*see* Chapter 22). It is controversial how long cessation must be before it can be termed irreversible, and there are pressures to make the determination as early as possible to maintain organ function. Second, anticoagulants and vasodilators may be administered to preserve the organs, and these drugs might hasten or cause death. Third, families may not have sufficient opportunity to be with dying patients.

In a second approach, potential non-heart-beating donors are patients in whom cardiopulmonary resuscitation fails or who are dead on arrival in the emergency department. Catheters are inserted into patients immediately after death is pronounced, and organs are perfused to keep them viable (11,12). Later, permission for transplantation is sought from relatives. This approach has been criticized because consent may not be obtained for insertion of catheters and perfusion of organs (2,12). Surveys show that the public strongly objects to such procedures being carried out without consent. Another criticism is that the vigor and duration of resuscitation attempts may be questioned (2,12).

Proposals to Increase the Donation of Organs

Mandated Choice

Individuals would be required to state their preferences regarding organ donation when renewing drivers' licenses, filing income taxes, or some other official task (14). This requirement would relieve relatives of the stress of making decisions about donation. In surveys, the vast majority of Americans support this policy.

Following Donor Cards

Physicians would retrieve organs from individuals who had signed donor cards, even if the next of kin objects. Legally, this policy would merely implement existing statutes. Ethically, it is consistent with respecting patient autonomy and advance directives.

Presumed Consent

Currently, organs are harvested only if the patient or family has given explicit consent. Under this proposed policy, organs would be harvested unless the patient or family specifically objects (15). However, fully 52% of respondents in a U.S. survey disapproved of presumed consent (16).

Changing the Definition of Death

Some advocate changing the definition of death to include adults in a persistent vegetative state or anencephalic infants in order to increase the number of potential organ donors (17). As discussed in Chapter 22, however, such changes would lead to serious problems.

Financial Incentives for Donation

In the United States, buying and selling of organs is illegal. There are proposals to pay donors or their families for organs or to pay funeral expenses (18). Pennsylvania adopted legislation to provide modest financial assistance to donor families for funeral costs (19). Critics charge that such proposals undermine altruism, treat organs as a commodity, and would result in exploitation, fraud, or coercion (20). Furthermore, commercially motivated renal transplantation in developing countries has a significantly higher rate of human immunodeficiency virus and hepatitis B infection (21).

Many of these proposals to increase the supply of organs may undermine trust in transplantation. The public may fear that physicians would shorten the lives of seriously ill patients or retrieve organs before patients are really dead. In the long term, such fears may make people less willing to donate and thereby worsen the shortage of organs.

SELECTION OF RECIPIENTS

Because the number of people needing transplants far exceeds the number of donated organs, difficult decisions about allocating organs are unavoidable.

Historical Background

When dialysis was first developed in the 1960s, selection of patients posed allocation dilemmas. At that time, committees assigned the limited number of dialysis machines according to the perceived social worth of candidates (22). Critics charged that some allocation decisions were based on prejudice and unwarranted value judgments. In response, Congress decided to fund the care of all patients with end-stage renal disease; the allocation problem was resolved by providing unlimited funding for renal dialysis. In transplantation, however, the limiting factor is a lack of organs, not funding.

Because people donate cadaveric organs without knowing who will receive them, a fair allocation procedure is essential to maintain public faith in transplantation (20,23). In the United States, rules for allocating cadaveric organs are set by the federal government and the United Network for Organ Sharing (UNOS), a nonprofit organization with whom the government contracts to operate the system for distributing organs.

Specific selection criteria are too detailed to be discussed here (1,6,24). The main ethical considerations are medical benefit and justice (25,26). Different considerations receive priority for different organs.

Beneficence

From a utilitarian perspective, scarce organs should go to those patients who will receive the greatest net medical benefit. Relevant factors include the likelihood and duration of survival and improvement in the patient's quality of life. Although this criterion appears objective, it actually involves complex value judgments. For example, if a subgroup of patients has a 20% lower 1-year graft survival rate than other patients, should they have lower priority for transplantation? Similarly, what probability of failure should disqualify a candidate as a recipient (27)?

Psychosocial factors such as poor adherence to medical regimens, substance abuse, and lack of family support may compromise outcomes of transplantation. Recent injection drug use and a history of nonadherence are commonly regarded as contraindications to transplantation (28–30). It seems pointless to transplant a scarce organ if it would be rejected because of nonadherence to immunosuppression drugs. Critics, however, contend that psychosocial factors might "cloak biases about race, class, social status, and other factors that, if stated openly, would not be tolerated" (23). Furthermore, such obstacles might be overcome with rehabilitation and psychosocial support (26).

Justice

The guideline that scarce resources should be distributed fairly or equitably is indisputable in the abstract but difficult to operationalize.

Time on the Waiting List

The precept of first-come, first-served seems intuitively fair if there are no other compelling reasons to distinguish among candidates. However, time on the waiting list can be manipulated by putting patients on the waiting list earlier in their illness (31) or by placing patients on the waiting list at several regional transplantation networks (20,32). Better educated and wealthier patients are more likely to be on multiple waiting lists.

Medical Urgency

In liver and heart transplantation, patients who would die soon without transplantation are given priority over more stable patients (24). This practice is justified by the maxim of assisting those in greatest need.

Ability to Pay

Transplantation is generally performed only on patients who can pay for it. Kidney transplantation is covered for all Americans by Medicare. For other transplantation procedures, however, coverage depends on the patient's insurance. Most private insurers and most state Medicaid programs cover liver and heart transplantation (33). For the 45 million Americans who lack health insurance, transplantation of organs other than kidneys is impossible unless they raise money, as through public appeals.

Allocating organs by ability to pay, although routinely practiced, has been strongly criticized (20). It seems unfair to ask all people, rich and poor alike, to be organ donors, if the poor or uninsured may not be eligible to receive a transplant. Also people may be less willing to donate organs if they perceive that the distribution system favors the wealthy. In a public opinion poll, only 8% of respondents agreed that persons who can afford transplantation should have priority (34).

Directed Donation

Patients may appeal to the public for an organ to be donated to them, rather than to the community pool. Critics contend that such designated donations undermine fairness by making an exception to rules that apply to other candidates (35,36).

Previous Transplantation

The success rate in transplanting a second organ after a transplanted organ fails is substantially lower than in first-time transplants (37). The guideline of promise-keeping or loyalty is often used to justify retransplantation: having made a commitment to the patient, the surgeons cannot now abandon her. Critics contend, however, that retransplantation may be "an obdurate, publicly theatricalized refusal" to accept the inevitable limits of human life and an unwillingness to say "enough is enough" (38).

Citizenship

Should people who are not long-term U.S. residents receive organs harvested in the United States (20)? Particular objections have been directed at foreigners who come to the United States specifically to obtain a transplant. It seems unfair, however, to exclude foreign nationals who contribute to the U.S. economy and would be asked to serve as organ donors.

Geographic Location

In response to significant disparities in waiting times for liver transplantation, it has been proposed that organs be allocated on a national basis to those with greatest medical need, with less emphasis on keeping organs in the geographic area where they are donated (39). This proposed change would provide more organs to large referral centers, which have sicker patients and better outcomes. However, opponents object that such geographical redistribution is unfair because it penalizes states that make efforts to increase donations (1).

Ethnic Background

African-Americans have less access to renal transplantation. They are less likely to be placed on waiting lists and are placed on the waiting lists less promptly as Caucasians (40). Furthermore, once on a waiting list, African-Americans do not receive transplants as promptly (40), even after immunological and demographic factors are taken into account (32). African-Americans are unlikely to be compatible with Caucasian donors because the prevalence of ABO and HLA antigens differs in the two ethnic groups. African-Americans are less likely to donate organs than Caucasians (41); this reluctance may be due to distrust of the medical establishment or to religious beliefs. Furthermore, African-Americans are more pessimistic about the outcomes of transplantation and more likely to have religious objections to transplantation or uneasiness at having a dead person's organs (42).

Conflicts between Guidelines for Organ Allocation

The ethical guidelines of beneficence and justice are balanced differently for different organs (24). For renal failure, dialysis is an effective alternative to transplantation, and HLA matching is a strong predictor of graft survival. Hence HLA matching is given most weight, and urgency is not considered. In contrast, in liver failure, because there is no alternative to transplantation, the highest priority is given to patients in the most critical condition. HLA matching is not considered because it has little impact on outcomes.

Different ethical considerations may conflict. For example, liver recipients with the most urgent need have worse outcomes and greater costs than more stable patients.

The Ambiguity of the Gift Relationship

The "gift of life" entails obligations and burdens (43). The gift of an organ is so extraordinary that it can never be repaid and may therefore become a "tyranny" (43). A live kidney donor may take a "proprietary interest" in the life of the recipient (43). The recipient's sense of indebtedness may make it difficult for him to remain independent of the donor.

These insights help explain two common procedures by transplantation teams. If a prospective live donor is deemed unsuitable for psychosocial reasons, they may be told they are not "compatible" with the recipient. Such misrepresentation is felt to be justified because pressure to donate, recrimination, and guilt might occur if the true reason were known (43). A second common practice is not to reveal the identities of donors and recipients to each other. Some programs have found that recipients, their kin, and donor families "become involved in each other's lives as if they were indebted and related to one another" (43).

Patient Behaviors that Cause Disease

Patients with end-stage alcohol-related liver disease initially were not considered for transplantation because it was believed that they would continue to drink and would not take immunosuppressive medications regularly. However, alcoholics who receive liver transplantation have survival rates comparable to those of patients with other liver diseases (44). Thus the issue is not whether such transplantation is medically feasible, but whether it should be done. One concern is the large number of persons with end-stage alcohol-related liver disease (45). Over 30,000 persons develop end-stage alcohol-related liver disease, far greater than the approximately 6000 organs donated each year. An additional argument for limiting transplantation in alcoholics is that patients who develop end-stage liver disease "through no fault of their own" should have higher priority (45). In this line of thinking, patients should be held responsible for behaviors that would deprive others of scarce resources. Others argue that the public may be less willing to donate organs if they are given to alcoholics.

On the other hand, restrictions on liver transplantation for alcoholics have been strongly criticized (46). Critics argue that because alcoholism has genetic and environmental components that are beyond the control of the individual, it would be unfair to hold people responsible for it. Furthermore, judgments of moral responsibility are not made for other illnesses. For example, smokers are not precluded from heart transplants. Moreover, investigations into the personal habits of potential recipients would be unworkable as well as intrusive.

COST OF TRANSPLANTATION

Because of the soaring cost of medical care, the cost effectiveness of organ transplantation cannot be ignored. In 1996, average billed charges for a kidney transplant were $94,000, for a liver transplant $290,000, and for a heart transplant $228,000 (39). Subsequent follow-up charges average $16,000 a year for kidneys and between $21,000 and $29,000 for liver, heart, and lung (39). The costs of transplantation need to be put in the context of other high-technology medical interventions. Hemodialysis costs $25,000 per year per case, and cancer chemotherapy costs $30,000 per year per case (33).

The cost of organ transplantation must also be viewed in the context of allocating resources in a health care system that denies many individuals access to basic care. Critics charge that "allowing ourselves to become too caught up in such problems as the shortage of transplantable organs while . . . millions of people do not have adequate or even minimally decent care, speaks to a values framework and a vision of medical progress that we find medically and morally untenable" (43).

In summary, organ transplantation can return patients with end-stage illness to active lives, yet transplantation raises difficult issues of informed choice in donation and fair allocation of scarce resources. These fundamental dilemmas will undoubtedly continue to generate difficult controversies.

REFERENCES

1. Committee on Organ Procurement and Transplantation Policy. *Organ procurement and transplantation: assessing current policies and the potential impact of the HHS final rule.* Washington, DC: National Academy Press, 1999.

2. Herdman R, Potts JT. *Non-heart-beating organ transplantation: medical and ethical issues in procurement.* Washington, DC: National Academy Press, 1997.
3. Spital A. The shortage of organs for transplantation: where do we go from here. *N Engl J Med* 1991;325: 1243–1246.
4. Perkins HS. Cultural differences and ethical issues in the problem of autopsy requests. *Tex Med* 1991;87:72–77.
5. Tolle SW, Bennett WM, Hickam DH, et al. Responsibilities of primary physicians in organ donation. *Ann Intern Med* 1987;106:740–744.
6. United States General Accounting Office. *Organ transplants: increased effort needed to boost supply and ensure equitable distribution of organs.* Washington, DC: US General Accounting Office, 1993:46–48.
7. Spital A. Ethical and policy issues in altruistic living and cadaveric organ donation. *Clin Transplant* 1997;11: 77–87.
8. Terasaki PI, Cecka JM, Gjertson DW, et al. High survival rates of kidney transplants from spousal and living unrelated donors. *N Engl J Med* 1995;333:333–336.
9. Caplan A. Must I be my brother's keeper? Ethical issues in the use of living donors as sources of liver and other solid organs. *Transplant Proc* 1991;25:1997–2000.
10. Sheil AGR. Ethics in organ transplantation: the major issues. *Transplant Proc* 1995;27:87–89.
11. Youngner SJ, Arnold RM. Ethical, psychosocial, and public policy implications of procuring organs from non-heart beating cadaver donors. *JAMA* 1993;269:2769–2774.
12. Institute of Medicine. *Non-heart-beating organ transplantation: protocols and practice.* Washington, DC: National Academy Press, 1999.
13. Youngner SJ, Arnold RM, Schapiro R, eds. *The definition of death.* Baltimore: Johns Hopkins University Press, 1999.
14. Council on Ethical and Judicial Affairs of the American Medical Association. Strategies for cadaveric organ procurement: mandated choice and presumed consent. *JAMA* 1994;272:809–812.
15. Kennedy I, Daar AS, Sells RA, et al. The case for "presumed consent" in organ donation. *Lancet* 1998;351: 1650–1652.
16. Kittur DS, Hogan MM, Thukral VK, et al. Incentives for organ donation? *Lancet* 1991;338:1441–1443.
17. Hoffenberg R, Lock M, Tilney N, et al. Should organs from patients in permanent vegetative state be used for transplantation? *Lancet* 1997;350:1320–1321.
18. Radcliffe-Richards J, Daar AS, Guttmann RD, et al. The case for allowing kidney sales. *Lancet* 1998;352: 1950–1952.
19. Stolberg SG. Pennsylvania set to break taboo on reward for organ donations. *New York Times*, May 6, 1999:A1.
20. Childress JF. Ethical criteria for procuring and distributing organs for transplantation. *J Health Politics Policy Law* 1989;14:87–113.
21. The Living Non-Related Renal Transplant Study Group. Commercially motivated renal transplantation: results in 540 patients transplanted in India. *Clin Transplant* 1997;11:536–544.
22. Fox RC, Swazey JP. *The courage to fail: a social view of organ transplants and dialysis*, 2nd ed. Chicago: University of Chicago Press, 1978.
23. Robertson JA. Patient selection for organ transplantation: age, incarceration, family support, and other social factors. *Transplant Proc* 1989;21:3431–3436.
24. Hauptmann PK, O'Connor KJ. Procurement and allocation of solid organs for transplantation. *N Engl J Med* 1997;336:422–431.
25. The UNOS statement of principles and objectives of equitable organ allocation. *Semin Anesth* 1995;14:142–166.
26. Council on Ethical and Judicial Affairs of the American Medical Association. Ethical considerations in the allocation of organs and other scarce medical resources among patients. *Arch Intern Med* 1995;155:29–40.
27. Monaco AP. Comment: a transplant surgeon views on social factors in organ transplantation. *Transplant Proc* 1989;21:3403–3416.
28. Evans RW, Manninen DL, Dong FB, et al. Heart transplantation recipient and donor selection criteria: the results of a consensus survey. In: Evans RW, Manninen DL, Dong FB, eds. *The National Cooperative Transplantation Study: final report.* Seattle: Battelle-Seattle Research Center, 1991:31-1–31-24.
29. Evans RW, Manninen DL, Dong FB, et al. Kidney transplantation recipient and donor selection criteria: the results of a consensus survey. In: Evans RW, Manninen DL, Dong FB, eds. *The National Cooperative Transplantation Study: final report.* Seattle: Battelle-Seattle Research Center, 1991:30-1–30-24.
30. Evans RW, Manninen DL, Dong FB, et al. Liver transplantation recipient and donor selection criteria: the results of a consensus survey. In: Evans RW, Manninen DL, Dong FB, eds. *The National Cooperative Transplantation Study: final report.* Seattle: Battelle-Seattle Research Center, 1991:32-1–32-24.
31. Jonasson O. Waiting in line: should selected patients ever be moved up? *Transplant Proc* 1989;21:3390–3394.
32. Sanfilippo FP, Vaughn WK, Peters TG, et al. Factors affecting the waiting time of cadaveric kidney transplant candidates in the United States. *JAMA* 1992;267:247–252.
33. Evans RW. Organ transplantation costs, insurance coverage, and reimbursement. In: Terasaki PI, ed. *Clinical transplants 1990.* Los Angeles: UCLA Tissue Typing Laboratory, 1990:343–352.
34. Evans RW. Public attitudes towards transplant recipient selection. In: Evans RW, Manninen DL, Dong FB, eds. *The National Cooperative Transplantation Study: final report.* Seattle: Battelle-Seattle Research Center, 1991: 35-1–35-16.
35. Boisaubin EV. Charity, the media, and limited medical resources. *JAMA* 1988;259:1375–1376.
36. Kluge EH. Designated organ donation: private choice in social context. *Hastings Center Rep* 1989;19:10–16.
37. Ubel PA, Arnold RM, Caplan AL. Rationing failure: the ethical lessons of the retransplantation of scarce organs. *JAMA* 1993;270:2469–2474.

38. Fox RC, Swazey JP. *Spare parts*. New York: Oxford University Press, 1992: 204–205.
39. Department of Health and Human Services. Organ Procurement and Transplantation Network; Final Rule. 42 CFR Part 121.
40. Alexander CG, Sehgal AR. Barriers to cadaveric renal transplantation among blacks, women, and the poor. *JAMA* 1998;280:1148–1152.
41. Callender CO, Hall LE, Yeager CL, et al. Organ donation and blacks: a critical frontier. *N Engl J Med* 1991;325: 442–444.
42. Ozminkowski RJ, White AJ, Hassol A, et al. Minimizing racial disparity regarding receipt of a cadaver kidney transplant. *Am J Kid Dis* 1997;30:749–759.
43. Fox RC, Swazey JP. *Spare parts*. New York: Oxford University Press, 1992:31–42, 208–209.
44. Kumar S, Stauber RE, Gavaler JS, et al. Orthotopic liver transplantation for alcoholic liver disease. *Hepatology* 1990;11:159–164.
45. Moss AH, Siegler M. Should alcoholics compete equally for liver transplantation? *JAMA* 1991;265:1295–1298.
46. Cohen C, Benjamin M, the Ethics and Social Impact Committee of the Transplant and Health Policy Center. Alcoholics and liver transplantation. *JAMA* 1991;265:1299–1301.

ANNOTATED BIBLIOGRAPHY

1. Council on Ethical and Judicial Affairs of the American Medical Association. Ethical considerations in the allocation of organs and other scarce medical resources among patients. *Arch Intern Med* 1995;155:29–40.
   Overview of the topic.
2. Committee on Organ Procurement and Transplantation Policy. *Organ procurement and transplantation: assessing current policies and the potential impact of the HHS final rule.* Washington, DC: National Academy Press, 1999.
   Review of proposed federal regulations to improve allocation of scarce organs (particularly livers) for transplantation.
3. Institute of Medicine. *Non-heart-beating organ transplantation: protocols and practice.* Washington, DC: National Academy Press, 1999.
   Analysis of protocols to harvest organs from patients who are declared dead by cardiorespiratory criteria rather than brain death criteria.
4. Cohen C, Benjamin M, the Ethics and Social Impact Committee of the Transplant and Health Policy Center. Alcoholics and liver transplantation. *JAMA* 1991;265:1299–1301.
   Moss AH, Siegler M. Should alcoholics compete equally for liver transplantation? *JAMA* 1991;265:1295–1298.
   These articles argue respectively for and against liver transplants in alcoholics.

45

Testing for Genetic Conditions

The Human Genome Project is a $3 billion initiative to sequence all human chromosomes. The ultimate goal is to develop tests and therapies for a variety of genetic illnesses. For some genetic diseases, such as sickle cell anemia, phenylketonuria, and Tay-Sachs disease, screening tests have been available for years. DNA-based testing has recently become available for such conditions as cystic fibrosis (CF), familial colon and breast cancer, Alzheimer's disease, hemochromatosis, and polycystic kidney disease.

It is important to distinguish testing for predisposition to adult-onset genetic diseases from carrier screening and prenatal testing. In adult-onset conditions, DNA testing raises dilemmas about what further diagnostic and therapeutic interventions are appropriate for the person being tested. In contrast, carrier screening has no therapeutic implications for the persons tested but may affect reproductive decision-making and the clinical care of children. This chapter focuses on genetic testing for adult-onset conditions.

With ongoing advances in molecular genetics, physicians in all specialties will increasingly be asked to advise patients about genetic testing. This chapter discusses important ethical issues in screening for genetic diseases. These include the clinical limitations of DNA-based screening tests, genetic discrimination, informed consent for genetic testing, and confidentiality of test results.

WHEN IS DNA-BASED GENETIC TESTING APPROPRIATE?

DNA-based testing for CF and inherited breast cancer illustrate the usefulness and limitations in DNA-based testing. The benefits and risks of testing will change as more knowledge about the condition is gained.

Cystic Fibrosis

CF is a common autosomal recessive condition. About 1 in 25 Caucasians are asymptomatic carriers of CF, and the disease occurs in about 850 homozygous infants born in the United States each year.

Multiple Alleles

Because more than 600 alleles are capable of causing CF, some carriers will not be identified by screening. The most common mutation accounts for about 70% of carriers in Caucasians. If 95% of mutations could be detected, 90% of couples at risk for bearing a child with CF could be identified. Current DNA-based tests for CF have a sensitivity of 90% in Caucasians, but a lower sensitivity in other groups (1).

Variable Expressivity of the Gene

Affected homozygotes for CF have a spectrum of clinical disease. Identification of the specific mutation in a homozygous individual has not been highly predictive of the severity of clinical pulmonary disease (1).

The prognosis of CF has improved substantially with recent advances in treatment. Most children who are homozygous for CF usually lead active, healthy lives into young adulthood. Hence, although DNA-based testing has become more sensitive, it has met limited public acceptance, except for prenatal testing and testing of individuals with a family history of CF (1).

Susceptibility to Breast Cancer

About 5% to 10% of cases of breast cancer are inherited in an autosomal-dominant manner. BRCA1 and BRCA2 are genes for susceptibility to breast cancer. In families with a high incidence of breast and ovarian cancer, mutations in BRCA1 are associated with a 85% lifetime risk of developing breast cancer and a 50% risk of ovarian cancer (2,3).

Lower Usefulness in Lower Risk Populations

Early longitudinal studies of the risk of BRCA1 mutations were carried out in women with strong family histories of early onset of breast and ovarian cancer. When testing was later offered to lower risk women who do not meet these strict criteria, the prevalence of BRCA1 mutations was found to be much lower than in the highly selected populations studied earlier (4,5). Hence early studies on highly selected populations may overestimate the yield of testing in a more general population,

False-Negative and False-Positive Results

Women with negative tests for BRCA1 may still be at increased risk. The clinical significance of a negative BRCA1 test usually is known only if a mutation has been identified in a family member with cancer. If no such family member can be identified, a negative result in an unaffected member may mean that a mutation was not detected by the test used or that the pattern of illness in the family is not caused by a BRCA1 mutation. Hence population-based screening may lead to many inconclusive results. Conversely, some BRCA1 polymorphisms may not be associated with an increased risk of cancer. In addition, the functional significance of many mutations is not worked out until long after they are identified.

Lack of Effective Prevention

Reliable tests for adult-onset genetic conditions will generally be available before effective preventive measures are discovered. Commercial tests for BRCA1 were available several years before studies found that prophylactic bilateral mastectomy may reduce short-term mortality (6). If future studies demonstrate convincingly that less drastic interventions, such as prophylaxis with selective estrogen receptor blockers, reduce the long-term incidence of breast cancer, there would be stronger reasons for BRCA1 testing.

The primary benefit of genetic testing in many adult-onset conditions will be to reassure those who are unaffected and to suggest increased surveillance for affected persons. In other clinical situations, earlier diagnosis alone is not considered a justification for population screening for risk factors. Instead, screening tests are recommended only if diagnosis and treatment in the presymptomatic stage have been shown convincingly to result in better outcomes than therapy initiated after the condition becomes symptomatic (7).

GENETIC DISCRIMINATION

Screening for genetic disorders may lead to stigmatization and discrimination. Persons susceptible to adult-onset genetic conditions may regard themselves, or be regarded by others, as impaired, unwhole, or flawed, even though they are healthy. Furthermore, stigmatization may result from the belief that it is "irresponsible and immoral for people who could transmit disability to their offspring to reproduce" (8). Persons with asymptomatic genetic abnormalities have been reported to suffer discrimination in employment or health insurance (8–12).

Because of past abuses in the United States, fears of discrimination resulting from genetic testing cannot be dismissed. In the early 1900's, eugenic laws were passed forbidding marriage or mandating sterilization of categories of persons deemed unfit, such as the feebleminded, insane, or certain criminals (13). During the 1970's, many states enacted sickle cell anemia screening programs that contained "blatant medical and scientific errors," including calling sickle cell anemia an infectious or sexually transmitted disease and confusing sickle cell disease with the trait (8). Persons with sickle cell trait, who have no impairment and no increased risk for disease, were denied employment, health insurance, and schooling. In addition, accusations of genocide were made, because many programs targeted African-Americans (14).

Insurers

In the current U.S. health care system, health and life insurance companies face pressures to use genetic testing to identify persons at risk and to avoid adverse selection. Patients who learn that they are at risk for genetic diseases naturally want to be well insured. Insurers argue that if they cannot identify such high-risk individuals, they would lose money by selling coverage at relatively low rates to individuals who know they are at increased risk for future illness. Insurers therefore want to know any pertinent medical information that the applicant knows. Insurers often refuse to insure individuals at risk for genetic diseases, exclude genetic diseases from coverage, or set prohibitive premiums. In response to such concerns, several states have prohibited genetic discrimination in health insurance (10).

Widespread genetic testing may be incompatible with the current system of risk rating and exclusion of high-risk persons from coverage (15). With widespread genetic screening, more and more individuals will be found to be at risk for some genetic disease. If all such persons were effectively excluded from coverage, the very purpose of health insurance, to pay for health care when illness strikes, would be negated.

Employers

Employers also have incentives to utilize genetic screening. Excluding employees who are likely to become sick will increase future productivity and cut health insurance premiums. Employers may also want to identify workers at genetic risk for occupational diseases, because it may be cheaper to exclude such individuals from the workplace than to reduce occupational exposure.

Genetic testing, however, could be a tragedy for employees identified as at risk for adult-onset conditions (16). They may be unable to find employment, even if they are asymptomatic and able to work productively. In turn, they would be unable to obtain employment-linked health insurance. Several states have enacted legislation banning employment discrimination on the basis of genetic information (16).

A more optimistic view is that genetic testing may heighten so many problems with the health care system that it will spur improvements (15). None of the above barriers to coverage would occur under a system of universal health insurance and community risk rating.

Antidiscrimination Law

The Americans with Disabilities Act (ADA) bans discrimination against persons who have conditions that result in significant impairment or who are regarded as having a significant impairment. Under the ADA, preemployment medical inquiries and examinations are prohibited until after a job offer has been made. Results may not be used to exclude an applicant unless the "exclusion is shown to be job related, consistent with business necessity, and not amenable to reasonable accommodation" (17). In regulations to implement the ADA, the Equal Employment Opportunity Commission (EEOC) has stated that the ADA covers persons who have suffered discrimination based on genetic information, for example, because of a genetic predisposition to a disease (12). However, this issue has not been adjudicated by the courts. Furthermore, the EEOC advisory interpretation does not cover carriers of recessive or sex-linked genetic diseases (15).

We next discuss how physicians can take steps to maximize the benefits of genetic testing, while minimizing the risks.

INFORMED CONSENT

DNA-based genetic testing differs from most other blood tests because it has significant psychosocial risks (18). Stigma and discrimination may occur. Even if they are asymptomatic, persons found to be at risk for adult-onset illness may regard themselves as abnormal or be regarded as such by as family members, teachers, or employers. In addition, patients may experience psychological distress after learning either positive or negative test results; the distress is generally mild, however (19). Furthermore, genetic information may be considered more sensitive than other clinical information because it also provides information about relatives.

Importance of Informed Consent

Informed consent is particularly important for genetic testing because individuals will differ on whether the benefits of testing outweigh the risks. Some persons at risk will want more prognostic information, even if the significance is uncertain and no proven therapy is available. Others will decline testing because they do not perceive themselves to be vulnerable or are concerned about losing health insurance (20).

Truly informed consent for genetic testing will be difficult to achieve. Genetic concepts and probability are difficult to comprehend. Misunderstandings about genetic testing and the interpretation of results are widespread among health professionals and laypeople alike (21). The availability of multiplex testing, which allows the detection of several genetic disorders from a single blood sample, will further complicate consent.

Nondirective Genetic Counseling

Nondirectiveness has been a core tenet in genetic counseling. People interpret this term differently. Commonly it means that all sides of an issue are presented in an unbiased manner, that the counselor's personal views should not influence the client's decision, and that the client's or couple's decision is respected (22). Historically, the ideology of nondirectiveness developed as a reaction to the eugenic goals of early genetic counseling and from the desire to distance prenatal genetic diagnosis from controversies over abortion (23).

Recent empirical studies question whether counselors are in fact nondirective. In one study, although almost all genetic counselors viewed nondirectiveness as important, 28% said they sometimes were directive (22). Fifteen percent would recommend testing or screening to a client (22). In another study, genetic counselors gave advice an average of almost 6 times per session (24). However, clients did not object. Fewer than 20% of clients thought they were definitely being steered in a particular direction. There was no association between directiveness and client satisfaction with counseling. Other writers argue that even when counselors do not explicitly direct their clients, the selection of topics and information discussed is never value free (25). In their view, the ideology of nondirectiveness merely hides unavoidable value choices. Still other writers suggest that most problems with nondirectiveness could be solved through better communication skills (26). Often counselors can respond to clients' direct questions about what to do by expressing empathy and suggesting issues to think about in making the decision. Moreover, advice can be framed tentatively as a suggestion, rather than as a certainty.

The stance of nondirectiveness is ethically problematical for several reasons. First, the nondirective counselor is powerless if clients make a decision that is ethically troubling (23). For example, clients may decide not to inform relatives that they may also be at risk for a serious genetic condition. Second, in some situations, effective measures to prevent the development of genetic illness will be available. For the physician not to recommend such genetic tests, as they would other clinical tests that are clearly beneficial, would violate the ethical guideline of beneficence.

Recommendations

Because of the shortage of formally trained genetic counselors (27), physicians will need to help patients make decisions about genetic testing. Genetic testing should not be regarded as just an ordinary blood test, like a cholesterol level.

Provide Pretest Counseling and Education

Before testing is carried out, physicians need to discuss the limitations of testing and the psychological and social risks, including possible discrimination in employment or insurance. Requiring written informed consent may highlight for patients that genetic testing differs from other blood tests. Physicians should also provide pretest counseling, for example, asking patients what they would do if the test results were positive, negative, or inconclusive.

Make a Recommendation Regarding Testing

Physicians should make a recommendation regarding genetic testing for adult-onset conditions. These recommendations should be guided by both evidence-based medicine and the patient's values and situation. In some situations, genetic tests are highly predictive of future disease, and effective prevention is available. Doctors should recommend such tests, just as they would for nongenetic screening tests that are similarly beneficial. In other situations, genetic testing will provide little or no guidance for clinical decisions. Physicians should recommend against such testing, just as they would for low-yield nongenetic tests. However, some patients may still want testing even though the physician does not recommend it (28); their informed choices should be respected.

CONFIDENTIALITY

Genetic testing provides information about relatives as well as about the individual tested. DNA-based genetic testing may have more predictive power than other types of genetic information. Persons identified as having a predisposition to an adult-onset genetic illness have a moral duty to inform relatives who might also be at risk. Similarly, persons identified as carriers of an autosomal recessive condition have a moral duty to disclose such information to their partner or spouse when making reproductive decisions. An ethical dilemma can arise for physicians when the patient objects to informing relatives.

When is Overriding Confidentiality Justified?

The guidelines in Chapter 5 for overriding confidentiality can be applied in the context of genetic testing (27). Suppose a breast cancer patient with a strong family history of breast and ovarian cancer is found to have a mutation for BRCA1 but refuses to inform her relatives. The potential harm to identifiable third parties is serious, and the likelihood of harm is high. There is no less invasive means for warning relatives at risk, because the presence of a BRCA1 mutation in this setting has much greater predictive power than just the family history of cancer. Breaching confidentiality allows relatives at risk to take effective steps to prevent harm. Relatives can be tested for BRCA1 themselves. If positive, they can obtain mammograms at an earlier age and consider preventive interventions such as prophylactic bilateral mastectomy. Thus there are good reasons to override confidentiality in this situation (29). If estrogen receptor blockers are found to be effective in preventing cancer and improving survival, the reasons for overriding confidentiality would be even stronger. On the other hand, the harms to the proband resulting from the breach of confidentiality may also be substantial. In partner notification or contact tracing in infectious diseases, the identity of the index case can be withheld. However, in genetic testing, the identify of the proband can almost always be inferred. Furthermore, the person notified may be harmed if she feels that her privacy has been violated or does not want to know that she is at risk (30).

In other cases of genetic predisposition to adult-onset conditions, the predictive power of the test may be less or there may be no effective preventive measures. The case for overriding confidentiality then is much weaker. If there is no effective prophylaxis or treatment, confidentiality should not be overridden (29). In autosomal recessive conditions such as CF, there are no compelling reasons to override confidentiality. Relatives who may be carriers have no risk for illness, and their offspring will be at risk only if their partners are also carriers.

Recommendations

Discuss Disclosure During Pretest Counseling

Most dilemmas about disclosure to relatives and spouses can be prevented by discussing the importance of disclosure during informed consent for testing.

Urge Disclosure of Positive Results to Relatives or Spouses

Physicians should urge patients to disclose positive results to relatives or spouses when the information is pertinent. In this situation, nondirective counseling is highly problematical. Physicians can elicit patients' concerns about sharing test results and help them resolve those concerns. For example, patients who do not want to have contact with estranged relatives may be willing to have the physician contact the relatives.

Disclosure Against the Wishes of the Patient Should be a Last Resort

In some situations, as we have discussed, there may be compelling reasons to disclose results of genetic testing to relatives over the objections of the patient. Such disclosure should be done only as a last resort after attempts have failed to persuade the patient to allow notification and after the physician has told the patient that notification will occur and given her the option to notify relatives directly. Furthermore, if the person at risk has indicated that he would not want to know the information, these wishes should be respected.

In summary, physicians will increasingly be asked to help patients weigh the benefits and risks of genetic testing. Physicians have an obligation to learn about the new applications of molecular genetics to clinical medicine. In advising patients about genetic testing, physicians need to be aware of the clinical limitations of testing, the risk of discrimination, the importance of informed consent, and the need for confidentiality. Physicians as well as society as a whole can take steps to maximize the benefits and promise of genetic testing while minimizing the harms.

REFERENCES

1. National Institutes of Health Consensus Development Conference Statement on Genetic Testing for Cystic Fibrosis. Genetic testing for cystic fibrosis. *Arch Intern Med* 1999;159:1529–1539.
2. Collins FS. BRC1—lots of mutations, lots of dilemmas. *N Engl J Med* 1996;334:186–188.
3. Weber B. Breast cancer susceptibility genes: current challenges and future promises. *Ann Intern Med* 1996;124: 1088–1090.
4. Malone KE, Daling JR, Thompson JD, et al. BRCA1 mutations and breast cancer in the general population. *JAMA* 1998;279:922–929.
5. Newman B, Mu H, Butler L, et al. Frequency of breast cancer attributable to BRCA1 in a population-based series of American women. *JAMA* 1998;279:915–921.
6. Hartmann LC, Schaid DJ, Woods JE, et al. Efficacy of bilateral prophylactic mastectomy in women with a family history of breast cancer. *N Engl J Med* 1999;340:77–84.
7. U.S. Preventive Services Task Force. *Guide to clinical preventive services.* Baltimore: Williams & Wilkins, 1989.
8. U.S. Congress Office of Technology Assessment. *Cystic fibrosis and DNA tests: implications of carrier screening.* Washington, DC: U.S. Government Printing Office, 1992:128–129.
9. Billings PR, Kohn MA, De Cuevas M, et al. Discrimination as a consequence of genetic testing. *Am J Hum Genet* 1992;50:476–482.
10. Hudson KL, Rothenberg KH, Andrews LB, et al. Genetic discrimination and health insurance: an urgent need for reform. *Science* 1995;270:391–393.
11. Lapham EV, Kozma C, Weiss JO. Genetic discrimination: perspectives of consumers. *Science* 1996;274:621–624.
12. Miller PS. Genetic discrimination in the workplace. *J Law Med Ethics* 1998;26:189–197.
13. Kevles DJ. *In the name of eugenics.* Berkeley: University of California Press, 1985:96–112.
14. Stoto MA, Almario DA, McCormick MC. *Reducing the odds: preventing perinatal transmission of HIV in the United States.* Washington, DC: National Academy Press, 1999:28.
15. Rothstein MA. Genetic privacy and confidentiality: why it's so hard to protect. *J Law Med Ethics* 1998; 26:198–204.
16. Rothenberg K, Fuller B, Rothstein M, et al. Genetic information and the workplace: legislative approaches and policy changes. *Science* 1997;275:1755–1757.
17. Americans with Disabilities Act of 1990, 42 USC §§12181,12182.
18. Grady C. Ethics and genetic testing. *Ad Intern Med* 1999;44:389–411.
19. Marteau TM, Croyle RT. Psychological responses to genetic testing. *BMJ* 1998;316:693–696.
20. Lerman C, Narod S, Schulman K, et al. BRCA1 testing in families with hereditary breast-ovarian cancer. *JAMA* 1996;275:1885–1892.
21. Giardiello FM, Brensinger JD, Petersen GM, et al. The use and interpretation of commercial APC gene testing for familial adenomatous polyposis. *N Engl J Med* 1997;336:823–827.
22. Bartels DM, LeRoy BS, McCarthy P, et al. Nondirectiveness in genetic counseling: a survey of practitioners. *Am J Med Genet* 1997;72:172–179.
23. Caplan AL. Neutrality is not morality: the ethics of genetic counseling. In: Bartels DM, LeRoy BS, Caplan AL, eds. *Prescribing our future: ethical challenges in genetic counseling.* New York: Aldine De Gruyter, 1993:149–165.
24. Michie S, Bron F, Bobrow M, et al. Nondirectiveness in genetic counseling: an empirical study. *Am J Hum Genet* 1997;60:40–47.

25. Gervais KG. Objectivity, value neutrality and nondirectiveness in genetic counseling. In: Bartels DM, LeRoy BS, Caplan AL, eds. *Prescribing our future: ethical challenges in genetic counseling.* New York: Aldine De Gruyter, 1993:119–130.
26. Kessler S. Psychological aspects of genetic counseling: nondirectiveness revisited. *Am J Med Genet* 1997;72:164–171.
27. Andrews LB, Fullarton JE, Holtzman NA, Motulsky AG, ed. *Assessing genetic risks: implications for health and social policy.* Washington, DC: National Academy Press, 1994.
28. Benkendorf JL, Reutenauer JE, Hughes CA, et al. Patients' attitudes about autonomy and confidentiality in genetic testing for breast-ovarian cancer susceptibility. *Am J Med Genet* 1997;73:296–303.
29. The American Society of Human Genetics Social Issues Subcommittee on Familial Disclosure. Professional disclosure of familial genetic information. *Am J Hum Genet* 1998;62:474–483.
30. Wickle JTR. Late onsent genetic disease: where ignorance is bliss, is it folly to inform relatives? *BMJ* 1998;317:744–747.

ANNOTATED BIBLIOGRAPHY

1. Marteau TM, Croyle RT. Psychological responses to genetic testing. *BMJ* 1998;316:693–696.
   Comprehensive review of patient responses to genetic testing.
2. Rothstein MA. Genetic privacy and confidentiality: why it's so hard to protect. *J Law Med Ethics* 1998;26:198–204.
   Thoughtful discussion of problems with measures to prohibit genetic discrimination within the current U.S. insurance system.
3. Rothenberg K, Fuller B, Rothstein M, et al. Genetic information and the workplace: legislative approaches and policy changes. *Science* 1997;275:1755–1757.
   Analyzes recent policy developments regarding workplace discrimination based on genetic information.
4. The American Society of Human Genetics Social Issues Subcommittee on Familial Disclosure. Professional disclosure of familial genetic information. *Am J Hum Genet* 1998;62:474–483.
   Position paper on whether genetic information should be disclosed to relatives over the objections of the patient.
5. Wickle JTR. Late onset genetic disease: where ignorance is bliss, is it folly to inform relatives? *BMJ* 1998;317:744–747.
   Analyzes the dilemma of whether to inform relatives at risk for late-onset genetic diseases.

Cases for Discussion

DISCUSSION SECTION 1

Physician-Assisted Suicide and Active Euthanasia

This session will help students understand:

1. The distinctions between physician-assisted suicide, active euthanasia, withdrawing or withholding life-sustaining interventions, and administering high-dose narcotics to terminally ill patients to palliate symptoms.
2. How physicians should respond to requests for assisted suicide by terminally ill patients.

CASE 1.1. *A 32-year-old man with the acquired immunodeficiency syndrome and a CD4 count of 7 has been hospitalized for* Pneumocystis *pneumonia and cryptococcal meningitis during the past 6 months. He has also developed refractory diarrhea, weight loss, and painful neuropathy that has persisted despite trials of carbamazepam, amitriptyline, and regular and increasing doses of narcotics. He says that he wants a prescription for a lethal dose of medications. He says that he does not want to wait for another opportunistic infection or to suffer increasing symptoms. His long-standing partner and his parents agree with his decision. He does not seem clinically depressed and is willing to see a psychiatrist to confirm the absence of major depression.*

Questions for Discussion

1. What are the common reasons patients make such a request?
2. What alternative responses can the physician make, other than giving the patient a prescription for a lethal dose of medication?
3. What actions should a physician who supports physician-assisted suicide take before deciding that it is appropriate to write a prescription for a lethal dose of medication in this case?
4. What actions should a physician who opposes physician-assisted suicide take in addition to refusing the patient's request?
5. How does the moral responsibility of the physician differ when writing a lethal prescription compared with injecting a lethal dose of medication, such as potassium?

CASE 1.1, continued. *Suppose the patient now presents to the emergency room with headache, fever, and altered mental status and is found to have multiple contrast-enhancing ring lesions on magnetic resonance scan, strongly suggestive of toxoplasmosis. He has com-*

pleted a durable power of attorney for health care, appointing his partner as proxy and refusing all life-prolonging interventions, even antibiotics for treatable infections. You agree not to treat his infection. He also has requested that he be placed on a high-dose morphine drip in case of a complication, because he would not want a prolonged death. Morphine and diazepam are started in the emergency department because he is restless and agitated, possibly because he has pain or delirium. On 10 mg morphine/hr and diazepam 2 mg/hr, the patient appears comfortable, without any twitching or myoclonus. His respiratory rate is 12/min. He does not respond when called or when an intravenous line is restarted. The partner and his parents request that you increase the drips, saying that he did not want a prolonged death.

Questions for Discussion

6. If the physician increases the rate of morphine or diazepam in this situation, is the intention to relieve suffering or to hasten death?

DISCUSSION SECTION 2

Refusal to Care for Patients

This session will help students understand:

1. The ethical reasons for and against allowing physicians to refuse to care for patients who seek care.
2. The legal restrictions on when physicians can refuse to care for patients who seek care.
3. Practical suggestions for improving difficult doctor–patient relationships.

CASE 2.1. *A 34-year-old man with human immunodeficiency virus (HIV) infection (CD4 level 180) is admitted to your service with his first episode of* Pneumocystis carinii *pneumonia. His intravenous line has infiltrated, and you are asked to restart it.*

Questions for Discussion

1. How would you feel if you suffered a needlestick injury while caring for an HIV-infected patient?
2. What is the risk to students and house staff who care for HIV-infected patients? How frequently do needlestick injuries occur and what is the risk of acquiring HIV infection from a needlestick?
3. One of the interns on the admitting team refuses to take care of this patient. What are the ethical considerations if:

   A. The intern says he is inexperienced at starting intravenous lines and thinks that a more experienced physician should care for the patient.
   B. The intern is a deeply religious person who believes that homosexuality is a sin. Because the patient is gay, the intern does not want to care for him.
   C. The patient is an injection drug user. The intern had been mugged by an injection drug user at the hospital earlier in his internship. The intern is still experiencing flashbacks about that earlier incident and does not want to be subjected to more stress.

CASE 2.2. *As a nephrologist, you have been caring for a 37-year-old injection drug user at your dialysis unit. She often misses scheduled dialysis appointments and later presents to the emergency department with uremic symptoms, requiring emergency dialysis. She does not adhere to dietary restrictions or take her medications regularly. She often comes to dialysis high on drugs or drunk, verbally abuses the nurses and other patients, and sometimes tries to hit them. You have tried unsuccessfully to have a family member or friend accompany her to dialysis and to refer her for drug rehabilitation and psychiatric counseling.*

Questions for Discussion

4. Can you ethically discharge her from your dialysis program? What are the pertinent ethical and legal considerations?
5. If you decide that it is appropriate to terminate the doctor–patient relationship, what steps should you take beforehand? What are the ethical reasons for doing so?
6. If the patient presents to the emergency department, are you and your dialysis staff obligated to perform emergency dialysis?

DISCUSSION SECTION 3

Ethical Dilemmas Facing Students and House Staff: Learning on Patients

This session will help students understand:

1. The ethical issues involved in learning invasive procedures.
2. The ethical issues involved in learning on unconscious or newly dead patients.
3. The ethical issues involved in whistleblowing when trainees observe clearly unethical behavior or substandard care.

CASE 3.1. *Suppose your favorite uncle has been recommended for cardiac bypass surgery by his primary care physician and cardiologist in New York. From your clinical epidemiology course you recall that the mortality rates for this operation vary from under 1% to over 8% and that New York State publishes mortality rates for hospitals and for individual surgeons.*

Questions for Discussion

1. Do you want to know the outcomes experience for the hospital or surgeon that would operate on your uncle? What are your reasons?

CASE 3.2. *Recall the first time you did a lumbar puncture (LP) (or central line, major suturing, or other major procedure).*

Questions for Discussion

2. How did you feel before doing your first invasive procedure?
3. One of your classmates says that by coming to a teaching hospital, patients have given implied consent to having students and residents do procedures. Thus, there is no need to tell the patient that a student will be performing a procedure. Do you agree, and why?
4. What would you do if before your first LP, the resident calls to say go ahead and do it yourself, because he and the interns are in the Emergency Room with critically ill new patients. The LP needs to be done today. How would you respond?

CASE 3.3. *On a clerkship, you observe what you consider flagrantly unethical behavior by one of your attending physicians. On several occasions, his speech is slurred and you smell alcohol on his breath. He also fails to round on his patients for days at a time, without having anyone cover for him, and does not return your pages or those of your resident.*

Questions for Discussion

5. What are the ethical reasons for reporting the situation to some appropriate person?
6. What are some of the risks in reporting the situation to more senior physicians?
7. In practical terms, how might you proceed?

DISCUSSION SECTION 4

Disclosing Mistakes

This session will help students understand:

1. The range of responses people in various roles have to mistakes in medicine.
2. The reasons to disclose serious mistakes to senior physicians, as well as the reasons not to disclose such mistakes.
3. The reasons to disclose serious mistakes to patients or family members, as well as the reasons not to disclose such mistakes.
4. Practical suggestions for responding to mistakes.

CASE 4.1. *A 42-year-old man is admitted to you with diabetic ketoacidosis. After treatment with intravenous fluids and an insulin drip, the patient's glucose declines from 745 to 289 ml/dl after 4 hours. However, the patient develops progressive leg weakness and difficulty breathing and requires transfer to the intensive care unit for mechanical ventilation. In reviewing the case, you check the computer for lab results and realize that the patient had a potassium of 2.7 mmol/L. No potassium replacement had been given during treatment of the ketoacidosis.*

Questions for Discussion

1. In your experience, how have colleagues reacted to mistakes?
2. If you were the subintern on the case, what would your feelings be?
3. Who is responsible for this mistake?
4. What would your concerns be about telling the attending physician about this mistake?
5. Would you tell the attending physician about the episode?

CASE 4.1, continued. *The family asks what happened. They say that the patient has been hospitalized several times for ketoacidosis and has never required mechanical ventilation.*

Questions for Discussion

6. What reasons might physicians give for not telling the patient and his family about this mistake?
7. What are reasons to disclose the mistake to the patient and his family?
8. A nurse asks what to tell the patient and family, saying that they are very concerned about what happened. How do you respond?

Subject Index

Page numbers followed by *t* denotes tables.

A

Abandonment, patient, 203–204
Abortion, 306
  providing information about, 303–304
Abuse
  child
    Baby Doe Regulations and, 291–292
    reporting, 48–49
  elder, reporting, 49
  partner, reporting, 49
  possibility of with physician-assisted suicide/
    active euthanasia, 159
  possibility of with psychiatric patients,
    310–311
  withholding tube and intravenous feedings
    and, 168–169, 171
Acquired immunodeficiency syndrome (AIDS).
  See HIV infection/AIDS
Active euthanasia, 156–166, 345–346
  abuse and, 159
  administering appropriate doses of narcotics/
    sedatives differentiated from, 157
  case study of, 345–346
  compassion for suffering patient and, 158
  de facto legalization of in Netherlands,
    161–162
  declining request for, 163–164
  definition of, 156
    physician confusion about, 161
  depression and, 159, 160
  improved palliative care affecting patient
    desire for, 163
  incidence of requests for, 160
  involuntary, 156
  justifiable situations and, 164
  legal status and practice of, 160–162
  manageability of suffering and, 158
  nonvoluntary, 156
  patient autonomy and, 158–159
  patient withdrawal of request for, 162
  physician role as healer and, 159
  policy options and, 162

  reasons against, 158–159
  reasons favoring, 158
  response to request for, 162–164, 162*t*
  safeguard violations and, 161–162
  sanctity of life and, 158
  voluntary, 156
  withholding/withdrawing medical interventions
    differentiated from, 157
ADA. *See* Americans with Disabilities Act
Adolescent patient, 288–289
  confidentiality issues and, 290
  parental consent for abortion and, 306
  reproductive health for, 304
Advance directives, 69, 94–102
  conflict with patient's best interests and, 98
  discussing with patient
    documenting, 102
    improving, 99–102, 100*t*
    ongoing evaluation in, 102
    problems with, 99
    rationale for, 98–99
  health care proxy/durable power of attorney
    for health care, 96–97, 108–110
  interpretation of, 97–98, 101–102
  limitations of, 97–98
  living wills, 96
  misunderstandings about, 97
  oral, 95–96
  physician-assisted suicide/active euthanasia
    requests and, 160
  trustworthiness of, 95–96, 96*t*
  types of, 95–97
  written, 96–97, 108–110
Advocate. *See* Patient advocate
Affirmative (positive) rights, 137
Agreement with physician
  decision-making capacity and, 81
  informed consent and, 20, 22
AIDS. *See* HIV infection/AIDS
Alcohol use
  liver transplantation and, 334
  during pregnancy, 307

Allocation of resources, 13, 236. *See also*
    Bedside rationing of health care
    cost of transplantation and, 334
    futility of interventions and, 75
    patient insistence on interventions and, 37
"Allowing to die," 157
Alternative approaches
    informed consent and, 20
        surgery and, 295
    out-of-plan interventions in managed care
        systems and, 252
American College of Physicians–Society for
    Internal Medicine, code of ethics of, 6
American Medical Association, code of ethics
    of, 6
Americans with Disabilities Act (ADA), 323,
    340
Anesthesia, for surgery and invasive procedures,
    suspension of DNR order and, 153
Artificial feedings, 167–172. *See also* Intra-
    venous feedings; Tube feedings
Assisted reproductive technologies, 303, 308
Automobile drivers, impaired, reporting to
    public officials, 47
Autonomy
    patient
        insistence on interventions and, 35
        potential for in children, 286
        refusal of treatment and, 89
            physician/hospital insistence on life-
                sustaining interventions and, 136
            respect for persons and, 11
    physician/caregiver
        insistence on life-sustaining interventions
            and, 136
        patient insistence on interventions and, 35

B

Baby Doe Regulations, 291–292
Barbiturates, for terminal sedation, 124–125
Battery, informed consent and, 24
Bedside rationing of health care, 236–243.
    See also Allocation of resources
    arguments against, 237
    arguments supporting, 237–239, 237*t*
    financial resources as basis for, 239–241
    notification of patient/surrogate and, 242
    suggestions for physicians considering,
        241–242, 241*t*
Beneficence, 12, 31–34. *See also* Best interests
    of patient
    patient insistence on interventions and, 36
        life-sustaining interventions and, 129–131

transplant recipient selection and, 331
    conflicts and, 333
Benzodiazepines, for terminal sedation, 124–125
Best interests of patient, 12–13, 30–41. *See also*
    Beneficence
    acting for patient benefit and, 35–36
    advance directive conflicting with, 98
    bedside rationing of health care and, 236–243
    children and, 285–286
    conflicts of interest and, 232, 234. *See also*
        Conflicts of interest
    deception/nondisclosure and, 53, 56
    decisions for incapacitated patients and, 13,
        104–105
    fiduciary relationship between doctor and
        patient and, 31–32
    futility differentiated from, 76
    maintenance of doctor–patient relationship
        and, 37
    medical paternalism and, 34
    negotiating mutually acceptable plan of care
        and, 39–40
    patient autonomy and, 35
    patient insistence on interventions and, 34–40.
        See also Futile interventions
        life-sustaining interventions and, 129–131
    patient refusal of beneficial interventions and,
        13, 30–34, 38, 39
    persuading patient to accept beneficial inter-
        ventions and, 38
    physician autonomy and, 35
    problems with, 32–33
    professionalism and, 32
    promotion of in shared decision-making,
        27–28, 37–40, 37*t*
    reaching agreement on, 37–40
    resource allocation and, 37
    substituted judgment conflicting with, 104
    treating patients against their wishes and, 92
Birth control, providing information about,
    303–304
Blood transfusions, refusal of by Jehovah's
    Witnesses, 90–91
    children and, 291
    increasing risk of surgery and, 298–300
Bonuses for reduced expenditures, as cost-
    containment measure, 256. *See also*
    Financial incentives
Brain death
    concept of, 177–178
    controversies regarding, 178–179
    definition of, 177–178
    higher brain/neocortical definition of, 178–179

legal status of, 179
organ transplantation and, 177, 179, 329
persistent vegetative state differentiated from, 174
practical suggestions regarding, 179
rejection of concept of, 179
whole-brain criteria for, 177–178
Breast cancer susceptibility, DNA-based testing for, 338–339

C

Cadaver donors
criteria for acceptability of, 329
non-heart-beating, harvesting organs from, 329–330
Capitation, as cost-containment measure, 256.
See also Financial incentives
Cardiopulmonary criteria, for brain death, 178
Cardiopulmonary resuscitation (CPR)
complications of, 147–148
effectiveness of, 147–148
discussing with patients, 150, 151
as futile intervention, 148–149
orders to withhold (DNR orders), 147–155
patient refusal of, 148
physician recommendations about, 151
surrogate refusal of, 148
Care. *See also* Doctor–patient relationship;
Health care resources; Health care
services; Interventions
goals of, futility defined in terms of, 74
incentives to decrease, 248–257
incentives to increase, 244–247
obligations to provide, 197–198
refusal to provide, 197–205
standard, unavailability of in managed care
system, 251–252
substandard, disclosing mistakes and, 263–270
termination of, sexual relationship between
physician and patient and, 215
Caregivers. *See also* Health care workers;
Physician
beliefs about withdrawing life-sustaining
interventions and, 136, 184
risk of acquiring HIV infection and, 199, 321–322
risk of transmitting HIV infection and, 322–326
Caring
ethic of, 16–17
tube and intravenous feedings as symbol of, 168, 170–171

Carrier screening, DNA-based testing for adult-
onset diseases differentiated from, 337
Case consultations, 9, 140–146
access to/requesting, 143
ethics committees for, 140, 144–145
ethics consultants for, 140, 145–146
goals of, 140–141, 141*t*
participants in, 143
problems with, 141–142, 141*t*
procedures for, 142–144
timeliness and, 142
Case law
definition of, 189
nature of, 189
Casuistry, 16
Cesarean section
emergency, consent and, 305
forced, 307–308
CF. *See* Cystic fibrosis
Child abuse/neglect
Baby Doe Regulations and, 291–292
reporting, 48–49
Childbirth. *See also* Obstetrics and gynecology
philosophical/religious questions about, 302
Children, 285–293
brain death determination in, 178
confidentiality and, 289–290
decision-making for
adolescents and, 288–289
disagreements between parents and
physicians and, 287–288
informed decisions and, 285
parental, 287
standards for, 286–287
disclosure of information to, 289
ethical issues in care of, 285–293
handicapped infants and, 291–292
interests of parents/family members and, 287
parental requests for treatment of, 289
physician as advocate for, 285–286
potential autonomy and, 286
preferences of, 286, 291
protecting best interests of, 285, 286
refusal of interventions and, 290–291
by child, 291
relationship of pediatrician to, 289–290
Citizenship, transplant recipient selection and, 333
Clinical ethics, 4–6. *See also* Decision-making,
ethical; Ethical dilemmas in patient care
law and, 5–6
as moral guidance source, 4–5
professional oaths/codes differentiated from, 6

Clinical ethics (*contd.*)
  theories of, 15
  use of by physicians, 6–7
Clinical interventions. *See* Interventions
Clinical protocols, in cost containment, 257
Clinical research ethics, 221–228
  academic rewards and, 225
  competing interests and, 225–227
  confidentiality of data from, 224
  conflicting interests and, 226–227
  constrained consent and, 222–223
  drug manufacturer funding and, 225–226
  fee-for-service research and, 226
  finder's fees and, 225–226
  informed consent and, 223–224, 223*t*
  Institutional Review Board and, 224
  participant selection and, 222–223
  patient lacking decision-making capacity and, 222
  research protocols and, 221–222
Clinical skills, basic, learning on patients, 278
Clinician-investigators. *See also* Clinical research
  academic rewards for, 225
  dual roles for, 225
Codes of ethics, clinical ethics and, 6
Coercion, informed consent and, 22
Comfort measures. *See also* Pain relief
  for patients refusing tube and intravenous feedings, 169
Commitment, involuntary. *See* Involuntary psychiatric commitment
Communicable diseases. *See* Infectious diseases
Communication, improvement of, ethics case consultations and, 141. *See also* Discussions
Competence, 69, 80–81. *See also* Decision-making capacity
  legal standards for, 81–82
  physician-assisted suicide/active euthanasia and, 159
Competing interests
  clinical research and, 225–227
  conflicting interests differentiated from, 233
Computerized medical records, confidentiality breaches and, 43
Conception, philosophical/religious questions about, 302
Conferences, drug companies paying for/sponsoring, 258–259
Confidentiality, 12, 42–51
  adolescents' requests for, 290
  difficulties in maintenance of, 42–43
  disclosure of information and, 43–44
    public figures and, 44

    to relatives and friends, 43–44
  exceptions to/overriding, 43*t*, 45–50
    child abuse and, 48–49
    domestic violence and, 49–50
    elder abuse and, 49
    genetic testing information and, 342
    justifications for, 45, 45*t*
    partner notification and, 47, 48
    patients who are dangerous to others and, 48, 314–315
    to protect patients, 43*t*, 48–50
    to protect third parties, 43*t*, 45–48, 45*t*
    public health reporting and, 46–47
    warning persons at risk and, 47–48
  genetic testing and, 342–343
  omission of information from medical record and, 44–45
  pediatric issues and, 289
  psychiatric conditions and, 311
    warning persons at risk of harm and, 48, 314–315
  reasons for, 42
  of research data, 224
  waivers of, 43
Conflicts of interest
  best interests of patient and, 13
  in clinical research, 226–227
  competing interests differentiated from, 233
  definition of, 232–233
  disclosure of, 234
  gifts from drug companies and, 258–262
    appearance of, 261
  health care rationing and, 236–243
  incentives to decrease services and, 248–257
  incentives to increase services and, 244–247
  managing, 233–235, 234*t*
  in nonmedical situations, 231–232
  overview of, 231–235
  perceived, 232–233
  protecting patients and, 234, 235
  reimbursement incentives and, 233, 244, 249–250
  self-referral and, 245–246
  students/house staff and, 277–282
  surrogate decision-making affected by, 114
Conscience, claims of, as justification of action, 4
Consent
  constrained, for clinical research, 222–223
  implied, 25
  informed. *See* Informed consent
  presumed, for organ donation, 330
Consent forms, 25
Consequentialist ethical theories, 15
Constitution, as source of law, 189

Consultations
   ethical, 9, 140–146. *See also* Case consultations
   neurologic, brain death declaration and, 179
Contact tracing, 47
Continuing medical education, drug companies
   paying for/sponsoring, 258–259
Contraception, providing information about,
   303–304
Cost-containment measures, in managed care,
   255–257. *See also* Health care costs
Counseling, genetic, nondirective, 340–341
Court-appointed guardian, as surrogate,
   111–112
CPR. *See* Cardiopulmonary resuscitation
Crimes, injuries involving
   determination of death and, 177
   reporting, 47
Cultural factors
   in deception/nondisclosure, 53
   insistence on life-sustaining interventions
     and, 132–133
Cystic fibrosis, DNA-based testing for, 337–338

D

Dead patient, learning procedures on, 279
Death
   brain
     concept of, 177–178
     controversies regarding, 178–179
     definition of, 177–178
     higher brain/neocortical definition of,
       178–179
     legal status of, 179
     organ transplantation and, 177, 179, 329
     persistent vegetative state differentiated
       from, 174
     practical suggestions regarding, 179
     rejection of concept of, 179
     whole-brain criteria for, 177–178
   definition/determination of, 177–180
     organ transplantation and, 177, 179, 329,
       330
     problems with cardiopulmonary criteria
       for, 177
     victims of crime and, 177
Deception
   avoidance of, 12, 52–61
     managed care systems and, 253
     secret information about patients and,
       219–220
   definition of, 52
   moral wrongness of, 53–54
   of patient, 53–56
     resolving dilemmas about, 54–56, 55*t*

   of third parties, 56–60
     resolving dilemmas about, 58–60, 58*t*
Decision-making
   for children
     adolescents and, 288–289
     disagreements between parents and
       pediatricians and, 287–288
     informed decisions and, 285
     parental, 287
     standards for, 286–287
   ethical
     approach to, 7–10, 7*t*
     areas of consensus and controversy and, 7
     clarifying issues and, 8
     conflicts of interest affecting, 232
     dilemma resolution and, 9
     guidelines for, 11–18
     identification of issues and, 6
     information gathering and, 7–8, 7*t*
     legal issues and, 5–6
     moral guidance sources and, 4–5
     professional oaths and codes and, 6
   patient. *See also* Decision-making capacity
     unwillingness and, 23, 26
     unwise/harmful
       best interests of patient and, 13, 30–41
       informed consent and, 23, 28
   shared
     approach to, 69–71
     best interests of patient and, 27–28, 37–40,
       37*t*
     informed consent and, 20, 26–28, 26*t*
     promoting, 26–28, 26*t*
     reasons for, 20–21
   surrogate, 111–117. *See also* Surrogate
   unilateral
     about cardiopulmonary resuscitation,
       148–149
     for children, 287–288
     justification of, 73–74
     problems with, 75–76
     safeguards and, 76–78, 77*t*
Decision-making capacity, 80–88. *See also*
     Competence
   assessment of, 84–86
     clinical context and, 83–84
   clinical standards for, 82–84, 82*t*
   comprehension of information and, 82–84
   delusions/distorted views of reality and, 83
   emergencies and, 86–87
   enhancing, 85
   ethical implications of, 81
   making/expressing choice and, 82

Decision-making capacity (*contd.*)
  mental illness and, 86, 310–311
    refusal of medical treatment and, 316
    refusal of psychiatric treatment and,
      315–316
  patient lacking, 69, 94–107, 95*t*
    advance directives and, 69, 94–102
    best interests of patient and, 13, 104–105
    caring for, 87
    clinical research and, 222
    informed consent and, 22, 25
    legal issues related to life-sustaining
        interventions and
      court involvement and, 191
      Cruzan case ruling and, 184–186
      Herbert case ruling and, 182–184
      Quinlan case ruling and, 181–182
    physician-assisted suicide/active euthanasia
        and, 159
    standards for decisions with, 94–107, 95*t*
    substituted judgment and, 102–104
  patient's values and goals and, 83
  reasoning and, 83
  religious beliefs and, 86
Delusions, decision-making capacity affected
    by, 83
Dementia, severe, persistent vegetative state
    differentiated from, 174
Deontological ethical theories, 15
Depression
  decision-making capacity and, 86
  requests for assisted-suicide/active euthanasia
    and, 159–160
Deselection, as incentive to provide fewer
    services, 257
Diabetes, prenatal testing for, 304
Diagnosis
  discussing bad news and, 60–61
  withholding. *See* Nondisclosure
Directed donation, 332
Disclosure. *See also* Nondisclosure
  benefits of, 54
  to children, 289
  discussing bad news and, 60–61
  of economic incentives of managed care
      systems, 251
  of genetic testing results, 342–343
  of gifts from drug companies, 262
  informed consent and, 21–22, 21*t*, 27
    standards for, 24–25
    surgery and, 295–297
  of mistakes, 263–270, 348
    case study of, 348
    other health care professionals and, 268–269

  to patient/surrogate
    ethical response and, 266
    reasons against, 263–264
    reasons for, 264–265, 264*t*
    situations not warranting, 266–267
  by trainees to attending physician, 267–268
  patient need for information and, 54
  to schools, 290
  of secret, to patient, 219–220
  surgery and, 295–297
    alternative approaches and, 295
    changes due to unanticipated findings and,
      296–297
    experience of surgeon and, 296
    provider-specific outcomes and, 295
Discrimination
  genetic, 339–340
    by employers, 339–340
    by insurers, 339
  against HIV-infected health care workers,
      323–324
  laws against, 340
Discussions
  about advance directives, 99–102
  bad news and, 60–61
  about decision-making capacity, 9, 85–86
  about difficult doctor-patient relationships,
      202–203
  about DNR orders, 149–151, 150*t*
  about family requests to withhold diagnosis
      from patient, 54–56
  about futile interventions, 77
  about health care rationing, 242
  about informed consent, 21–22, 21*t*, 24–25, 27
  with Jehovah's Witnesses, 91
  about persuading patients to accept beneficial
      interventions, 38–40
  about requests for life-sustaining interven-
      tions, 130–131
  with surrogates of patients, 115–116
  about uncovered/experimental treatment
      options, managed care restrictions on
      (gag rules), 250–251
Diversion programs, for impaired colleagues,
    273–274
DNR/DNAR orders. *See* Do Not Resuscitate
    (DNR)/Do Not Attempt Resuscitation
    (DNAR) orders
"Do no harm," principle of, 31
  restrictions on HIV-infected health care
      workers and, 323
Do Not Resuscitate (DNR)/Do Not Attempt
    Resuscitation (DNAR) orders, 147–155

anesthesia for surgery and invasive procedures and, 153
  discussing with patients, 149–151, 150*t*
  Emergency Medical Services and, 153
  implementing, 151–153
  implications of for other treatments, 152
  interpretation of, 152–153
  justifications for, 148–149
  "limited" or "partial," 152
  nursing home residents and, 153
  preventing misunderstandings regarding, 152
  slow or show codes and, 152–153
  writing, 151–152
Doctor–patient relationship, 195–196
  abuse of, sexual relationships with patients and, 214, 216
  with child, 289–290
  clinical research and, 221–228
  context of, 197–198
  difficult, 202–204
    improving, 202–203, 202*t*
  emergency care provision and, 201–202, 204
  ethical obligations to care for patients and, 197–198
  fiduciary nature of, 31–32
  gifts from patients and, 206–211. *See also* Gifts
  legal definition of, 198
  maintenance of
    patient insistence on interventions and, 37
    physician insistence on life-sustaining interventions and, 138
  managed care organizations affecting, 250–251
  occupational risks to physician and, 198–201
    HIV infection and, 199, 321–322
    responding to, 199–201, 200*t*
  overview of, 195–196
  with parents of patient, 289–290
  patient transfers and, 201–202
  physician-assisted suicide affecting, 161
  refusal of care and, 197–205
  sexual contact and, 212–218. *See also* Sexual contact between physicians and patients
  terminating, 203–204
Domestic violence, reporting, 49
Donation, organ, for transplantation. *See* Organ donation
Donor cards, 328–329, 330
Double effect doctrine, 123–124
  legal rulings and, 187–188
Drinking/liquids, patients refusing, 125, 167–172. *See also* Intravenous feedings; Tube feedings
Drivers, potential impairment of, reporting to public officials, 47

Drug manufacturers
  gifts from, 258–262
    continuing medical education/conferences as, 258–259
    objections to accepting, 260–261, 260*t*
    objectivity affected by, 260
    reasons for accepting, 259–260
    reasons for offering, 259
    reciprocity and, 260
    recommended solutions and, 261–262
    small, 258
    types of, 258–259
  research funded by, 225, 226
Durable power of attorney for health care (health care proxy), 96–97, 108–110. *See also* Surrogate
Duty, 15. *See also* Guidelines

E
Eating/food, patients refusing, 125, 167–172. *See also* Intravenous feedings; Tube feedings
Elder abuse, reporting, 49
Electroencephalogram, in brain death determination, 178
Emancipated minors, 288–289
Embryos, frozen, 303
Emergencies
  implied consent and, 25, 87
  obstetrical, 305
  parental permission and, 287
  questionable decision-making capacity and, 86–87
Emergency care, obligation to provide, 201–202, 204
Emergency departments, DNR orders and, 153
Emergency Medical Services, DNR orders and, 153
Emotional reactions
  to patient, patient insistence on interventions and, 39–40
  to physician-assisted suicide, 161
  to withdrawing/withholding life-sustaining interventions, 125–126
Emotional stress, surrogate decision-making affected by, 114
Emotional support, ethics case consultation and, 141
Ethical dilemmas in patient care, 3–10. *See also* Decision-making, ethical; Ethical issues
  approach to in clinical medicine, 7–10, 7*t*
  clinical ethics and, 4–6
    use of by physicians, 6–7
  clinical research and, 221–228

Ethical dilemmas in patient care (*contd.*)
  ethics committees and, 9, 140–146
  resolving, 9–10. *See also* Case consultation
    case consultation in, 140–146
    guidelines for, 11–18
    students and house staff and, 277–282
Ethical issues
  areas of consensus and controversy about, 7
  clarification of, 8
    case consultation in, 140–141
  HIV transmission as, 321–327
  identification of, 6
  in obstetrics and gynecology, 302–309
  in organ transplantation, 328–336
  in pediatrics, 285–293. *See also* Children
  in psychiatry, 310–317
  in surgery, 294–301
Ethics
  caring, 16–17
  clinical, 4–6. *See also* Clinical ethics;
    Decision-making, ethical
  casuistry and, 16
  guidelines for, 11–18
    conflicting, 14
    exceptions to, 14
    interpretation of, 14
    use of, 13–14
  morality differentiated from, 5
  theories of, 15
  virtue, 16
Ethics committees, 144–145
  for case consultation, 9, 140–146. *See also*
    Case consultations
  advantages of, 144–145
  disadvantages of, 145
  composition of, 144
  delays in arranging meeting with, 145
  demystification of ethics by, 145
  diffusion of responsibility in, 145
  group dynamics affecting decisions of, 145
  interdisciplinary membership of, 144
  primary data gathering by, 143–144
  recommendations made by, 144
Ethics consultants, 9, 145–146
  for case consultation, 9, 140–146. *See also*
    Case consultations
  advantages of, 145
  disadvantages of, 145–146
  expertise of, 145
  individual bias affecting, 146
  primary data gathering by, 143–144
  recommendations made by, 144
  timeliness/detail of consultation with, 145
  undue deference to, 145

Ethnic background
  insistence on life-sustaining interventions
    and, 132–133
  transplant recipient selection and, 333
Euthanasia
  active. *See* Active euthanasia
  passive, 157
Extended care facilities, DNR orders for
  residents of, 153
Extraordinary care, 122. *See also* Life-sustaining
  interventions

F

Family planning, providing information about,
  303–304
Family/significant others
  active euthanasia requests by, 160, 161, 164
  concerns of about disclosure, 55
  disclosure of mistakes to
    case study of, 348
    ethical response and, 266
    other health care workers and, 268–269
    reasons against, 263–264
    reasons for, 264–265, 264*t*
    situations not warranting, 266–267
  disclosure of patient information to, 43–44
  discussion of DNR orders with, 149–151, 150*t*
  discussion of futile interventions with, 77
  meeting with, decision-making and, 9
  as surrogate, 112–113. *See also* Surrogate
    legal issues regarding, 113
Fee-for-service reimbursement
  conflicts of interest and, 233
  increases in services and, 244
  problems with, 244
Fee-for-service research, 226
Feeding problems, tube and intravenous feedings for, 167–168. *See also* Intravenous
  feedings; Tube feedings
Feeding tube. *See* Tube feedings
Fertilization, *in vitro*, 303
Fetus
  as patient, 303
    maternal/fetal conflict and, 306–308
  prevention of harm to, 303, 306–308
    compelled treatment of pregnant woman
    and, 91–92
    routine prenatal testing and, 304–305
Fiduciary relationship, between doctor and
  patient, 31–32. *See also* Best interests
  of patient
  conflicts of interest and, 234
  definition of, 32

Financial incentives
    balanced, 250, 256
    bedside rationing of health care and, 239–241
    conflicts of interest and, 233
    decreasing services and, 233, 249–250, 250,
        256
    increasing services and, 233, 244, 245–246
    for organ donation, 330–331
    research ethics and, 226
Finder's fees, for research subject, 225–226
Food
    as gift from drug company, 258
    patients refusing, 125, 167–172. *See also*
        Intravenous feedings; Tube feedings
Formulary restrictions, bedside rationing and, 241
Friends. *See* Family/significant others
Frozen embryos, 303
Futile interventions, 72–79
    best interests differentiated from, 76
    cardiopulmonary resuscitation as, 148–149
    definition of
        loose, 74–75
        strict, 73–74, 73*t*
    discussion of, 77–78
    guidelines for, 77
    legal cases involving, 72–73
    mistakes in judgments of, 75–76
    "no medical indications" and, 78
    problems with concept of, 75–76
    refusal to operate and, 297
    safeguards and, 76–78, 77*t*

G

Gag rules, in managed care, 250–251
Gamete donation, 303
Gatekeeper, physician as, 249, 256
Genetic counseling, nondirective, 340–341
Genetic testing, DNA-based, for predisposition
        to adult-onset disease, 337–344
    appropriate instances for, 337–339
    confidentiality and, 342–343
    discrimination and, 339–340
    informed consent and, 340–341
    nondirective counseling and, 340–341
    prenatal testing and carrier screening differ-
        entiated from, 337
    pretest counseling and, 141
    recommendations for, 341
Gift relationship, transplantation and, 333–334
Gifts
    from drug companies, 258–262
        continuing medical education/conferences
            as, 258–259
        objections to acceptance of, 260–261, 260*t*

objectivity affected by, 260
reasons accepted, 259–260
reasons offered, 259
reciprocity and, 260
recommended solutions and, 261–262
small, 258
types of, 258–259
    from patients, 206–211
        clinical judgment affected by, 208
        cultural significance for patient and, 207
        declining, 210
        doctor–patient relationship affected by,
            207–208
        erosion of public trust and, 208
        as expression of appreciation ("thank you"),
            206
        problems with, 207–209
        psychological needs of patient and, 206
        reasons for giving, 206–207
        responding to, 209–211
        sharing, 210
        soliciting, 208–209
        special treatment/unethical requests and,
            207, 210–211
Goals
    of care. *See also* Interventions
        futility defined in terms of, 74
    patient, decisions consistent with, 83
Gonorrhea
    prenatal testing for, 304
    public health reporting of, 46
Group dynamics (groupthink), ethics committee
        decision affected by, 145
Guardian, court-appointed, as surrogate, 111–112
Guidelines
    ethical, 11–18
        conflicting, 14
        exceptions to, 14
        interpretation of, 14
        use of, 13–14
    practice, in cost containment, 257
Gynecology. *See* Obstetrics and gynecology

H

Handicapped infants, 291–292
Harm
    bedside rationing of health care and, 238–239
    disclosure of mistakes and, 264–266
    physician–patient sexual relationship and,
        213–214
    preventing
        deception and nondisclosure in, 53
        "do no harm" principle and, 31
        impaired colleagues and, 272, 274

Harm, preventing (*contd.*)
    restrictions on HIV-infected health care
      workers and, 323
    treating patients against their wishes and, 92
Health care costs
    bedside rationing and, 236–243
    gifts from drug companies affecting, 260
    managed care systems decreases in services
      and, 248–257
    resource allocation and, 13, 37, 75, 236
    transplantation costs and, 334
Health care institution/organization
    mission of, insistence on life-sustaining inter-
      ventions and, 136
    responsibility of for incentives to decrease
      services, 250–251
Health care proxy/durable power of attorney for
    health care, 96–97, 108–110. *See also*
    Surrogate
Health Care Quality Improvement Act, 274
Health care resources. *See also* Health care
    services
    allocation of, 13, 236
      cost of transplantation and, 334
      futility of interventions and, 75
      patient insistence on interventions and, 37
    bedside rationing of, 236–243
      arguments against, 237
      arguments supporting, 237–239, 237*t*
      financial resources as basis for, 239–241
      notification of patient/surrogate and, 242
      suggestions for physicians considering,
        241–242, 241*t*
Health care services. *See also* Health care
    resources
    direct limitations on, in cost containment, 257
    incentives to decrease, 248–257
      cost-containment measures in managed
        care and, 255–257
      ethical concerns about, 249–250
      financial incentives and, 233, 249–250,
        250, 256
      patient requests for interventions and,
        253–254
      responses of physicians to, 251–253
      responsibility of health care organizations
        and, 250–251
    incentives to increase, 244–247
      fee-for-service reimbursement, 244
      nonfinancial, 247
      self-referral, 245–246
    unavailability of in managed care system,
      251–252
Health care team, in decision-making, 8, 9

Health care workers
    beliefs about withdrawing life-sustaining
      interventions and, 136, 184
    risk of acquiring HIV infection and, 199,
      321–322
    risk of transmitting HIV infection and,
      322–326
Health maintenance organizations (HMOs),
    255. *See also* Managed care systems
Heroic care, 122
Higher brain death, 178–179. *See also* Brain
    death
    versus whole brain death, 178
Hippocratic Oath
    clinical ethics and, 6
    confidentiality addressed in, 42
HIV infection/AIDS
    partner notification and, 45, 47, 48
    prenatal testing for, 305
    public health reporting of, 46
    transmission of in health care settings, 321–327
      from health care workers to patients,
        322–326
        CDC guidelines and, 324
        exposure of patients to health care
          worker's blood and, 325
        impairment of health care worker and,
          325–326
        patients' questions about physician's
          HIV status and, 324–325
        policy dilemmas and, 324
        public health dilemmas and, 323
        public perception of risk of, 322–323
        restrictions on seropositive health care
          workers and, 323–324
        risk of, 322–323, 323
      from patients to health care workers, 199,
        321–322
HIV testing, consent and, 321–322
HMOs. *See* Health maintenance organizations;
    Managed care systems
Hospital, mission of, insistence on life-sustaining
    interventions and, 136
Hospital ethics committees. *See* Ethics committees
Hospitalization, involuntary. *See* Involuntary
    psychiatric commitment
House staff
    ethical dilemmas facing, 277–282
      learning on patients and, 277–279, 347
      case study of, 347
      in gynecological and obstetrical care,
        279, 308
      suggestions for, 281

taking too much clinical responsibility and,
280
unethical behavior/substandard care by other
physicians and, 280–281, 347–348
case study of, 347–348
mistakes by, disclosure of, 267–268
Human Genome Project, 337
Human immunodeficiency virus infection.
See HIV infection/AIDS
Hunger. *See also* Intravenous feedings; Tube
feedings
in patients refusing oral intake, 169

I

Impaired colleagues, 271–276
causes of impairment/incompetence, 271
concerns about intervening with, 272–273
dealing with, 274–275, 274t
legal issues regarding, 273–274
protecting patient from, 272, 274
reasons for intervening with, 271–272, 272t
Impaired drivers, reporting to public officials,
47
Implied consent, 25
In vitro fertilization, 303
Incompetence. *See* Decision-making capacity,
patient lacking
Incompetent physician, 274. *See also* Impaired
colleagues
Infants, handicapped, 291–292
Infectious diseases
contact tracing/partner notification and, 47, 48
public health reporting of, 46
treating against patient's wishes, 91
warning persons at risk and, 47, 48
Infertility treatment, 303, 308
Information
comprehension of, decision-making capacity
and, 84
patient need for
disclosure and, 54
informed consent and, 21–22, 21t, 24–25, 27
provision of to third party
deception and, 56–60
no legal right to information and, 59
overriding confidentiality and, 43t, 45–48, 45t
Informed consent, 12, 19–29
agreement with physician and, 20, 22
assent of children, 286
choices among alternatives and, 20
surgery and, 295
for clinical research, 223–224, 223t
definition of, 19–20
disclosure of role of trainees, 308

disclosure of experience of surgeon, 296
emergencies and, 25, 305
exceptions to, 25–26
for genetic testing, 340–341
information discussed with patient and, 21–22,
21t, 24–25, 27
for invasive procedures by trainees, 278–280
legal aspects of, 24–25
as legal requirement, 21
objections to, 23
in obstetrics and gynecology, 303–306
patient lacking decision-making capacity and,
22, 25
patient refusal of interventions and, 20, 90
patient self-determination and, 20
patient well-being and, 20–21
reasons for, 20–21
requirements for, 21–22, 21t
shared decision-making and, 20, 20–21,
26–28, 26t
for surgery, 295–297
therapeutic privilege and, 25–26
waiver of right of, 26
Insistence on treatment
best interests of patient and, 34–37, 38,
39–40. *See also* Futile interventions
life-sustaining interventions and. *See also*
Life-sustaining interventions
caregiver insistence and, 135–139
patient insistence, 128–134
managed care and, 253–254
Institutional Review Board, for clinical
research, 224
Insurers
genetic discrimination by, 339
deception of, 56–60
Interventions (treatment). *See also* Care; Health
care resources; Health care services
Baby Doe Regulations and, 291–292
best interests of patient and
children and, 285, 286, 290–291
negotiating mutually acceptable plan of
care and, 39–40
patient insistence on, 34–40, 128–134. *See
also* Interventions (treatment), futile
patient refusal of, 13, 30–34, 38, 39
persuading patient to accept, 38
shared decision-making and, 26–28, 26t,
37–40, 37t
caregiver insistence on, 135–139
children's preferences and, 285, 286, 291
futile, 72–79
cardiopulmonary resuscitation as, 148–149
handicapped infants and, 291–292

Interventions (treatment) (*contd.*)
  incentives to decrease, 248–257
  incentives to increase, 244–247
  informed consent regarding
    agreement and, 19, 22
    choosing among alternatives and, 20
      surgery and, 295
    information discussed with patients and,
      21–22, 21*t*, 24–25, 27
    making recommendations and, 27
    patient lack of decision-making capacity
      and, 22, 25
    patient lack of understanding of information
      and, 23
    patient refusal of treatment and, 20, 90
    patient unwillingness to make decision
      and, 23
    shared decision-making and, 20–21,
      26–28, 26*t*
    unwise/harmful choices and, 23, 28
  life-sustaining. *See* Life-sustaining interventions
  medical indications for, futility and, 78
  parents refusal of, 290–291
  patient insistence on, 34–40, 128–134. *See
    also* Interventions (treatment), futile
  managed care and, 253–254
  patient refusal of
    best interests of patient and, 13, 30–34,
      38–39
    children and, 290–291
    by competent/informed patients, 89–93
    decision-making capacity and, 80–88
    informed consent and, 20, 90
    life-sustaining interventions and, caregiver
      insistence and, 135–139
      patient transfer and, 138–139
  shared decision-making about
    approach to, 69–71
    best interests of patient and, 26–28, 26*t*,
      37–40, 37*t*
    informed consent and, 20, 20–21, 26–28,
      26*t*
  surgical. *See* Surgery
  unilateral decisions about. *See also* Inter-
    ventions (treatment), futile
    cardiopulmonary resuscitation and, 148–149
    children and, 287–288
    justification of, 73–74
    problems with, 75–76
    safeguards and, 76–78, 77*t*
Intravenous feedings, 167–172
  burdens/benefits of, 170
  clinical recommendations regarding, 171–172
  for comfort and symptom alleviation, 168
  defining goals of care and, 167–168
  legal status of, 171
  as life-sustaining intervention, 168
  as ordinary care, ethical distinctions regarding,
    122, 168–170
  prolonging dying and, 169
  prolonging life and, 168
  reasons for providing, 168–169
  as symbol of care, 168, 170–171
  withdrawing
    legal rulings on, Herbert case, 182–184
    versus withholding, 168, 170
  withholding
    abuses and, 168–169
    hunger and thirst symptoms and, 169
    legal issues and, 171
    reasons for, 169–171
    starvation and, 168
    versus withdrawing, 168, 170
Invasive procedures
  HIV transmission from seropositive health
    care workers and, 322, 324
  suspension of DNR order for, 153
  trainees performing, 278–279
Involuntary euthanasia, 156
Involuntary psychiatric commitment, 311–312
  abuses and, 311
  decision-making capacity and, 86, 310, 311
  procedures for, 311–312
  rationale for, 311
  refusal of treatment and, 315–316
  standards for, 311
  for suicidal patient, mitigating adverse
    consequences of, 313
IRB. *See* Institutional Review Board
IVF. *See In vitro* fertilization

J

Jehovah's Witnesses, refusal of blood trans-
    fusions by, 90–91
  children and, 291
  increasing risk of surgery and, 298–299, 300
Judgment
  conflicts of interest affecting, 232
  gifts from drug company and, 259
  gifts from patient and, 208
  substituted. *See* Substituted judgment
Justice
  allocation of health care resources and, 13
  transplant recipient selection and, 332–333
  conflicts and, 333

L

Law. *See also under Legal*
  clinical ethics and, 5–6

on life-sustaining interventions, 189–192
  case law and, 189–191
  judicial discretion and, 190
  legal rulings, 181–188
  myths regarding, 191–192
  precedents and, 190
  state by state variations and, 190–191
  sources of, 189
Legal issues/status. *See also* Law
  active euthanasia and, 159–160, 160–161, 161–162
  brain death and, 179
  clinical ethics and, 5–6
  competence standards and, 81–82
  family/significant other as surrogate and, 113
  futile interventions and, 72–73
  impaired colleagues and, 273–274
  information provision to third party and, 59
  informed consent and, 21, 24–25
  life-sustaining interventions and, 181–188, 189–192
  oral advanced directives and, 95
  tube and intravenous feedings and, 171
Legal rulings. *See also* Law
  Abortion cases, 306
  Bouvia case, 137
  Baby K case, 73
  Cruzan case, 184
  Gilguun case, 72
  Herbert case, 182
  on life-sustaining interventions, 181–188
  Moore case, 227
  Physician-assisted suicide cases, 186
  Quinlan case, 181
  Tarasoff case, 314
  Wanglie case, 78
Life-sustaining interventions, 69–70. *See also* Advance directives
  Baby Doe Regulations and, 291–292
  cardiopulmonary resuscitation as, withholding, 147–155
  confusing ethical distinctions regarding, 121–127
  distinction between withholding and withdrawing and, 121–122
  handicapped infants and, 291–292
  insistence on
    caregiver (physician/hospital), 135–139
      arguments for, 135–136
      objections to, 136–138, 136*t*
      payment for unwanted services and, 138
      timely and clear notification of patients and, 138

transferring patient and, 138–139
    patient/surrogate, 128–134
      clinical considerations and, 128–129
      ethical considerations and, 129–131
      patient suffering and, 131
      recommendations for response to, 131–133, 131*t*
      religious-based, 130–131
      requests that "everything" be done and, 130
  intravenous feedings as, 168. *See also* Intravenous feedings
  legal issues and, 189–192
    case law and, 189–191
    judicial discretion and, 190
    legal rulings, 181–188
    myths regarding, 191–192
    precedents and, 190
    sources of law and, 189
    state by state variations and, 190–191
  parents refusal of, 290–291
  payment for, caregiver insistence and, 138
  tube feedings as, 168. *See also* Tube feedings
    withdrawal of, negative vs. positive rights and, 137
  withholding/withdrawing
    assisted suicide/active euthanasia differentiated from, 157
    cardiopulmonary resuscitation and, 147–155
    confusing ethical distinctions regarding, 121–122
    criminal liability for, 191–192
      Herbert case and, 182–184
    differentiating between withholding and withdrawing and, 121–122
    discussing with physician, 98–102
    emotional reactions to, 125–126
    health care proxy and, 96–97
    legal rulings on, 181–188
    living wills regarding, 96
    negative vs. positive rights and, 137
    terminal sedation and, 124–125
Limit setting, patient insistence on interventions and, 40
Live donors, 329
Liver transplantation, for alcoholics, 334
Living wills, 96
Locked-in syndrome, persistent vegetative state differentiated from, 174
Lying
  definition of, 52
  moral wrongness of, 53–54

M

Macroallocation. *See* Health care resources,
     allocation of
Malpractice, informed consent and, 24
Managed care systems
     compromises in quality of care and, 249
          informing patients of, 251–252
     cost-containment measures in, 255–257
     financial reimbursement in, conflicts of inter-
          est and, 233, 249–250, 256
     incentives to decrease services and, 248–257
     out-of-plan interventions and, 252
     physician as gatekeeper in, 256
     physician as patient advocate in, 252–253
Manipulation, informed consent and, 22
Maternal/fetal conflict, 306–308
Mature minors, 288
Meals, as gift from drug company, 258
Mechanical ventilation, withdrawal of, 121
     emotional responses to, 126
     legal rulings on
          Herbert case, 182–184
          Quinlan case, 181–182
Medical indications for interventions, futility
          and, 78
Medical interventions. *See* Interventions
Medical paternalism, 34
Medical records
     advance directive discussions documented in,
          102
     confidentiality of, 42–50. *See also* Confi-
          dentiality
     DNR orders written in, 152
     omitting sensitive information from, 44–45
Mental illness. *See* Psychiatric patient
Mental status testing, decision-making capacity
          assessment and, 84–85
Mercy killing, 156. *See also* Active euthanasia
Microallocation. *See* Health care resources,
          bedside rationing of
Minimally acceptable standard of conduct,
          legal vs. ethical actions and, 5
Minors
     consent for treatment by, 288–289
     emancipated, 288–289
     mature, 288
     parental consent for abortion and, 306
Misrepresentation. *See also* Deception;
          Nondisclosure
     definition of, 52
     resolving dilemmas about, 54–56, 55*t*
Mistakes, disclosure of, 263–270, 348
     case study of, 348
     other health care workers and, 268–269

     to patient/surrogate
          ethical response and, 266
          reasons against, 263–264
          reasons for, 264–265, 264*t*
          situations not warranting, 266–267
     by trainees to attending physician, 267–268
Moral exhortation, physician response to
          occupational risks and, 199–200
Moral guidance, clinical ethics as source of, 4–5
Moral values, personal, dilemmas in clinical
          ethics and, 4
Morality, ethics differentiated from, 5

N

Needlestick exposure of health care worker,
          321–322
Negative rights, 137
Neglect, child
     Baby Doe Regulations and, 291–292
     reporting, 48–49
Negligence, informed consent and, 24
Negotiation, of mutually acceptable plan of
          care, 39–40
No CPR order, 147. *See also* Do Not Resuscitate
          (DNR)/Do Not Attempt Resuscitation
          (DNAR) orders
Nondisclosure, 53–56. *See also* Deception;
          Disclosure
     avoidance of, 12, 52–61
          discussing bad news and, 60–61
     definition of, 52
     of mistake, harm to physician and, 265
     resolving dilemmas about, 54–56, 55*t*
Nonmaleficence, 12, 31
     restrictions on HIV-infected health care
          workers and, 323
Nonvoluntary euthanasia, 156
"Not medically indicated," futility and, 78
Nurses/nursing staff, beliefs about withdrawing
          life-sustaining interventions and, 136, 184
Nursing homes, DNR orders for residents of, 153
Nutrition. *See* Feeding problems; Intravenous
          feedings; Tube feedings

O

Obstetrics and gynecology, ethical issues in,
          302–309
     abortion and, 306
          providing information and, 303–304
     adolescent patients and, 304
     alcohol use during pregnancy and, 307
     assisted reproductive technologies and, 303,
          308
     compelled treatment and, 91–92

family planning information and, 303–304
forced cesarean section deliveries and,
    307–308
informed consent in, 303–306
life-sustaining interventions for brain dead
    mother until delivery and, 178
mother and fetus as patients and, 303
    maternal/fetal conflict and, 306–308
obstetrical emergencies and, 305
philosophical/religious questions and, 302
prenatal testing and
    HIV, 305
    routine, 304–305
sterilization and, 305–306
student/trainee participation in, 279, 308
substance abuse during pregnancy and, 307
third party influences and, 302
Occupational risks for health care workers,
    198–201
    HIV infection and, 199, 321–322
    reducing, 200
    responding to, 199–201, 200*t*
Operating room. *See* Surgery
Opioids, high doses of for symptom relief, 123–124
    emotional responses and, 126
Oral directives (advanced), 95–96
    legal status of, 95
    limitations of, 95
    statements to family/friends, 95–96
    statements to physicians, 96
    trustworthiness of, 95–96, 96*t*
Oral intake, patients refusing, 125, 167–172. *See
    also* Intravenous feedings; Tube feedings
Ordinary care, 122
    tube and intravenous feedings as, ethical dis-
        tinctions regarding, 122, 168–170
Organ donation, 328–331
    criteria for acceptable cadaver donors and, 329
    current system for, 328–330
    definition/determination of death and, 177,
        179, 329–330
    directed, 332
    donor card choices and, 330
    ethical concerns about, 328
    financial incentives for, 330–331
    gift relationship and, 333–334
    harvesting organs from non-heart-beating
        cadaver donors and, 329–330
    live donors and, 329
    mandated choice and, 330
    presumed consent and, 330
    proposals to increase, 330–331
    required request laws and, 329
    routine notification laws and, 329

Organ Procurement Organizations, 329
Organ transplantation, 328–336
    cost of, 334
    gift relationship and, 333–334
    organ donation and, 328–331. *See also* Organ
        donation
        definition/determination of death and, 177,
            179, 329–330
        recipient selection and, 331–334. *See also*
            Transplant recipient
    repeat, after rejection, 332

P
Pain relief
    high doses of opioids/sedatives for, 123–124
        emotional responses and, 126
    for patients refusing tube and intravenous
        feedings, 169
Paramedics, DNR orders and, 153
Parental decision-making, 287
    disagreements with pediatrician and, 287–288
Partner abuse, reporting, 49
Partner notification
    by physicians, 48
    by public health officials, 47
Passive euthanasia, 157
Paternalism, medical, 34
Patient
    advance directives of, 69, 94–102
        surrogate selection and, 100, 112
    best interests of. *See* Best interests of patient
    cardiopulmonary resuscitation refused by, 148
    deceiving, avoidance of, 12, 52–61
    disclosure of mistakes to
        case study of, 348
        ethical response and, 266
        other health care workers and, 268–269
        reasons against, 263–264
        reasons for, 264–265, 264*t*
        situations not warranting, 266–267
    discussion of bad news with, 60–61
    discussion about decision-making capacity
        with, 9, 85–86. *See also* Decision-
        making capacity
    discussion of DNR orders with, 149–151, 150*t*
    discussion of futile interventions with, 77
    discussion of health care rationing with, 242
    discussion of information with, informed
        consent and, 21–22, 21*t*, 24–25, 27
    gift-giving to physician by, 206–211. *See
        also* Gifts
    identification of trainee to, 277–278
    incompetent. *See* Decision-making capacity,
        patient lacking

Patient (*contd.*)
  learning procedures on, 277–279, 347
    case study of, 347
    in gynecological and obstetrical care, 279,
      308
    in managed care system, physician as advocate
      for, 252–253
  preferences/values of, surrogate decisions
    inconsistent with, 114
  refusal to care for, 197–205, 346–347
    case study of, 346–347
    doctor–patient relationship and, 197–198
      difficult, 202–204, 202*t*
    obligations to provide emergency care and,
      201–202, 204
    occupational risks to physicians and,
      198–201, 200*t*
    surgery and, 297–298
  relationship of with physician. *See* Doctor–
    patient relationship
  respect for, 11–12
    confidentiality and, 42
  sexual contact with physician and, 212–218.
    See also Sexual contact between physi-
    cians and patients
  surrogate selection by, 100, 112
  unwillingness of to know diagnosis, deception/
    nondisclosure and, 53
Patient abandonment, 203–204
Patient advocate
  for children, pediatrician as, 285–286
  physician in managed care system as, 252–253
Patient autonomy. *See* Autonomy
Patient care, ethical dilemmas in, 3–10. *See also*
  Decision-making, ethical
Patient confidentiality. *See* Confidentiality
Patient self-determination, respect for, informed
  consent and, 20
Patient transfer
  obligations to provide emergency care and,
    201–202
  refusal of life-sustaining interventions and,
    138–139
Patient well-being, enhancing, informed consent
  and, 20–21
Pediatrics, ethical issues in, 285–293. *See also*
  Children
Pelvic examination, by student/trainee, on
  patient under anesthesia, 279, 308
Persistent vegetative state, 173–176
  appropriate treatment in, 174–175
  clinical features of, 173–174
  definition of, 174
  tube feedings and, 174, 175

  withholding/withdrawing interventions and,
    174–175
    Cruzan case ruling and, 184–186
    Quinlan case ruling and, 181–182
Persuasion, patient acceptance of beneficial
  interventions and, 38
Physician
  attending, disclosure of trainee mistakes to,
    267–268
  as gatekeeper, 249, 256
  HIV status of
    CDC guidelines for practice and, 324
    discrimination and, 324
    impairment and, 325–326
    patient exposure to blood and, 325
    patient questions about, 324–325
    public health dilemmas and, 323
    restrictions and, 323–324
    risk of transmission to patients and, 322–323
  impaired, 271–276. *See also* Impaired
    colleagues
  as patient advocate
    for children, 285–286
    in managed care system, 252–253
  sexual contact with patient and, 212–218. *See*
    also Sexual contact between physicians
    and patients
  solicitation of gifts from patients by,
    208–209. *See also* Gifts
Physician-assisted suicide, 156–166, 345–346
  abuse and, 159
  actual use of prescribed drugs and, 161
  administering appropriate doses of narcotics/
    sedatives differentiated from, 157
  case study of, 345–346
  compassion for suffering patient and, 158
  de facto legalization of in Netherlands,
    161–162
  declining request for, 163–164
  definition of, 156–157
    physician confusion about, 161
  depression and, 159, 160
  doctor–patient relationship and, 161
  emotional impact of on physician, 161
  improved palliative care affecting patient
    desire for, 163
  incidence of requests for, 160
  justifiable situations and, 164
  legal rulings on, 186–188
  legal status and practice of, 159–162
  legalization of in Oregon, 159–160
  manageability of suffering and, 158
  patient autonomy and, 158–159
  patient withdrawal of request for, 162

physician role as healer and, 159
policy options and, 162
practice of in United States, 160–161
reasons against, 158–159
reasons favoring, 158
response to request for, 162–164
safeguard violations and, 161–162
sanctity of life and, 158
withholding/withdrawing medical inter-
    ventions differentiated from, 157
Physician autonomy
    patient insistence on interventions and, 35
    physician/caregiver insistence on life-
        sustaining interventions and, 136
Physician–patient relationship. *See* Doctor–
    patient relationship
Positive rights, 137
Power of attorney for health care, durable
    (health care proxy), 96–97, 108–110.
    See also Surrogate
PPOs. *See* Managed care systems; Preferred
    provider organizations
Practice guidelines, in cost containment, 257
Precedents, case law and, 190
Preferred provider organizations (PPOs), 255.
    See also Managed care systems
Pregnancy. *See also* Obstetrics and gynecology
    compelled treatment and, 91–92
    ethical issues in, 302–309
    life-sustaining interventions for brain dead
        mother until delivery and, 178
    philosophical/religious questions about, 302
    substance and alcohol abuse during, 307
Prenatal testing
    differentiation of from DNA-based testing for
        adult-onset diseases, 337
    for HIV, 305
    routine, 304–305
Preventing harm. *See* Harm, preventing
Principles, 14–15. *See also* Guidelines
Privacy, sexual relationship between patient and
    physician and, 212
Product recognition, drug company gifts and, 259
Professional oaths/codes, clinical ethics differ-
    entiated from, 6
Professionalism. *See also* Doctor–patient
    relationship
    gifts from drug companies affecting, 260–261
    impaired colleagues and, 272
    nature of, best interests of patient and, 32
    nondisclosure of mistake affecting, 265
    physician-patient sexual relationship and, 214
    self-referral and, 245–246
        AMA standards and, 246

Promise-keeping, 12, 62–65
    ethical significance of, 62–63
    exceptions to, 63
    guidelines for, 64–65
Protection of victims, overriding confidentiality
    and, 48, 314–315
Protocols, in cost containment, 257
Provider-specific outcomes, disclosure of, 295
Proxy, for health care (durable power of attorney
    for health care), 96–97, 108–110.
    See also Surrogate
Psychiatric patient
    decision-making capacity and, 86, 310, 311
        refusal of psychiatric treatment and,
            315–316
    ethical issues in care of, 310–317
        confidentiality and, 311
        danger to others and, 313–315
        impairment and, 310
        involuntary commitment and, 311–312
            mitigating adverse effects of, 313
        refusal of treatment and
            medical treatment, 316
            psychiatric treatment, 315–316
        risk of abuses and, 310–311
        suicide threats and, 312–313
    violence by, 313–315
        warning persons at risk and, 48, 314–315
Psychiatrists, consultation by, decision-making
    capacity assessment and, 85
Psychosocial issues, dealing with in ethical
    dilemmas, 9
Public figures, release of information about, 44
Public health issues, transmission of HIV from
    seropositive health care workers and, 323
Public health officials
    partner notification by, 47
    reporting patient information to, 46–47
PVS. *See* Persistent vegetative state

Q

Quality of life
    assessment of, 33
    best interests of patient and, 33
    futility of interventions and, 75, 76
        cardiopulmonary resuscitation and, 149
Queuing, as cost containment measure, 257
Quinlan case, 181–182

R

Randomization, in clinical research, 222
Randomized controlled trials, 221–222

Rationing health care. *See* Allocation of resources; Bedside rationing of health care
Reality, distorted views of, decision-making capacity affected by, 83
Reasoning, use of, decision-making capacity and, 83, 84
Reciprocity, gifts from drug company and, 260
Refractory symptoms/suffering
  high doses of opioids/sedatives for symptom relief and, 123–124
    emotional responses and, 126
  responses to, 124–125
Refusal to care for patient, 197–205, 346–347
  case study of, 346–347
  doctor–patient relationship and, 197–198
    difficult, 202–204, 202*t*
  obligations to provide emergency care and, 201–202, 204
  occupational risks to physicians and, 198–201, 200*t*
  surgery and, 297–298
Refusal of treatment
  best interests of patient and, 13, 30–34, 38–39
  by competent/informed patients, 89–93
  decision-making capacity and, 80–88
  informed consent and, 20, 90
  by Jehovah's Witnesses, 90–91
    children and, 291
    increasing risk of surgery and, 298–299, 300
  of life-sustaining interventions. *See also* Advance directives; Life-sustaining interventions
    caregiver insistence and, 135–139
    patient transfer and, 138–139
  by parents for children, 290–291
  by psychiatric patients
    medical treatment, 316
    psychiatric treatment, 315–316
  respecting, 89
  restrictions on, 91–92
  scope of, 89–90
  surgery and, 299–300
Regulations, as source of law, 189
Reimbursement incentives. *See also* Financial incentives
  as conflicts of interest, 233
    decreases in services and, 249–250
    increases in services and, 244–246
Relatives. *See* Family/significant others
Religious beliefs
  insistence on life-sustaining interventions and, 130–133
  unconventional decisions based on, 86

Reporting
  child abuse, 48–49
  crimes involving injuries, 47
  domestic violence, 49
  drug/alcohol use during pregnancy, 307
  elder abuse, 49
  impaired automobile driver, 47
  impaired colleagues, 273, 275
  to public health officials, 46–47
  unethical behavior/substandard care by senior physician, 280–281
Reproductive technologies, assisted, 303, 308
Research ethics, 221–228
  academic rewards and, 225
  competing interests and, 225–227
  confidentiality of data from, 224
  conflicting interests and, 226–227
  constrained consent and, 222–223
  drug manufacturer funding and, 225–226
  fee-for-service research and, 226
  finder's fees and, 225–226
  informed consent and, 223–224, 223*t*
  Institutional Review Board and, 224
  participant selection and, 222–223
  patient lacking decision-making capacity and, 222
  research protocols and, 221–222
Research protocols, design of, 221–222
Resources
  allocation of, 13, 236
    cost of transplantation and, 334
    futility of interventions and, 75
    patient insistence on interventions and, 37
  bedside rationing of, 236–243
    arguments against, 237
    arguments supporting, 237–239, 237*t*
    financial resources as basis for, 239–241
    notification of patient/surrogate and, 242
    suggestions for physicians considering, 241–242, 241*t*
Respect for persons, 11–12
  confidentiality and, 42
Retransplantation, 332
Rh type, prenatal testing for, 304
"Right to die." *See* Active euthanasia; Life-sustaining interventions; Physician-assisted suicide
Rights, claims of, as justification of action, 4–5
Rubella, prenatal testing for, 304
Rule, 15. *See also* Guidelines

S
Safeguards
  assisted suicide/active euthanasia and, 161, 162

futile interventions/unilateral decision-making and, 76–78, 77*t*

Salary, as cost-containment measure, 256. *See also* Financial incentives

Schizophrenia, decision-making capacity and, 86

Schools, disclosure of information to, 290

Second opinion, futile interventions and, 77

Secrets, physician's response to, 219–220

Sedation, terminal, 124–125

Sedatives, high doses of for symptom relief, 123–124
  emotional responses and, 126

Self-determination, patient, informed consent and, 20

Self-referral by physicians, 245–246

Sexual contact between physicians and patients, 212–218
  abuse of doctor–patient relationship and, 214
  justifications for, 212–213
  legal issues and, 215
  objections to
    current patients and, 213–215, 213*t*
    former patients and, 215–216
  prevalence of, 212
  responding to advances by patients and, 217
  suggestions for physicians considering, 216–217

Sexually transmitted diseases, partner notification and, 47, 48

Shortness of breath, high doses of opioids/sedatives for relief of in terminal patients, 123

Show code, 152–153

Significant others. *See* Family/significant others

Slippery slope argument
  physician-assisted suicide/active euthanasia and, 159
  withholding tube and intravenous feedings and, 168–169, 171

Slow code, 152–153

Spousal abuse. *See* Domestic violence

Standard of conduct, minimally acceptable, legal vs. ethical actions and, 5

Standards for disclosure, informed consent and, 24–25

Starvation, withholding tube and intravenous feedings and, 168

State constitutions, as source of law, 189

Statutes, 189

Sterilization, informed consent and, 305–306

Students
  ethical dilemmas facing, 277–282
    introducing students to patients, 277
    learning on patients and, 277–279, 347
      case study of, 347

    in gynecological and obstetrical care, 279, 308
    suggestions for, 281
    taking too much clinical responsibility and, 280
    unethical behavior/substandard care by other physicians and, 280–281, 347–348
      case study of, 347–348
  mistakes by, disclosure of, 267–268

Substance abuse, during pregnancy, 307

Substituted judgment, 102–104
  conflict with patient's best interests and, 104
  inaccuracy of, 103
  inconsistency of, 103
  problems with, 103–104

Suffering, requests for interventions causing, 131

Suicidal patients, 312–313
  identification of, 313
  interventions for prevention and, 312–313
  involuntary hospitalization of, mitigating adverse consequences of, 313

Suicide, assisted. *See* Physician-assisted suicide

Surgeon, disclosure of experience of, 296

Surgery
  ethical issues in, 294–301
    disclosure of information and, 295–297
    informed consent and, 295–297
    patient requests that increase risk and, 298–300
    refusal to operate and, 297–298
    refusal of surgery and, 299–300
  suspension of DNR order for, 153

Surrogate, 69, 111–117. *See also* Family/significant others
  active euthanasia requests by, 160, 161, 164
  cardiopulmonary resuscitation refused by, 148
  court-appointed guardian as, 111–112
  decision-making by, 111–117
    conflicts of interest and, 114
    disagreements among family members and, 114
    discussing with patient, 101–102
    emotional stress affecting, 114
    improving, 115–116, 115*t*
    inconsistency with patient preference/values and, 114
    legal issues regarding, 113
    misconceptions about, 115
    problems with, 113–115
    unacceptable reasons and, 114
  disclosure of mistakes to
    case study of, 348
    ethical response and, 266

Surrogate, disclosure of mistakes to (*contd.*)
    other health care workers and, 268–269
    reasons against, 263–264
    reasons for, 264–265, 264*t*
    situations not warranting, 266–267
discussion of DNR orders with, 149–151, 150*t*
discussion of futile interventions with, 77
discussion of health care rationing with, 242
family member as, 112–113
insistence on life-sustaining interventions by,
    128–134
for patient with no family member available,
    113
selection of, 111–113
    by patient, 100, 112
suspicion of, 115
Surrogate motherhood, 303
Syphilis, prenatal testing for, 304

T
Tarasoff case, 314
Teaching hospital, implied consent for trainee
    care and, 277–278. *See also* Trainees
Terminal illness
    refractory symptoms/suffering and
        high doses of opioids/sedatives for relief
            of, 123–124
        emotional responses and, 126
        responses to, 124–125
    voluntary stopping of eating and drinking
        and, 125, 167–172. *See also* Intravenous
        feedings; Tube feedings
Terminal sedation, 124–125
Therapeutic privilege, 25–26
Third parties
    deception of, 56–60
        no legal right to information and, 59
        resolving dilemmas about, 58–60, 58*t*
    influence of on reproductive health, 302
    protection of
        bedside rationing of health care and,
            237–238
        overriding confidentiality and, 43*t*, 45–48,
            45*t*
    treating patients against their wishes and, 92
Thirst. *See also* Intravenous feedings; Tube
        feedings
    in patients refusing oral intake, 169
Tiered formulary benefits, bedside rationing
        and, 241
Trainees
    ethical dilemmas facing, 277–282
        learning on patients and, 277–279, 347
            case study of, 347

in gynecological and obstetrical care,
    279, 308
suggestions for, 281
taking too much clinical responsibility and,
    280
unethical behavior/substandard care by other
    physicians and, 280–281, 347–348
    case study of, 347–348
mistakes by, disclosure of, 267–268
Transfusions (blood), refusal of by Jehovah's
        Witnesses, 90–91
    children and, 291
    increasing risk of surgery and, 298–299, 300
Transplant recipient, selection of, 331–334
    beneficence and, 331
    conflicts between guidelines and, 333
    gift relationship and, 333–334
    historical background of, 331
    justice and, 332–333
    patient behaviors causing disease and, 334
Transplantation, 328–336
    cost of, 334
    gift relationship and, 333–334
    organ donation and, 328–331. *See also* Organ
        donation
        definition/determination of death and, 177,
            179, 329, 330
    recipient selection and, 331–334. *See also*
        Transplant recipient
    repeat, after rejection, 332
Treatment. *See* Interventions
Truth-telling, 52. *See also* Deception; Misrepre-
        sentation
Tube feedings, 167–172
    burdens/benefits of, 170
    clinical recommendations regarding,
        171–172
    for comfort and symptom alleviation, 168
    defining goals of care and, 167–168
    legal status of, 171
    as life-sustaining intervention, 168
    as ordinary care, ethical distinctions regarding,
        122, 168–170
    persistent vegetative state and, 174–175
    prolonging dying and, 169
    prolonging life and, 168
    reasons for providing, 168–169
    as symbol of care, 168, 170–171
    withdrawing
        Cruzan case ruling and, 184–186
        negative vs. positive rights and, 137
        versus withholding, 168, 170